MEDICAL LIBRARY
WATFORD POSTGRADUATE
MEDICAL CENTRE
WATFORD GENERAL HOSPITAL
VICARAGE ROAD
WATFORD WD1 8HB

KT-175-180

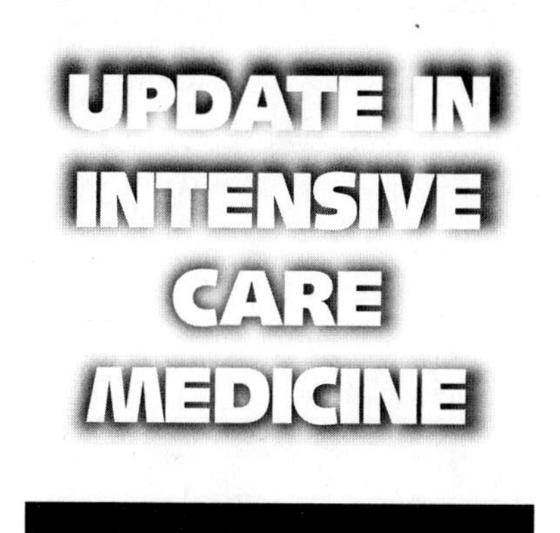

Series Editor: Jean-Louis Vincent

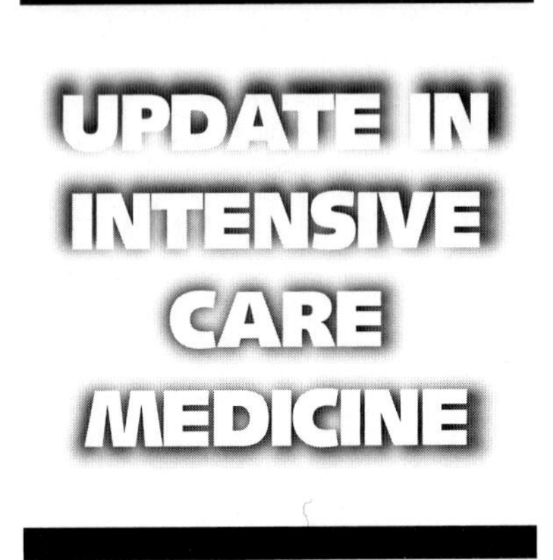

Springer
New York
Berlin
Heidelberg
Barcelona
Hong Kong
London
Milan
Paris
...kyo

EVALUATING CRITICAL CARE

Using Health Services Research to Improve Quality

Volume Editors:

William J. Sibbald, MD, FRCPC, FCCHSE
Professor of Medicine, Critical Care
University of Toronto
and
Physician-in-Chief, Department of Medicine
Sunnybrook and Women's College Health Sciences Centre
Toronto, Ontario, Canada

Julian F. Bion, FRCP, FRCA, MD
Reader and Regional Advisor in Intensive Care Medicine
Department of Anesthesia and Intensive Care Medicine
University of Birmingham
Queen Elizabeth Hospital
Birmingham, UK

Series Editor:

Jean-Louis Vincent, MD, PhD, FCCM, FCCP
Head, Department of Intensive Care
Erasme University Hospital
Brussels, Belgium

With 46 Figures and 49 Tables

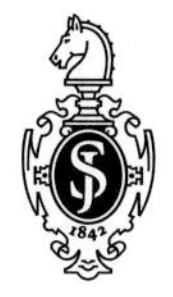

Springer

William J. Sibbald, MD, FRCPC, FCCHSE
Professor of Medicine, Critical Care
University of Toronto
and
Physician-in-Chief, Department of Medicine
Sunnybrook and Women's College
Health Sciences Centre
Toronto, Ontario M4N 3M5
Canada

Julian F. Bion, FRCP, FRCA, MD
Reader and Regional Advisor in
Intensive Care Medicine
Department of Anesthesia and
Intensive Care Medicine
University of Birmingham
Queen Elizabeth Hospital
Birmingham B15 27H
UK

Series Editor:
Jean-Louis Vincent, MD, PhD, FCCM, FCCP
Head, Department of Intensive Care
Erasme University Hospital
Route de Lennik 808
B-1070 Brussels
Belgium

Library of Congress Cataloging-in-Publication Data applied for

Printed on acid-free paper.

Hardcover edition © 2001 Springer-Verlag Berlin Heidelberg.

Softcover edition © 2002 Springer-Verlag Berlin Heidelberg.

All rights reserved. This work may not be translated or copied in whole or in part without the written permission of the publisher (Springer-Verlag New York, Inc., 175 Fifth Avenue, New York, NY 10010, USA), except for brief excerpts in connection with reviews or scholarly analysis. Use in connection with any form of information storage and retrieval, electronic adaptation, computer software, or by similar or dissimilar methodology now known or hereafter developed is forbidden.

The use of general descriptive names, trade names, trademarks, etc., in this publication, even if the former are not especially identified, is not to be taken as a sign that such names, as understood by the Trade Marks and Merchandise Marks Act, may accordingly be used freely by anyone.

While the advice and information in this book are believed to be true and accurate at the date of going to press, neither the authors nor the editors nor the publisher can accept any legal responsibility for any errors or omissions that may be made. The publisher makes no warranty, express or implied, with respect to the material contained herein.

Production managed by PRO EDIT GmbH, Heidelberg, Germany.
Typeset by TBS, Sandhausen, Germany.
Printed and bound by Mercedes-Druck, Berlin, Germany.
Printed in Germany.

9 8 7 6 5 4 3 2 1

ISSN 0933-6788
ISBN 3-540-42606X SPIN 10851550

Springer-Verlag New York Berlin Heidelberg
A member of BertelsmannSpringer Science+Business Media GmbH

Contents

Techniques for Acquiring Information

Application and Interpretation: Using Data to Improve Outcomes

List of Contributors

D.C. Angus
Critical Care Medicine
University of Pittsburgh
Pittsburgh, Pennsylvania
USA

J.F. Bion
Department of Anesthesia and Intensive Care Medicine
University of Birmingham
Queen Elizabeth Hospital
Birmingham
UK

S. Brimioulle
Department of Intensive Care
Erasme University Hospital
Free University of Brussels
Brussels
Belgium

H. Burchardi
Department of Anesthesiology
University Hospital
Göttingen
Germany

J. Carlet
Department of Intensive Care
Hospital Saint-Joseph
Paris
France

D.J. Cook
Department of Medicine
Division of Critical Care
St. Joseph's Hospital
Hamilton, Ontario
Canada

E.A. Draper
FMAS Corporation
Rockville, Maryland
USA

G. Ellrodt
Berkshire Health Systems
Pittsfield, Massachusetts
USA

A. Flabouris
Division of Critical Care
Liverpool Hospital
Sydney, New South Wales
Australia

A. Frutiger
Department of Intensive Care
Kantonsspital
Chur
Switzerland

M. Garrouste-Orgeas
Department of Intensive Care
Hospital Saint-Joseph
Paris
France

M.K. Giacomini
Center for Health Policy Analysis
McMaster University
Hamilton, Ontario
Canada

M. Goedee
Free University of Brussels
Brussels
Belgium

J.B. Hall
Section of Pulmonary and Critical Care Medicine
Department of Critical Care
University of Chicago Hospitals
Chicago, Illinois
USA

D.K. Heyland
Departments of Medicine and Community Health and Epidemiology
Queen's University
Kingston General Hospital
Kingston, Ontario
Canada

K. Hillman
The Simpson Centre for Health Service Innovation
The University of New South Wales
and
The Liverpool Hospital
Liverpool, New South Wales
Australia

M. Imhoff
Department of Surgery
Städtische Klinik
Dortmund
Germany

M. Jegers
Center for Economics and Management
Free University of Brussels
Brussels
Belgium

W.A. Knaus
Department of Health Evaluation Science
The University of Virginia School of Medicine
Charlottesville, Virginia
USA

D.J. Kutsogiannis
Department of Public Health Sciences
Division of Critical Care Medicine
The University of Alberta
Edmonton, Alberta
Canada

J.U. Leititis
University Hospital
Gottingen
Germany

J. Lomas
Canadian Health Services Research Foundation
Ottawa, Ontario
Canada

J.C. Marshall
Department of Surgery and Interdepartmental Division of Critical Care Medicine
Toronto General Hospital
University of Toronto
Toronto, Ontario
Canada

D.R. Miranda
Health Services Research Unit
University Hospital
Groningen
The Netherlands

L. Montuclard
Department of Intensive Care
Hospital Saint-Joseph
Paris
France

R. Moreno
Department of Intensive Care
Hospital de Santo António dos Capuchos
Lisbon
Portugal

T. Noseworthy
Department of Community Health Sciences
University of Calgary
Calgary, Alberta
Canada

M. Parr
Intensive Care Unit
Liverpool Hospital
University of New South Wales
Sydney, New South Wales
Australia

P. Pronovost
Department of Surgery and Anesthesiology and Critical Care Medicine
Johns Hopkins University
Baltimore, Maryland
USA

S.A. Ridley
Department of Anaesthetics and Intensive Care
Norfolk and Norwich Acute NHS Trust
Norwich, Norfolk
UK

G.D. Rubenfeld
Division of Pulmonary and Critical Care Medicine
University of Washington
Seattle, Washington
USA

W.J. Sibbald
Department of Medicine, Critical Care
University of Toronto
and
Department of Medicine
Sunnybrook and Women's College
Health Sciences Centre
Toronto, Ontario
Canada

L.G. Thijs
Medical Intensive Care Unit
Free University Hospital
Amsterdam
The Netherlands

J.L. Vincent
Department of Intensive Care
Erasme University Hospital
Brussels
Belgium

D.P. Wagner
Department of Health Evaluation Sciences
School of Medicine
University of Virginia
Charlottesville, Virginia
USA

A.R. Webb
Department of Intensive Care
University College London Hospitals
London
UK

G.K. Webster
London Health Sciences Centre
University of Western Ontario
London, Ontario
Canada

J.E. Zimmerman
Department of Anesthesiology and Critical Care Medicine
The George Washington University Hospital
Washington, District of Columbia
USA

Abbreviations

AIDS	Acquired immunodeficiency syndrome
APACHE	Acute physiology and chronic health evaluation
ARDS	Acute respiratory distress syndrome
CIS	Clinical information systems
CME	Continuing medical education
CQI	Continuous quality improvement
EBM	Evidence-based medicine
EKG	Electrocardiogram
GCS	Glasgow coma score
GNP	Gross national product
HIS	Hospital information systems
HMO	Health maintenance organization
HRQL	Health related quality of life
HSR	Health services research
ICU	Intensive care unit
LODS	Logistic organ dysfunction score
LOS	Length of stay
MOD	Multiple organ dysfunction
MPM	Mortality prediction model
QUALY	Quality adjusted life year
R&D	Research and development
RCT	Randomized controlled trial
SAPA	Simplified acute physiology score
SMR	Standardized mortality ratio
SOFA	Sequential organ failure assessment
TISS	Therapeutic intervention scoring system
tPA	Tissue plasminogen activator
TQM	Total quality management
VAP	Ventilator associated pneumonia

Overview

Introduction – Critical Care: Problems, Boundaries and Outcomes

J.F. Bion and W.J. Sibbald

"Men make history, and not the other way around. In periods where there is no leadership, society stands still. Progress occurs when courageous, skillful leaders seize the opportunity to change things for the better." (Harry S Truman).

As we enter a new millennium and complete almost half a century since the first intensive care units were developed, the conjunction is an opportune occasion on which to reflect on past achievements and future goals for critical care. From one point of view, the extent of development has been enormous. The discipline has evolved from a service provided opportunistically in ward areas set aside for polio victims receiving cuirasse ventilation (the iron lung), to a speciality managing complex patients with multiple organ failure in purpose-built units. Critical care complexes are now the focal point of many modern hospitals, and have an important rate-limiting effect on complex surgery and overall patient throughput. There have been many achievements during this period in the fields of pathophysiology, therapeutics, technology, epidemiology and clinical measurement, including case mix adjustment. Intensive care has become a multidisciplinary speciality and accounts for a substantial proportion of health care expenditure in many countries [1].

However, closer inspection of this story raises many questions, particularly in relation to outcomes from critical illness. Despite initial enthusiasm, the promise of laboratory studies into sepsis, metabolism and the inflammatory response has not been translated into consistent improvements in clinical outcomes. A decade of research and interventions targeted at the cytokine cascade [2], nitric oxide [3], and growth hormone [4], for example, have not only failed to improve outcome, but in some instances have actually increased mortality. Studies demonstrating better survival rates using lower thresholds for blood transfusion [5], lower tidal volumes for mechanical ventilation [6], and non-use of pulmonary artery catheterization [7] (for higher oxygen delivery goals?) could be interpreted as showing that, in intensive care, more is worse. In contrast, non-pharmacological interventions such as semi-recumbent positioning of ventilated patients [8], daily ward rounds by an intensivist [9], and ensuring that patients are not discharged from the ICU to the ordinary wards during the night [10], demonstrate the power of simple organizational arrangements to improve outcomes and reduce complications. This view is supported by the extensive literature on preventing critical illness by optimizing the high risk surgical patient, which supports the approach of reconfiguring the intensive care service as an early-intervention medical emergency team. The powerful methods for case mix adjustment in intensive care have also revealed substantial local and regional variations in outcomes from critical illness which cannot be explained by severity of disease. Governments and health care purchasers are unlikely to accept spiraling costs in the absence of evidence of cost-efficacy and cost-efficiency, and patients will demand greater humanity and autonomy from intensive care practitioners.

Resolving these issues requires a different mindset from that fostered by conventional research, where ideas are frequently generated and tested within a single scientific discipline. It requires a much broader approach, involving collaboration between many fields of enquiry including those not traditionally part of the medical scientific frame such as health service managers and administrators, the public, and non-medical disciplines. What is missing are the *links* between the diverse activities of laboratory science, epidemiology, clinical research, organization, education and ethics. We term this activity of association or *integration* 'health services research'. Health services research has been defined as "a multidisciplinary field of inquiry, which examines the use, costs, quality, accessibility, delivery, organization, financing and outcomes of health care services, to increase knowledge and understanding of the structure, processes and effects of health services for individuals and populations. It involves studying cost-effectiveness, cost-benefit and other economic aspects of health care, health status and quality of life, outcomes of health technology and interventions, practice patterns, data and information management, health care decision making, health planning and forecasting" [11]. Health services research is therefore a domain, not a single discipline.

Intensive care lends itself to the type of activity envisaged by the term 'Health Services Research'. Indeed, the costs and consequences to any health care jurisdiction of the provision of intensive care require the immediate development and dissemination of a vibrant infrastructure to undertake this type of measurement and evaluation. As society ages and the prospect of an increasing need for intensive care resources looms large, the need for an aggressive health services research agenda in this hospital sector is imperative. Collaborating on an international scale, learning from others and integrating approaches already known to work, is the only sensible approach in this time of rapid change. It was with this background that the 2000 Brussels Roundtable Meeting was convened, bringing together experts from a range of disciplines and from many countries, to discuss and debate the topic: '*Evaluating Critical Care: Using Health Services Research to Improve Quality*'.

What follows is just the beginning of an important dialogue that must lead to change. This Roundtable concluded with agreement on many key learning points and recommendations for our political, health policy and medical leadership regarding an agenda for health services research in the world's intensive care units and critical care training programs. Members of this Roundtable committed themselves to providing *leadership* in the promotion of a forum for integrating the health services research message and skillsets in intensive care medicine, with key aims that must include: supporting the development of an open-architecture; a common minimum data set describing the acutely ill patient independent of context; a common taxonomy for standards in critical care; and the inclusion of HSR principles in medical education at undergraduate and postgraduate level.

References

1. Angus DC, Sirio CA, Clermont G, Bion JF (1997) International comparisons of critical care outcome and resource consumption. Crit Care Clin 13:389–407
2. Baue AE (1997) Multiple organ failure, multiple organ dysfunction syndrome, and systemic inflammatory response syndrome. Why no magic bullets? Arch Surg 132:703–707
3. Dellinger RP, Zimmerman JL, Taylor RW, et al (1998) Effects of inhaled nitric oxide in patients with acute respiratory distress syndrome: results of a randomized phase II trial. Inhaled Nitric Oxide in ARDS Study Group. Crit Care Med 26:15–23
4. Takala J, Ruokonen E, Webster NR, et al (1999) Increased mortality associated with growth hormone treatment in critically ill adults. N Engl J Med 341: 785–792
5. Hebert PC, Wells G, Blajchman MA, et al (1999) A multicenter, randomized, controlled clinical trial of transfusion requirements in critical care. Transfusion Requirements in Critical Care Investigators, Canadian Critical Care Trials Group. N Engl J Med. 340:409–417
6. Anonymous (2000) Ventilation with lower tidal volumes as compared with traditional tidal volumes for acute lung injury and the acute respiratory distress syndrome. The Acute Respiratory Distress Syndrome Network. N Engl J Med 342: 1301–1308
7. Connors AF Jr, Speroff T, Dawson NV, et al (1996) The effectiveness of right heart catheterization in the initial care of critically ill patients. SUPPORT Investigators. JAMA 276: 889–897
8. Cook D, Giacomini M (2000) The integration of evidence based medicine and health services research in the ICU. In: Bion J, Sibbald W (eds) Evaluating Critical Care: Using Health Services Research to Improve Quality. Springer, Heidelberg, pp 185–197
9. Pronovost P, Jenckes M, Dorman T, et al (1999) Organizational characteristics of intensive care units related to outcomes of abdominal aortic surgery. JAMA 281:1310–1317
10. Goldfrad C, Rowan K (2000) Consequences of discharges from intensive care at night. Lancet 355: 1138–1142
11. Field MJ, Tranquada RE, Feasley JC (1995) Health services research: Work force and educational issues, Institute of Medicine. National Academy Press, Washington

Health Services Research: A Domain where Disciplines and Decision Makers Meet

J. Lomas

Learning Points

- Health services research is a field of inquiry not a discipline
- Health services research is interdisciplinary between health and social scientists
- Health services research is driven by the management and policy questions of those running the health care system
- Health services research is about both producing new knowledge and encouraging its use by decision makers
- Applied health services research involves decision makers in the research process and researchers in the decision process
- Future trends in health services research will move it into increased consideration of values and equity, broader use of methods, and integration into transdisciplinary teams

Introduction

"Flood of Patients Overwhelms Quebec Emergency Rooms" [1]. In many jurisdictions this type of headline is common every January and February. Variously, shortages of money, nurses, doctors, beds or equipment are blamed. Less commonly, if ever, lack of research and planning are identified as the culprits. Yet flu-induced emergency room overcrowding seems to happen every year and raises the question as to why, if it is so predictable, it generates a crisis anew every winter.

Figure 1 documents the recurrent nature of the overcrowding phenomenon [2]. It plots the 'occupancy rate' of emergency rooms across each month from 1994/95 to 1998/99 for the Canadian province of Quebec. The data were analyzed and plotted following a spate of newspaper headlines, like the one above, in early 1999. The January/February 'bulge', largely attributable to diagnoses of respiratory disorders, is present in each and every year. (The particularly pronounced bulge in 1997/98 was the add-on effect of a severe ice-storm that winter.) These data are, from a planning perspective, ideal as they show a predictable not random 'peak load'.

The numbers are readily available to any hospital wishing to plan carefully for emergency room loads on a monthly basis. The analysis and plotting of the num-

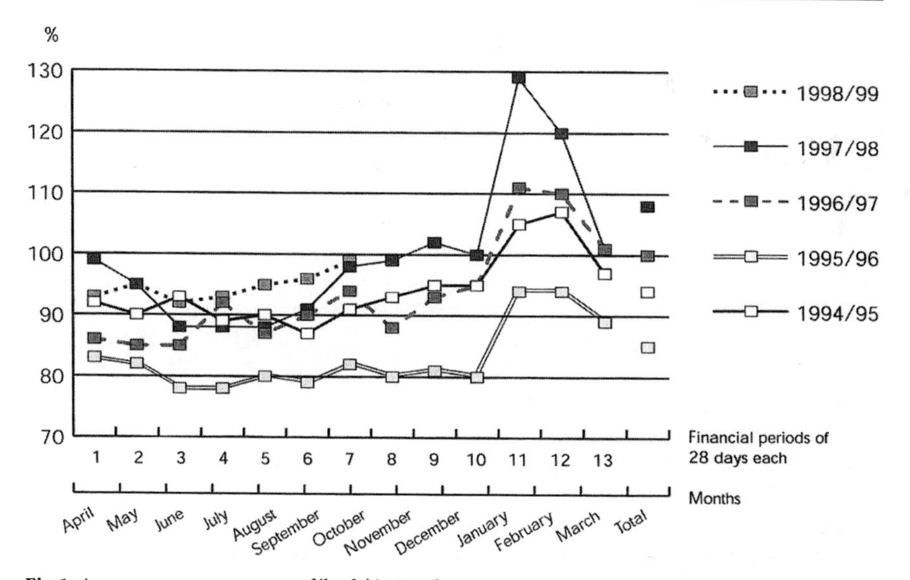

Fig. 1. Average occupancy rate of 'beds' in Quebec emergency rooms 1994–1998. (Source: M Breton, Clinical Organization Division, Quebec Ministry of Health and Social Services)

bers are introductory-level health services research. Yet few hospitals undertake such basic health services research and, therefore, treat every year as a renewed crisis without the additional staffing, equipment, or contingency plans needed to accommodate. Research on health services clearly has a long way to go, at least in Canada, before it becomes well integrated with the delivery of health services! This chapter reviews health services research and how to improve its integration with decision making.

What is Health Services Research?

Health services research serves the scientific needs of those who finance, organize, manage and deliver health services. It is therefore concerned with the three E's of health care: effectiveness, efficiency and equity. The Institute of Medicine (IOM) in the United States provides a more formal definition [3]:

"A multi-disciplinary field of inquiry, both basic and applied, that examines the use, costs, quality, accessibility, delivery, organization, financing and outcomes of health care services to increase knowledge and understanding of the structure, processes, and effects of health services for individuals and populations."

Health services research is usually distinguished from biomedical and clinical research. For instance, a 1979 definition by the IOM required two criteria to be met, one of which was "... [the research] is related to a conceptual framework other than that of contemporary applied biomedical science" [4].

However, UK definitions contrast with at least two aspects of the IOM's North American approach to health services research: the focus on individuals versus on populations, and the applied and basic versus applied-only research orientation. In a discussion of the UK's recent research and development (R & D) approach, Long agrees with the separation from biomedical research but not with the focus on individuals: "a clear demarcation is evident between biomedical and clinical research, where the focus lies at the individual level, and epidemiologic or health systems (or services) research , *where interest lies at the population level*" [5] (emphasis added). In the 1988 House of Lords Select Committee report that spawned the UK's R & D strategy in the 1990s, health services research is defined as "*all strategic and applied research* concerned with the health needs of the community as a whole, including the provision of services to meet those needs" [6] (emphasis added). Note here the exclusion of basic research from the remit of health services research.

There are, therefore, some cultural differences in what is considered health services research. In the UK and most of Europe it has become the 'R & D arm' of the health service, with concomitant expectations for relevance and a target audience of those who make policies for and manage the services. Individuals are neither the object of, nor the audience for, the research, and the basic science underpinning investigations is drawn from without, emerging from the discipline-specific efforts of some of its contributing practitioners.

In the US, where it has more of a stand-alone status, the field claims its own methods development, while recognizing that these new methods often have their origins in discipline-specific activity. Although still driven by the perceived needs of the managers and policymakers, health services researchers operate as more than a support service for the health care sector.

Nevertheless, practitioners of health services research in the US reflect the context of their culture: a greater focus on individual rights, consumer choice and the role of markets, and a less clearly defined, even fragmented, locus of decision making for health services. They are, therefore, necessarily less concerned with impacts on the overall health of the population, more concerned with individual health impacts, and more likely to see the public as an audience for their work.

For instance, performance measurement report cards in the US are driven as much, or more, by the need to provide information for consumer choice as they are by the need to do administrative benchmarking for accountability and managerial effectiveness. Development of capitation formulae in the US focus more on adjusting for individual-level health status anomalies than they do on designing a system with incentives to maximize the health status of the population/s served. As one critic has put it "health services research in the United States looks at the branches of the trees but never at the forest (i.e., the macro forces that shape the nature of medicine) and the relationship between the trees and the forest" [7].

Cultural differences aside, these definitions do agree on much and highlight a number of important features about health services research. First, it is not a discipline. Rather, it is a field of inquiry, a domain, where many disciplines and many methodologies meet. A corollary to this is that it is neutral about methods, using multiple methods derived from different disciplines, and matched to the nature of the research question and the pragmatics of the context. For instance, recent work highlights that life-support technology in intensive care units (ICUs) is not only about saving lives (initiation of life-support) but also about ending life (discontinuation of life-support). This challenges traditional clinical trial approaches, with their focus on a single primary outcome. A recent study commented on "understanding the ICU as a social world .... biomedical, evaluative, ethical and social science studies of life-support technology remain poorly integrated. .... combined disciplinary perspectives can be used to examine the diverse purposes of life-support technologies as they are used in practice" [8].

Second, it is driven either directly or indirectly by the questions and issues encountered by those working in health services. Put another way, it is more mission-oriented and less curiousity-driven than biomedical research. Careful assessment of research priorities is therefore a central part of health services research. Furthermore, whereas clinical research is often concerned with efficacy studies ("will this work under ideal circumstances?"), health services research is largely concerned with effectiveness questions ("will this work under real-world circumstances?"). This mission-oriented focus is also driven by the structure of research funding which, in the health services research area, is increasingly demanding reassurance on relevance and potential impact as part of the grant adjudication process, even using contracts and commissioning rather than granting to ensure this.

Third, and a corollary to the last feature, health services research is not only concerned with the production of the research but also with its use by those working in health care. Rather than academic colleagues being the sole audience for the work done by health services researchers, its communication to and use by decision makers without a research background is also important. The emergence of practice guidelines, the Cochrane Collaboration, Bandolier, and other digests and syntheses of research reflects this focus [9]. Indeed, there is a commitment within health services research to a research agenda on implementation of findings [10, 11].

These common features emphasize that health services research, even more than other categories of investigation, really is a process rather than a product. It involves:

- assembling an inter-disciplinary team skilled in the variety of methodologies likely needed
- gaining input from non-researchers in health services to refine and make relevant the questions under investigation, i.e., to help set the research agenda
- linking with those non-researchers during conduct of the research to keep them informed and to keep the research relevant and 'on-track', and
- communicating and disseminating the findings in formats and venues of relevance to the non-researchers who can use the findings in their health service decision-making.

These features are not completely compatible with the incentives faced by most university-based researchers, pressured as they are to publish in academic journals and to treat the decision making world of the health system as a peripheral rather than central concern in their lives. Perhaps this is why, after an investigation of the sources used by policymakers in three countries for their research needs, Gwatkin concluded "If one wants research of the sort that [policymakers] find relevant for their problems, independent or ministry-affiliated research institutes and consulting firms appear much more promising places to look than universities" [12]. Nevertheless, linkage and exchange between those in the two processes of research and decision making for health services is central to relevant, effective and useable health services research.

In a subsequent section, I will provide some examples of past and current health services research that use this 'linkage and exchange' model, highlighting the importance of the inter-disciplinary team, the linkage with decision makers to set agendas and keep relevance at the forefront, and the attention to appropriate dissemination strategies. First, however, I discuss health services research in the context of the related areas of technology assessment, clinical epidemiology and social sciences more generally.

Health Services Research and....

From the first section it is obvious that fuzzy boundaries surround health services research. The precise borders depend on culture, funding mechanisms, health system structure, historical era and so on. This provides much grist for the epistemological mills of academe. Is technology assessment a sub-branch of health services research or a separate field of study? Is clinical epidemiology part of or separate from health services research? What role, if any, do the social sciences play in health services research?

Figure 2 provides my idiosyncratic attempt to relate these fields of study and disciplines one to the other. Health services research is separated from clinical epidemiology to respect the former's origins as an offshoot from medical or clinical research [13]. In this diagram, clinical trials of a specific intervention, even those assessing effectiveness rather than efficacy, are an input to, but are not part of, health services research. Conversely, development work on outcome measures

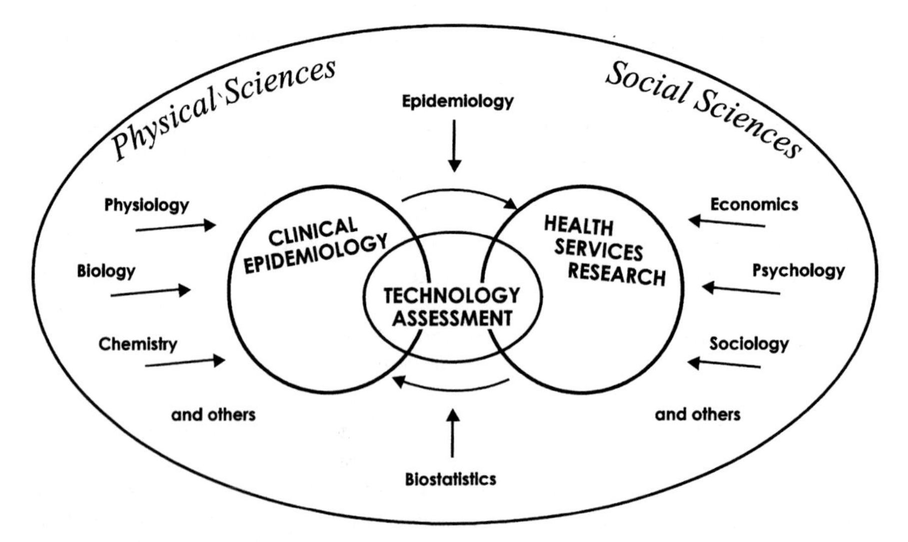

Fig.2. Health services research and related domains

such as QUALYs or other quality-of-life adjustments is done within health services research as an input to, but not as part of, clinical epidemiology. This view is obviously not universally held; there are 'lumpers' who would prefer to fuzz the boundaries more [14], but as an inveterate 'splitter' the distinction seems important to me, at least to respect the field's historical origins and, in the view of others, to prevent the medicalization of health services research [7].

Technology assessment is portrayed as overlapping with both clinical epidemiology and health services research, thus acting as a bridge between the two. Although in theory technology assessment is about a lot more than purchasing decisions, in practice it has become rather narrowly dedicated to this function in most health care systems. The UK's Health Technology Assessment program "encapsulates several strands of activity ... notably health services research, clinical epidemiology and health economics", in order to inform coverage and purchasing decisions [15]. Unlike health services research, technology assessment clearly includes the conduct of clinical trials.

Social science informs all three areas, although clearly relevant to a lot more than just the health sector. Economics generates the basis for cost-effectiveness and cost-benefit studies in health services research and technology assessment [16]. Psychology provides the basis for much of the outcome measurement tools developed in health services research and used in clinical epidemiology and for the underpinnings of medical decision making [17]. Sociology has refined many of the survey instruments used in health services research, developed qualitative methods (along with anthropology), and provides some of the tools for analyzing power relationships between health professionals [18]. The list could go on, but the general point is that health services research provides a 'melting pot' for the social sciences where not just multi- and inter-disciplinary work are possible, but also where transdisciplinary work can be developed, "where disciplines can build on their distinct traditions and coalesce to become a new field of research" [19].

This emerging transdisciplinarity is already seen in the complementary use of quantitative and qualitative methods within the same study [20, 21], and will be needed more and more as 'values' – those of providers, patients, and entire populations – play an increasingly important role in the delivery of health services [22]. Social science tools have much to offer health services research as it explores the role of values in such things as end-of-life or rationing decisions [23,24]. The role for social sciences will grow even more in the future because "these questions of value are on a different plane from the ones that usually engage health services researchers ... They lie not completely in the field of the clinical researcher, nor of the economist, nor of the decision analyst, nor of the psychologist, nor of the ethicist. They are boundary-crossing questions ... and they drive almost everything else" [22]. They are part of the future agenda for health services research.

The 'Linkage and Exchange' Model of Health Services Research

Health services research is increasingly seen, especially under the R & D approach of the UK, as the tool to improve the scientific basis of decisions made by those working in health services. Consequently health services research is evolving into a new partnership linking researchers and decision makers: "the promotion of a knowledge-based health service is the central aim of the R & D strategy as a whole. For this to succeed, research activities must be defined by the needs of decision makers, and it is ownership by, and responsiveness to, the needs of the NHS that singles out the R & D strategy from other research enterprises" [15].

This new paradigm for research will not be easy to achieve. Writing a decade ago on assignments for health services research in the 1990s, Berwick noted that "few of even the most distinguished investigators have experience in managing health care. And few managers, health care executives, policymakers, or leading clinicians have drawn extensively upon the results of health services research to guide their decisions. Health services research has apparently dangled just out of reach of those who make health care happen" [22].

During the 1990s, however, some have built the ongoing linkage and exchange between these two worlds with new models of the research process [25–29]. These focus on joint agenda-setting for the research, incorporation of decision makers into the research, and collaborative dissemination of results that exploits venues and formats friendly to the decision making world.

Joint Agenda-Setting

The main advantage claimed for involving decision makers in setting research priorities is that health services research will be based on the actual rather than the perceived needs of patients, providers and managers.

Matched against this are some concerns. First, that front-line managers and providers are so caught up in day-to-day issues that their suggested research agenda reflects current crises rather than future needs. Research, after all, usually takes years not months to come to fruition and should feed off tomorrow's needs not today's crises. Second, it is not clear whom you ask for their research priorities; how does one ensure that those you involve are representative decision makers?

A recent exercise in the UK answers at least the second of these concerns. The Intensive Care National Audit and Research Centre generated a large pool of suggested research topics from a survey of the staff in 187 ICUs. After categorizing and removing duplicates, 100 were left. These were then reduced to 37 priority topics by a nominal group process involving a geographically and occupationally representative sample of 10 ICU practitioners. When these priorities were presented back to a larger sample of 244 ICUs they validated the ordering of the priorities, with both significant Mann-Whitney U test values for the ordering, and significant Pearson Product Moment Correlation values for the degree of association. It would appear that "the views of a small nominal group can represent those of the wider community from which they are drawn" [30].

Some of the high priorities concerned clinical or technology issues, e.g., "does early enteral feeding improve outcome?". Interestingly, however, 24 of the 37 priorities were concerned with organizational aspects of critical care, e.g., "does regionalisation of paediatric intensive care improve outcomes?"; "does inter-hospital transfer, due to a shortage of available beds, affect patient outcome?" or "does the nurse : patient ratio affect patient outcomes?". This organizational rather than clinical/technological 'bias' in the priority research questions may be one of the major differences between a decision maker-initiated agenda and one initiated by researchers on their own.

The emerging use of good quality clinical databases or registries, such as the Intensive Care National Audit and Research Centre [31], also facilitates agenda-setting by decision makers. Contributing to the registry, maintaining the quality of the data inputs, and dedicating resources to the task, all motivate the decision maker to specify and demand output that is relevant for his or her work. As Black points out, this also enables health services research "to become more cost-effective ... [with] cheaper and faster research by adding on both randomised and non-randomised studies" [32].

Incorporating Decision Makers into the Research

There are at least two advantages claimed for involving decision makers in the conduct and interpretation of health services research. First, their involvement will generate ownership in the research results. Second, the managers and providers best able to implement implied changes from the research will have 'inside' knowledge of its strengths and limitations. Indeed, they will be in a better position to interpret the results than researchers who are unconnected to 'the field'.

These advantages appear to be corroborated by the experience of Stiell and colleagues who are working with managers in the Ontario Ministry of Health in Canada to assess the impact on cardiac arrest survival of fully optimized emergency response and defibrillation programs. The Ontario Ministry of Health was inundated with requests from communities for various enhancements to ambulance and emergency services. They are collaborating with university researchers to answer the questions in pilot form before committing to full province-wide implementation of potentially expensive but unproven programs. The first assessment proved that "improving dispatch methods, better deploying existing EMS [emergency medical services] vehicles, and using first-responder defibrillation" increased the survival to hospital discharge rate by 33% [33]. On the basis of this research these changes to optimize emergency response are now being implemented on a province-wide basis. As a result of the fruitful collaboration in this initial research, assessment of further potentially beneficial enhancements such as Advanced Life Support programs is now underway – again with pilot assessment prior to potentially expensive province-wide implementation [34].

In intensive care the frequent debate about growing shortages of dedicated beds was addressed in a novel way by decision makers in the UK's Intensive Care Society. Using registry databases, investigators compared night time discharges from ICUs for the periods 1988-90 and 1995-98 under the assumption that night time discharges represented sub-optimal performance and would be avoided unless there was significant pressure on available beds. The study confirmed the latter assumption; premature discharge being commoner at night (42.6% of night time and 5% of day time discharges being judged 'premature'), and the odds ratio for hospital mortality following night discharges compared to day discharges being 1.46 (1.33 when case-mix adjusted). These data also confirmed the anecdotal impressions of shortage, with more than double the rate of night time discharges in 1995-98 than in 1988-90 (6% versus 2.7%) [35]. This type of analysis relies heavily on the front line knowledge of ICU decision makers who are able to interpret and suggest proxy measures such as those used in this study. These results are now being used by ICU practitioners to underpin requests for increased numbers of dedicated beds in the UK.

In some instances the linkage with decision makers is for more than a single project. In the Canadian province of Manitoba the Centre for Health Policy and Evaluation (MCHPE) has an ongoing collaborative relationship with the provincial Ministry of Health. Over the last ten years results from a series of health services research projects have been incorporated into provincial health policy [27]. For instance, when hospital beds in main urban areas were closed the assumption was that expansion would be needed for hospitals in the rural areas. When actual utilization patterns were analyzed by MCHPE they showed that shorter lengths of stay in the urban areas had more than accommodated to the reduced bed numbers, and expansion of rural facilities was not required [36].

The researchers report that this ongoing collaboration is very valuable, noting that "one of the intriguing things about this process is that the research we have done under the Centre's auspices is very similar to what we had been doing, and publishing, for the previous 20 years ... The combination of popular press coverage and interest from key policymakers meant that differences in costliness of hospitals and differences in lengths of stay suddenly became meaningful and of interest ... within the government or within the institutions" [37].

Work by Singer and colleagues on 'end-of-life' decisions illustrates the value of involving patients and their families as decision makers. Using quantitative and qualitative methods they uncovered little quantitative impact of a 'living will' on their measured outcomes, but after discussion with the families involved in the study they came to understand that the *process* of considering the living will options made most families feel better equipped to handle and more satisfied with the end-of-life crisis they faced [21]. Similarly, understandings about the providers' experience of the decision to withdraw life support emerged from studies with health care workers by Cook and colleagues [38].

Health services research on intensive and critical care can, therefore, profitably involve non-researchers such as families, clinicians, managers and policy makers, in addition to the usual academic disciplinary mix.

Disseminating Results

The approach of involving decision makers in the conduct of the research actually improves dissemination. Instead of treating the dissemination process as a final activity that starts only when results become available, this approach gives warning to decision makers about the impending results and allows time for them to come to understand implications. As one observer has stated "if it takes a research team two years to get hold of its study, conceptually speaking, why would we assume that the reading of a single research report in a few days ... will bring enlightenment to the decision maker" [39].

All decision makers, however, do not have the same needs for information or the same preferences for how they receive research results [40]. Table 1 outlines these different information needs and preferences by type of decision maker: legislative, administrative, clinical or industrial. None of these formats are compatible with scholarly journal articles – the 'unit of transfer' most favored by academics – and will require additional work beyond the university publication paradigm.

In constructing persuasive communication of results [41], health services researchers would do well to remember the words of Eleanor Chelimsky, who for many years headed the General Accounting Office in the US that was charged with doing and reporting requested research to Congress: "We use the style of reporting that is most natural to legislative policymakers and their staffs: the anecdote. This may seem somewhat ironic, given that by conducting an evaluation in the first place one has moved deliberately away from the anecdote ... to disseminate findings to policymakers it seems that one of the most effective ways to present them is to rediscover the anecdote – but this time an anecdote that represents the broader evaluative evidence" [42]. In our own organization, the Canadian Health Services Research Foundation, we require researchers to use the '1:3:25 rule' when reporting their research, i.e., one page of bullet points for the main messages, three page executive summary, and a maximum of 25 pages double-spaced for the full report [43].

This collaborative model of linkage and exchange illustrated above is relatively new to the health services research field. Areas such as agriculture or education

Table 1. A summary of audience types, their research needs, and preferred information formats

Audience	Type of Decision Maker	Research Needs	Preferred Format
LEGISLATIVE	politician bureaucrat interest group	* problem definition * affirmation of assumed causes * policy 'ideas' (health policy analysis)	* person-to-person * overview in brief memo * media
ADMINISTRATIVE	program manager regional administrator hospital executive	* program evaluation * practice variation * cost-effectiveness (health services research)	* 'special' contacts * summary report * dedicated seminar
CLINICAL	practitioner professional society expert panel member	* effectiveness * ethics * patient preference (clinical research)	* colleagues * action-oriented synthesis
INDUSTRIAL	company scientist corporate executive venture capitalist	* marketable product (biomedical, information technology research)	depends on scientist vs non-scientist

have longer histories of this approach and have informed some of these developments in health services research. The value of the approach is put succinctly by Huberman who, after many years of working collaboratively with decision makers in the education sector, concluded that "interpersonal links, spread through the life of a given study, are the key to research use. They allow non-researchers to find their niche and their voice while a study is still young .... There are reciprocal effects, such that we are no longer in a conventional research-to-practice paradigm, but in more of a conversation among professionals bringing different expertise to bear on the same topic" [39].

Looking to the Future

Although it is not a new field, health services research has seen tremendous growth in both Europe and north America during the 1980s and 1990s. In addition to the emerging importance of 'linkage and exchange' between decision makers and researchers, the increasing role for values in defining the questions or underpinning analyses, and the move toward transdisciplinary teams, in what other ways is it likely to evolve in the next decade?

First, the disciplines upon which it draws will widen still further. "Recognition of qualitative methods and their rigour taken together with the limited generalizability of the findings of RCTs to routine practice suggests the need for both a hierarchy of qualitative and quantitative models of evidence" [5]. This increasing incorporation of qualitative methods will likely draw in not only the social scientists but also the business schools, law schools and public administration faculties where case studies have long been a mainstay of teaching and research.

Second, health services research's roots in the analysis of medical care will be increasingly left behind and supplanted by a broader remit around overall health-related services, including those social services with demonstrable impacts on health. Under pressure from emerging professional groups and with technology making ever more sophisticated choices available (in institutions and outside in the community) research agendas and results will be driven more by the managers and the policy makers than by the clinicians. The emergence in the UK of the new R & D program on Service Delivery and Organization (SDO) is a recognition that prior programs focused on the needs of clinicians and clinician managers and left largely unserved the broader needs of those who manage health services as professional administrators [44].

Third, issues of access and equity will come more to the fore. As population-based data systems allow us to focus on those not being served as well as those who do receive service [45], the unmet needs of defined population groups will receive attention. The potential conflict between these unmet needs and maintaining the affordability of health services will necessarily drive health services research increasingly into issues of equity, an area of investigation poorly served by health services research in the past. As Navarro comments on the US scene "The micro focus of health services research, excluding the macro structural concerns, reproduces a health care system that is profoundly unjust, inefficient and inhuman ... one must understand and try to change the socio-economic and political forces that are responsible for these inequities" [7].

Finally, health services researchers will clarify their relative roles in dissemination versus implementation of findings. Concomitant with, if not caused by, the rise in funding for health services research has been the expectation that researchers will not only communicate their findings more effectively, but also they will fill the 'implementation gap' and help bring about changes in providers', managers' and policy makers' behaviors. Black has noted that "despite our limited knowledge of implementation methods, it seems reasonable to assume that the skills required for implementation may not be the same as those needed to carry out good research ... Implementation is largely concerned with bringing about change in health care. But this, surely, is the essence of operational management, the basic task of most health service managers" [46].

The growing interest of management in the health sector in developing its own capacity to acquire, appraise and apply health services research to decision making should generate a 'pull' from the potential users to match the now well-developed 'push' from dissemination of findings. This should relieve the researchers of the unreasonable expectation to be scientists, disseminators, *and* change agents. The future of health services research looks dynamic as it not only develops its own domain, but encourages complementary developments in the related domains of health sector decision making and university academic disciplines.

Acknowledgment. I would like to thank Nick Black and Mita Giacomini for providing some of the examples of health services research in critical care.

References

1. Clark C (1999) Flood of patients overwhelms Quebec ER. National Post 1:A6
2. Anonymous (1999) Emergency room overcrowding: Predictable or not? Quid Novi, The Newsletter of the Canadian Health Services Research Foundation 2:12
3. Institute of Medicine (1995) Health services research: Work force and educational issues. National Academy of Sciences, Washington DC
4. Institute of Medicine (1979) Health services research. National Academy of Sciences, Washington DC
5. Long A (1998) Health services research – a radical approach to cross the research and development divide. In: Baker M and Kirk S (eds) Research and development for the NHS. Evidence, evaluation and effectiveness, 2nd edn. Radcliffe Medical Press, Oxford, pp 87–100
6. House of Lords Select Committee on Science and Technology (1988) Priorities in medical research. HMSO, London
7. Navarro V (1993) Health services research: What is it? Int J Health Serv 23:1–13
8. Cook D, Giacomini G, Johnson N, Willms D (1999) Life support in the intensive care unit: A qualitative investigation of technological purposes. Can Med Assoc J 161:1109–1113
9. Kirk S (1998) Developing, disseminating and using research information. In: Baker M, Kirk S (eds) Research and development for the NHS. Evidence, evaluation and effectiveness, 2nd edn. Radcliffe Medical Press, Oxford, pp 43–52
10. Haines A, Jones R (1994) Implementing the findings of research. Br Med J 308:1488–1492
11. Lomas J (1993) Diffusion, dissemination and implementation: Who should do what? In: Warren K, Mosteller F (eds) Doing more good than harm: The Evaluation of health care interventions. Ann NY Acad Sci 703:226–234

12. Gwatkin D (1996) How can research influence health policy. Reports from policymakers in three countries. Occasional paper, International Health Policy Program, Washington DC
13. White K (1993) Comments on Navarro's review of health services research: An anthology. Int J Health Serv 23:603–605
14. Naylor CD, Basinski A, Abrams H, Detsky A (1990) Clinical and population epidemiology: Beyond sibling rivalry. J Clin Epidemiol 43:607–611
15. Stein K, Milne R (1998) The NHS R&D Health Technology Assessment Programme. In: Baker M, Kirk S (eds) Research and development for the NHS. Evidence, evaluation and effectiveness, 2nd edn. Radcliffe Medical Press, Oxford, pp 67–86
16. Drummond M, Stoddart G, Torrance G (1987) Methods for the economic evaluation of health care programmes. Oxford University Press, Oxford
17. Tversky A, Kahneman D (1982) Judgement under uncertainty: Heuristics and biases. Cambridge University Press, Cambridge
18. Pope C (1992) What use is material sociology to health services research? Medical Sociology News 18:25–27
19. Rosenfield P (1992) The potential of transdisciplinary research for sustaining and extending linkages between health and social science. Soc Sci Med 35:1343–1357
20. Baum F (1995) Researching public health: behind the qualitative-quantitative methodological debate. Soc Sci Med 40:459–468
21. Singer P, Martin DK, Kelner M (1999) Quality end-of-life care: Patients' perspectives. JAMA 281:163–168
22. Berwick D (1989) Health services research and quality of care. Assignments for the 1990s. Med Care 27:763–771
23. Zussman R (1992) Intensive care. University of Chicago Press, Chicago.
24. Giacomini MK (1999) The "which" hunt: assembling health technologies for assessment and rationing. J Health Polit Policy Law 24:715–758
25. Brownlee A (1986) Applied research as a problem–solving tool: Strengthening the interface between health management and research. J Health Adm Educ 4:31–44
26. Lilford R, Harrison S (1994) Health services research – what it is, how to do it, and why it matters. Health Serv Manage Res 7:214–219
27. Roos NP (1999) Establishing a population data-based policy unit. Med Care 37:JS15–JS26
28. Lomas J (2000) Connecting research and policy. Isuma: Cana J Policy Res 1:140–144
29. Lomas J (2000) Using linkage and exchange to move research into policy at a Canadian foundation. Health Aff (Millwood) 19:263–240
30. Vella K, Goldfrad C, Rowan K, Bion J (2000) Use of consensus development to establish national research priorities in critical care. Br Med J 320:976–980
31. Rowan K (1994) Intensive Care National Audit and Research Centre – past, present and future. Care of the Critically Ill 10:148–149
32. Black N (1997) Health services research: saviour or chimera? Lancet 349:1834–1836
33. Stiell I, Wells G, Field B, et al (1999) Improved out-of-hospital cardiac arrest survival through the inexpensive optimization of an existing defibrillation program. OPALS study phase II. J AMA 281:1175–1181
34. Stiell I, Spaite D, Wells G, et al (1998) The Ontario prehospital advanced life support (OPALS) study: Rationale and methodology for cardiac arrest patients. Ann Emerg Med 32:180–190
35. Goldfrad C, Rowan K (2000) Consequences of discharges from intensive care at night. Lancet 355:1138–1142
36. Black C, Burchill C (1999) An assessment of the potential for repatriating care from urban to rural Manitoba. Med Care 37:JS167–JS186
37. Roos NP, Shapiro E (1999) From research to policy: What have we learned? Med Care 37:JS291–JS305
38. Cook D, Guyatt G, Jaeschke R, et al (1995) Determinants in Canadian health care workers of the decision to withdraw life support from the critically ill. JAMA 273:703–708
39. Huberman M (1994) Research utilization: The sate of the art. Knowledge and Policy 7:13–33

40. Lomas J (1997) Improving research dissemination and uptake in the health sector: Beyond the sound of one hand clapping. McMaster University Centre for Health Economics and Policy Analysis, Hamilton, Ontario.
41. Winkler J, Lohr K, Brook R (1985) Persuasive communication and medical technology assessment. Arch Intern Med 145:314–317
42. Chelimsky E (1994) The politics of dissemination on the hill: what works and what doesn't. In: Sechrest L, Bakker T, Rogers E, Campbell T, Grady M (eds) Effective dissemination of clinical and health information. US Department of Health and Human Services, Agency for Health Care Policy and Research, AHCPR Pub No 95-0015, Washington DC, pp 37–40
43. Canadian Health Services Research Foundation (1998) Communications Primer. Ottawa, Ontario
44. Culyer A (1998) Foreword. In: Baker M, Kirk S (eds) Research and development for the NHS. Evidence, evaluation and effectiveness, 2nd edn. Radcliffe Medical Press, Oxford, pp vi–x
45. Roos NP, Black C, Roos LL, et al (1999) Managing health services. How the population health information system (POPULIS) works for policymakers. Med Care 37:JS27–JS41
46. Black N (1996) What is 'development'? J Health Serv Res Policy 1:183–184

Methods of Measurement in Intensive Care

The Structure of Intensive Care

G.D. Rubenfeld

Learning Points

- Structure is an important measure of critical care quality
- The structure of critical care is extremely variable and the terminology for describing it has not been well established
- The evidence base for ascribing specific outcomes to specific intensive care unit (ICU) structures is lacking
- The most studied areas of ICU structure are the effect of the use of pharmacists in the ICU and the effect of closing the ICU to specially trained practitioners
- Although more difficult to measure, teamwork, collaboration, and ICU governance play an important role in ICU structure

A fellow visiting Seattle from Europe was on a tour of an academic ICU in the United States. At every turn she was amazed, surprised, and even shocked at the differences in the structure of the unit compared to where she was trained. Many aspects of care she took for granted from her experience. Nurses and doctors were not specially gowned in the rooms. Patients' families seemed to be allowed to visit at all times – and even children were allowed to visit. Each patient had their own room. Most surprising of all was the notion that different physicians, many not certified in critical care, could admit patients to the ICU and that there was no attending intensivist physically in the ICU at night. In response to her surprise, her tourguide observed, "Well, when you've seen one ICU's organization, you've seen one ICU's organization."

> "Structure denotes the attributes of the settings in which care occurs. This includes the attributes of material resources (such as facilities, equipment, and money), of human resources (such as the number and qualifications of personnel), and of organizational structure (such as medical staff organization, methods of peer review, and methods of reimbursement)."
>
> Donabedian 1988 [1]

Introduction

Measuring the quality of a complex service like critical care that combines the highest technology with the most intimate caring is a challenge. Recently, consumers, clinicians, and payers have requested more formal assessments and comparisons of the quality and costs of medical care [2]. Donabedian [1] proposed a framework for thinking about the quality of medical care that separates quality into three components: structure, process, and outcome. An instructive analogy for understanding this framework is to imagine a food critic evaluating the quality of a restaurant. The critic might comment on the decoration and lighting of the restaurant, how close the tables are to each other, the extent of the wine list and where the chef trained. These are all evaluations of the restaurant structure. In addition, the critic might comment on whether the service was courteous and timely – measures of process. Finally, the critic might comment on outcomes like customer satisfaction or food poisoning. Similarly, to a health care critic, structure is the physical and human resources used to deliver medical care. Processes are the actual treatments offered to patients. Finally, outcomes are what happens to patients, for example, mortality, quality of life, and satisfaction with care (Table 1).

There is a debate about which of these measurements is the most important measure of quality. A compelling argument, and, in fact, one source of the growing 'outcomes research' movement, is that, ultimately, what happens to patients is the most important measure of medical care quality. To live up to the definition, better quality medical care must improve patient outcomes. Several attempts have been made at judging the quality of intensive care based on an important outcome, mortality adjusted for severity of illness [3-5]. Nevertheless, there are two good reasons to consider measurements of structure and process as measures of quality of care.

First, the only aspects of medical care that clinicians can directly influence are its structure and process. Therefore, to effect change in practice, studies of medi-

Table 1. Domains of ICU Structure

1. Material resources • Physical Layout • Technology
2. Human Resources • Physicians • Nurses • Non–physician clinicians
3. Organizational Structure • Admission policy – closed versus open • Governance style • Specialty units and teams

cal care must be operationalized in terms of structure or process. A randomized controlled trial (RCT) of the effect of a new drug for sepsis on mortality is an example of a study of the effect of a process on outcome. An observational cohort study of the effect on family satisfaction of increasing nursing continuity in the ICU is a study of the effect of structure on outcome. Studies that evaluate structure and process are important precisely because they are the factors that can be changed at the bedside. To link structure causally to outcomes and processes, clinicians draw on the tools of evidence-based medicine (EBM). The extent to which the science will justify a claim between a given structure or process and improved outcome is the strength of evidence supporting that claim.

Of course, some structures and processes are important even in the absence of empiric evidence that they change outcome. For example, one can decide that having oxygen available at the bedside in an ICU is a measure of quality without a RCT showing that it reduces mortality. Once a process of care is accepted as improving patient outcome, it is more efficient to measure the process as a marker of quality than the outcome [6]. Because of the modest effect many medical processes have on outcome, it is easier to demonstrate the improvement in a process measure in a small sample size than an improvement in the outcome. For example, if the goal is to reduce the outcome of deep venous thrombosis (DVT) in the ICU, it is easier and less expensive to show that a given intervention has increased the number of patients receiving DVT prophylaxis than to show a reduction in the number of DVTs.

Studies of ICU structure are complicated by the variable nature and elusive definition of critical care. One must decide whether one is studying the structure of the ICU as a geographic location (as all existing studies have done) or of critical care as a service to a particular patient population. Are patients on prolonged ventilatory support in a nursing home in an ICU? Are patients being weaned in a post-anesthesia care area after cardiac bypass surgery receiving intensive care? Is the emergency department an 'ICU' because critically ill patients are cared for there for various periods of time? The answers to these questions will determine which special care areas and which processes of care constitute critical care.

In thinking about measuring ICU structure it is important to consider the instruments used to study structure. Some aspects of ICU structure are simple to identify and measure objectively: for example, the number of ICU beds, availability of bedside electrocardiographic (EKG) monitoring, or presence of respiratory therapists. Other aspects of ICU structure are more difficult to measure and require special qualitative or quantitative assessment [7,8]. Examples include how well the multidisciplinary providers in the ICU work as a team, the extent to which the ICU is managed by a core group of intensivists, and whether the ICU incorporates concepts of continuous quality improvement. Several investigators have developed explicit survey tools to measure these variables [8-10].

There is a limited number of studies describing ICU structure and its relationship to outcome. Four large studies deserve special mention because they compose most of the available data. Shortell, Zimmerman and their colleagues were involved with a number of studies using the APACHE database [8, 10, 11]. Three descriptive studies describe, in varying degrees of detail, the structure of ICUs in the US and Europe. In 1991, Groeger and colleagues surveyed ICU medical directors and used American Hospital Association data to describe ICUs in the US [12]. Recently, the COMPACCS (Committee on Manpower for Pulmonary and Critical Care Societies) produced a report that relied on a survey of critical care physicians and ICU directors to generate data on ICU structure in the US [13]. Finally, Vincent et al., used survey data from European ICUs participating in the European Prevalence of Infection in Intensive Care (EPIC) study to produce a picture of ICU structure in Europe [14] (Table 2).

While the best data available, these studies are difficult to summarize and compare because they did not use identical data elements or comparable definitions. Models for organizing critical care services are extremely variable and even the definition of which beds constitute 'intensive care' beds varies. Distinctions are subtle in separating a 'step down' or 'intermediate care' bed from other beds and many hospitals use flexible staffing and moveable technology to convert emergency room and post-anesthesia care areas into critical care beds. Finally, these descriptive studies of ICU structure were based on the results of surveys filled out by ICU directors with varying response rates and incomplete attempts to verify the reported data.

Information about ICU structure can be gleaned from published recommendations. The Society of Critical Care Medicine (SCCM) has published a number of guidelines on these topics [15, 16]. The American College of Surgery's criteria for trauma center designation contains very explicit recommendations for the organization of critical services [17]. This detailed document lists criteria for four levels of trauma center designation. It includes specific structural criteria for human and material resources as well as their organization. Recognizing the significance of the physical layout, this document even recommends where individuals should stand during evaluation of the trauma patient and where instruments should be placed in a resuscitation bay. Of note, this document also recommends that Level I trauma centers use a dedicated ICU team run by an appropriately credentialed critical care surgeon. Because of the lack of data to guide

Table 2. Structure of US and Western European ICUs

	US 1992 [12]	US 1998 [13]	Western Europe 1997 [14]
Affiliation			
University or university affiliated	31%	43%	49%
Community	69%	57%	51%
Size	Average 11.7 beds	48% > 10 beds 40% 6–10 beds 12% <6 beds	25% > 10 beds 57% 6–10 beds 18% < 6 beds
Mixed medical surgical	45%	66%	74.4%
Closed unit	22%	29%	NR
24-hr critical care specialist available	5%	NR	71.7%

NR: not reported.

the optimal structure for critical care, published guidelines and recommendations are, for the most part, based on expert opinion and common sense.

It is not surprising that the issue of structure is very important to intensivists. At its core, the ICU is a structural creation [18]. The ICU was born when the material and human resources devoted to caring for severely ill patients were focused in one part of the hospital. Two important themes emerge from a review of the literature on ICU structure. With one or two important exceptions, there is little evidence on which to base structural recommendations, and there is enormous variability in the structure and organization of ICUs around the world. Many important questions remain about the optimal structure for the ICU and the relationship between structure and process and structure and outcome.

Measuring the Structure of Critical Care

Material Resources

Physical Layout. The physical plant and layout of the ICU have not received much attention in the academic literature. There have been two sets of recommendations by the SCCM for the layout and resources necessary for an ICU [16, 19]. Although there are recommendations from a number of bodies and a variety of regulatory requirements, there is little empiric evidence that a particular physical layout for the ICU leads to better process or outcome. Many of the recommendations come from common sense and basic concepts of human performance engineering [20].

Hospital designers frequently stress the relationship between layout and clinician performance. It is essential that the function of the ICU room and personnel be considered when placing the electrical outlets, the monitors, and even the windows. The layout of the ICU rooms and their relation to a central control area has been stressed [21]. Equally important, even for the ICU, is the effect of the room, its layout, and design on the patient and visitors [22]. In fact, ICU designers must consider a variety of users who spend time in the ICU including clinicians, patients, visitors, janitorial staff, radiology staff, engineering support personnel, etc. Optimal design of the ICU for any one of these groups may compromise the design for another group. Therefore, it is essential that design of new units or modification of existing units be a collaborative process [23–25].

Technology. Perhaps nothing defines the modern ICU more than its armamentarium of sophisticated technology for monitoring, supporting, and changing human physiology, as well as organizing and displaying the collected data. This technology is in constant evolution as new devices are developed or adapted for use in the ICU from other areas in the hospital. Although the exact level of monitoring that is required for any given type of ICU patient falls under the category of process of care, the SCCM guidelines recommend, at a minimum, "the analysis and display of one or more electrocardiographic leads, at least two fluid pressures, and direct or indirect measures of arterial oxygen levels." [19] . Other guidelines and recommendations have been published based on expert panel recommendations. For example, the SCCM breaks critical care services into three levels of care (Ia – comprehensive and teaching, Ic – comprehensive, and II – limited to single organ failure and stabilization) [15]. This document makes specific recommendations for the technology that should be available to provide a specified level of care. For a Ia unit this includes extensive monitoring capability, intracranial pressure monitoring, in-house computed tomography (CT) scanning, Doppler, and echocardiography.

Technology has a profound effect on the organization and process of care in the ICU. Non-invasive measurements of blood pressure, arterial hemoglobin saturation, and respiratory rate allow the patient's status to be evaluated by a nurse at a central station that is not physically at the bedside [26-28]. Theoretically, sophisticated 'smart' alarms would allow one nurse to care for more patients. Unfortunately, while it seems intuitive that trading technology for human labor will result in lower costs, there is little evidence that substituting technology for nurses can result in significant cost savings. The effect of advanced technology on patient outcome is itself a controversial area [29-31]. Some studies suggest that having advanced technology available leads to better outcome, other studies do not [8]. Certainly, these analyses are complicated by the possibility that availability of advanced technology may be highly correlated with other aspects of ICU structure, for example, better skilled clinicians seeking environments with cutting edge equipment, and therefore the observed associations may not be causal ones. Curiously, and perhaps not unexpectedly, one study found that higher levels of technologic availability was associated with a decreased ability to meet family needs, raising the possibility that a focus on technology may lead ICU providers to neglect the human needs of their patients [8].

One aspect of ICU technology should be discussed separately. An enormous amount of information is gathered on critically ill patients: physiologic data, laboratory data, and clinical documentation present an overwhelming database. Organizing and presenting this information in a cohesive format was, and still is in many ICUs, relegated to large paper flowsheets. Computerized databases that integrate the clinical laboratory and bedside data promise several advantages [32, 33]. Data can be processed and organized to facilitate detection of trends and facilitate diagnosis. Data can be collected and used for clinical research and quality improvement and pooled to provide data on large populations of critically ill patients [34]. Objective prognostic data can be calculated and presented to clinicians. Medication errors can be flagged automatically. A number of commercially available ICU information management systems exist to fill this role.

Human Resources

Intensive care may be one of the most multi-disciplinary areas of medicine. Every specialty of medicine sees patients in the ICU, from psychiatry to surgery and from neonatology to geriatrics. In addition to physicians and nurses, a large number of 'non-physician clinicians', allied health personnel, and support staff contribute to the care of critically ill patients. Workforce issues related to critical care are extremely important [13, 35]. Recent health care reforms in the US have had a profound effect on the deployment of human resources throughout the health care delivery system [35]. Future needs for physicians, nurses, and other providers are hotly debated. The ability of mathematical models to predict future needs of different types of clinicians has been criticized. Recent data on actual marketplace demand for specialists suggests that health care reforms have reduced the need for various specialists [36]. The aging world population, the demonstrated efficacy of life prolonging treatments in the elderly, and society's unwillingness to withhold treatments on the basis of age or ability to pay will undoubtedly increase demand for critical care services [13].

Physicians. Although there is a great deal of data on the impact of the organization of the ICU on outcome which will be discussed below, there is relatively little data on the effect of subspecialty physician training on knowledge, process of care or outcome in the ICU. Studies evaluating patient outcome and physicians' knowledge in cardiology and acquired immunodeficiency syndrome (AIDS) care show benefit of specialty training [37, 38]. Critical care is an additional specialty certification in North America and Western Europe. The traditional routes to critical care board certification are through internal medicine (particularly pulmonary medicine), surgery, anesthesiology, and pediatrics. In a recent survey of self-described adult intensivists in the US, 38% were pulmonologists, 18% were anesthesiologists, 9% were surgeons, and 35% were internists [13]. In this survey, a high proportion of the intensivist respondents were board certified in critical care, ranging from 59.5% of the anesthesiologists to 88.1% of the pulmonologists. Specific studies addressing the effect of board certification on knowledge and outcome in critical care are lacking. Similarly, the optimal number of physicians needed to care for a given number of critically ill patients has not been assessed.

Nurses. The critical care nurse is the center of the ICU. In many ways, intensive 'care' is intensive 'nursing care'. The education and allocation of nursing staff in an ICU is an important job for ICU leaders [39, 40]. There is relatively little data available to guide clinicians as to the optimal nurse:patient ratio for critically ill patients. In one study the nurse:patient ratio was not associated with outcome or efficiency of ICU care [8]. It may be that the actual nurse:patient ratio has less of an effect on care than how the patient needs are assessed and how tasks are assigned. A number of quantitative staffing scores have been developed to assess patients and their nursing needs [41, 42].

Non-physician clinicians. A number of non-physician clinicians participate in the care of critically ill patients. These include physician assistants, nurse practitioners, advanced practice nurses, respiratory therapists, and pharmacists. These providers have demonstrated efficacy in a number of practice areas outside of the ICU [43]. There is some experience using non-physician clinicians to replace housestaff in neonatal intensive care [44]. There is also some reported experience with physician-assistants in critical care [45]. Experience within the adult ICU is limited and a recent ICU survey suggests that less than 10% of adult ICUs use physician assistants or nurse practitioners [13]. Nevertheless, a growing body of literature indicates that removing physicians from the decision loop can facilitate decision-making and make care more efficient [46-48]. In these settings, non-physician clinicians are empowered to make independent judgements within the confines of a decision tree. Finally, although virtually every ICU in the US employs respiratory therapists, very little is known about the organization and delivery of respiratory care in ICUs [49].

The role of pharmacists in critical care deserves special mention. Given the polypharmacy that is routine in the care of the critically ill, and the complications imposed by drug interactions and the impairments of metabolism and excretion seen in multiple organ failure, it is not surprising that adverse drug events are common in this patient population. A recent report on the effect of medical errors on patient outcomes identified adverse drug events as a major component of preventable hospital mortality and morbidity [50]. There is a compelling body of evidence that routine use of pharmacists in the ICU and computerization of drug ordering can reduce these negative outcomes [51-57].

Organizational Structure

Organization is a somewhat less tangible aspect of ICU structure than either human or material resources. It describes how the individual pieces of the ICU interact to form a whole. In business schools, there are entire texts and courses devoted to organizational structure and psychology as it is well recognized that these aspects of collaborative enterprises determine the quality and efficiency of the product. In critical care, two texts focus on organizational management issues in critical care [58, 59]. Perhaps one of the most controversial areas of ICU structure, and the one area in ICU structure that has generated the most data, revolves around admitting policies, which is a question of ICU organization.

Methodological Challenges. Studies of organizational structure on outcome are complicated for several reasons. From a study design standpoint, the unit of analysis, the 'intervention', is at the level of the ICU [60]. Therefore, in a study of the effect of five different organizational structures in five ICUs, the study power is affected by the fact that only five ICUs were observed even if data on 5,000 patients' outcomes were collected. This makes studies of ICU organization different from studies that clinicians are used to, for example, RCTs of drugs, where the unit of analysis is the individual. Simply evaluating patients admitted to different 'teams' within a single ICU is a weaker design because it ignores the effect of the ICU organization on all patients admitted there. This hierarchical design issue, that is, studying the effect on individuals within larger organizational units, is a common one in the social sciences and there are sophisticated statistical techniques to evaluate it assuming there are enough units to observe [61]. Failing to account for the hierarchical nature of the research question in studies of ICU organization can lead to biased study results. RCTs of ICU organization are also difficult because they would require patients to be randomized to admission at different ICUs [2].

Generalizing the results of studies of organizational change to any individual setting is problematic. Because organizational change is multifactorial and depends on the individuals involved, it can be difficult to identify which aspect of the care is responsible for changes in outcome. For example, numerous studies have shown the benefits of having an on-site intensivist, however, it is unclear what specific interventions account for the improved outcome. Does the intensivist offer specific novel treatments, or does the intensivist avoid errors, or does a single responsible team allow for more effective quality improvement? This makes it more difficult for institutions hoping to reproduce the findings of these studies to know which aspect of organization actually improved outcome.

For the purposes of this chapter, organizational questions in the ICU fall into three general categories: admission policies, governance style, and specialization.

Admission policy. While most ICUs have a physician medical director, the responsibility of this person for the actual care of patients varies considerably between ICUs [12]. Although there is no standard terminology, admission policies to ICUs are described as 'open' (physicians admit their own patients to the ICU and direct their care), 'closed' (admission to the ICU is restricted, physicians must transfer primary care of their patients on admission to a designated ICU team that is responsible for order writing), or 'semi-closed' (patients receive mandatory consultation from a select group of physicians but primary care of the patient is not transferred). Obviously, these are points along a continuum and a variety of intermediate admitting models exist. In some hospitals different units will be run under different admitting policies [12]. Obviously, the supervision of the ICU and identifying the optimal admitting policy is a question of intense interest to critical care specialists and has generated a considerable number of studies and editorials on the topic [62, 63].

Because there is no standard set of terms to describe these policies in ICUs, it is difficult to compare results from different studies and therefore difficult to understand what the admitting policies are in various ICUs around the world. Vincent et al. [14], found that 72% of Western European ICUs had a "committed 24-hour doctor" but did not specifically comment on their responsibility. Groeger and colleagues [12], in the largest reported survey of critical care in the US, found that only 22% of ICUs in 1991 were closed. A study of the effect of ICU organization on abdominal aortic surgery found that 87% of the study ICUs had daily rounds by an ICU physician but only 5% of the ICUs used an intensivist other than the operating surgeon to care for the patients [64].

Although there is tremendous variability in admitting policy, it is not random variability. Larger hospitals with larger ICUs, academic hospitals, medical units (as opposed to surgical), and ICUs with predominantly managed care patients, all tend to have closed units [12, 13]. These data suggest that the impediments to an organized critical care service may be due to insufficient ICU activity to support a full-time service, reimbursement strategies that provide incentives to care for one's own patients in the ICU, and the reluctance of operating surgeons to relinquish control over care of their patients.

At least 16 studies have tackled, in one form or another, the question of the effect of admitting policy and authority on ICU outcome (Table 3). Although the admitting policies in these studies and the methods are too heterogeneous to allow a formal quantitative meta-analysis, some general themes emerge. Generally, the studies show an improvement in outcome with a reduction in mortality or in the standardized mortality ratio (the ratio of the number of deaths observed to

Table 3. Studies of organization on ICU outcome

	Design	Population	Organizational model(s) studied	Effect
Teres et al, 1983 [81]	Comparison of 2 ICUs	Med-Surg	Mandatory admission to ICU team compared to private attending	Reduction in mortality
Li et al, 1984 [82]	Before-after in 1 ICU	Medical	On-site physician staffing of ICU	Reduction in mortality Increased use of invasive monitoring
Pollack et al, 1988 [83]	Before-after in 1 ICU	Pediatric	No pediatric intensivist to pediatric intensivist with daytime ICU team	Reduction in monitor-only patients Reduction in adjusted mortality
Reynolds et al, 1988 [84]	Before-after in 1 ICU	Medical	No intensivist attendings to staffing by intensivists	Reduction in mortality
Brown and Sullivan, 1989 [85]	Before-after in 1 ICU	Medical	No critical care consultation to mandatory consultation	Reduction in ICU and hospital mortality
Marshall et al, 1992 [86]	Before-after in 1 ICU	Surgical	Reduction in ICU beds, no critical care service	Bed allocation decisions not based on medical suitability or severity of illness
Pollack et al, 1994 [87]	Cohort in 16 ICUs	Pediatric	Presence of pediatric intensivist	Reduction in mortality
Mallick et al, 1995 [88]	Cohort in 2879 ICUs	Mixed	Greater day to day involvement by medical directors	Improved ICU utilization
Carson et al, 1996 [89]	Before-after in 1 ICU	Medical	Mandatory critical care consultation changed to mandatory admission to critical care team led by intensivist	Improvement in standardized mortality ratio No effect on resource use Increased use of invasive monitoring
Kollef and Ward, 1996, 1999 [90,91]	Cohort in 1 ICU	Medical	Absence of private attending providing care in ICU	Dying patients more likely to have active withdrawal of treatments and shorter process of dying
Manthous et al, 1997 [92]	Before-after in 1 ICU	Medical	No ICU director to optional consultation by full-time ICU director	Reduction in mortality Reduction in length of stay Improved housestaff performance on critical care examination
Multz et al, 1998 [93]	Before-after in 1 ICU Prospective cohort 2 ICUs	Medical	Optional critical care consultation changed to mandatory admission to critical care team led by intensivist	No effect on mortality Reduction in ICU and hospital length of stay

Table 3. *Continued.*

	Design	Population	Organizational model(s) studied	Effect
Tai et al, 1998 [94]	Before-after in 1 ICU	Medical	Open admission to mandatory admission to critical care team led by intensivist	No effect on mortality Reduction in ICU length of stay for survivors Increased use of invasive monitoring
Hanson et al, 1999 [95]	Prospective cohort in 1 ICU	Surgical	Care managed primarily by intensivists compared to care managed primarily by attending surgeon	No effect on mortality Reduction in length of stay and resource use
Ghorra et al, 1999 [96]	Before-after in 1 ICU	Surgical	Consulting critical care team to mandatory admission to critical care team led by intensivist	Reduction in morbidity Reduction in mortality not statistically significant No effect on length of stay Reduction in consultations and use of low-dose dopamine
Pronovost et al, 1999 [64]	Cohort of 39 ICUs	Surgical	Daily ICU rounds by intensivist	Reduction in mortality and morbidity

the number of deaths predicted by a standardized formula usually APACHE). None of the studies show worsening mortality with a move toward a controlled admission policy. Almost all of the studies show some improvement in the way the ICU is used: reductions in monitor-only patients, reduction in length of stay, or reduction in ineffective treatments.

Governance style. Older, hierarchical models of medical care where a single physician autocratically determines management are no longer tenable. As medicine becomes more complex and inter-disciplinary, newer, collaborative models of governance are required [58, 59, 65]. Modern quality improvement techniques rely on empowering all workers to identify novel solutions and work towards improving the process of care. Critical care epitomizes team-based, multi-disciplinary care and it seems fairly obvious that teams that communicate well, that empower all members to contribute ideas, and where responsibility is shared, will provide better care.

Baggs et al. [7], found that better measures of nurse-physician collaboration were associated with better outcomes in a medical ICU population and, interestingly, have also shown that nurses and physicians do not always have the same perception of the amount of collaboration that exists in a given decision [66]. Daly and her colleagues [67, 68] have explored extensively the impact of a novel model of governance for chronically critically ill patients that relies on a shared governance model and uses a nurse case-manager to direct many decisions.

Shortell and colleagues [8, 10] used instruments developed to assess organization to measure a variety of aspects of the ICU. Many of the variables studied under their heading of caregiver interaction fall under the category of governance (Table 4). Interestingly, there was no association of these variables with mortality; however, better caregiver interaction was associated with lower ICU length of stay, lower rates of nursing turnover, higher quality of care as assessed by providers, and better ability to meet family member needs as assessed by providers [8, 10]. Similarly, Mitchell and colleagues [9] showed that organizational variables were associated with higher levels of provider satisfaction and lower nurse turnover but were unable to show an association with mortality or length of stay.

Many of the modern tools for improving outcome and efficiency in medical care work by minimizing the direct input of physicians at every part of the decision loop. This allows routine decisions like extubation, weaning, DVT prophylaxis, and even ventilator management of acute respiratory distress syndrome (ARDS) to occur without the specific involvement of the intensivist. To realize these efficiencies alternative governance styles are essential. It turns out that empowering team members increases their sense of job satisfaction and may improve patient and family satisfaction with care [8]. Governance style and its measurement does not fit easily into the standard biophysiologic paradigm of critical care medicine but may have as important an impact on outcome as any aspect of technologic monitoring or intervention.

Specialty units and teams. One of the most reproducible observations in health services research is called the 'volume-outcome' relationship [69]. Across a broad range of medical treatments, the more experience a provider or hospital has with a particular disease or procedure, the better the outcomes appear to be [70-73]. By focusing resources and experience on a particular problem, clinicians become skilled with its management. Two models have been explored: 1) bringing the patient to the experienced providers (specialized ICUs); and 2) bringing the experienced providers to the patient (special consult teams within a general ICU).

By far, the most common type of ICU in the US is the mixed medical/surgical ICU [12]. To meet specific needs, a variety of specialized ICUs have been created including: neonatal, pediatric, cardiac, post-operative cardiac, neurological, neu-

Table 4. Measures of ICU sStructure (adapted from references [8, 10])

Measure	Definition
Technological availability	Specific devices available for use in the ICU
Task Diversity	Range of diagnoses that are cared for in a single ICU
Staffing	Nurse to patient ratio
Caregiver interaction	How do providers work with each other?
culture	self-expression, achievement, and cooperation
leadership	emphasize standards of excellence, communicate goals
communication	timeliness
coordination	coordination between ICU and other hospital areas
conflict management	open collaboration problem solving

rosurgical, trauma, burn, chronically critically ill, palliative care, step-down or intermediate care, and long-term ventilator. Some of these units work by focusing material resources, for example, non-invasive monitoring units or intermediate care units attempt to substitute less expensive material resources for human resources [74]. Some of these units capitalize on reimbursement opportunities, for example, in the US, certain long-term ventilator units were afforded exemptions from billing limitations. Primarily, the goal of the specialized unit is to bring patients with unique needs in contact with providers with expertise in their care. These specialty units are uncommon and tend to be in larger hospitals. In addition to the general volume-outcome observation, there are some data to support the use of specialized ICUs; for example, ICUs with greater diagnostic diversity are associated with worse mortality [8].

Alternatively, expertise can be brought to the patient in the form of a multi-disciplinary consult team. A variety of consult teams for critically ill patients have been reported including ventilator weaning, palliative care, nutrition, rehabilitation medicine, and psychiatry [75, 76]. Although individual groups have reported promising outcomes, there are little comparative data to justify broad attempts to institute specialized consultation teams in critical care.

Novel Structures

A number of technological innovations may profoundly affect the organization of critical care over the next decade. These may lead to novel structures for ICUs or may lead to the dissolution of the ICU as we currently know it. In most hospitals, patients are moved to the ICU when they become critically ill. Another possibility is to move the technology and the nurse to the patient [77]. With mobile monitoring equipment and sufficiently equipped rooms this is a possibility. Rather than move the technology to the patient or the patient to the ICU, modern telemedicine and remote monitoring technology may allow clinicians to care for critically ill patients at a distance [78]. Of course, this technology further raises concerns of the dehumanization of the ICU and it is not too difficult to imagine a patient surrounded by a nest of monitoring equipment with no human contact. Although the feasibility of these techniques have been evaluated, their ability to improve patient outcome has rarely been tested [79].

Thus far, we have dealt with the ICU as a structural entity in isolation. However, there are important organizational issues in how the ICU relates to the rest of hospital care and, more broadly, how critical care is incorporated into a regional health care system. The 'hospitalist', a new specialty of physician, has been proposed in part to meet the specialized needs of an increasingly complex and severely ill population of hospitalized patients [80]. These patients exist on a continuum of severity of illness with critically ill patients. How hospitalists and intensivists will share responsibility for critically ill patients as they move from the emergency room, operating room, or hospital ward to the ICU and back has not been carefully worked out. Trauma and transplant care have benefited from regionalization. Regionalization of intensive care services within a health care system may improve outcomes by focusing expertise on the critically ill.

Conclusion

The modern ICU is a structural entity. In it are focused specific human and material resources organized to deliver care to critically ill patients. While some improvements in ICU structure have face validity and may not merit extensive empiric validation, many questions about the optimal organization of critical care remain. Studies demonstrating an effect of ICU structure on process of care or outcome are challenging because they do not lend themselves to RCTs, present hierarchical data analysis problems, and may not generalize beyond the ICU where they were studied. Regardless of these limitations, ample data exist that the structure of health care has a profound effect on process of care and outcome. Identifying which structural and organizational improvements apply in different ICU settings and linking these to specific patient outcomes is a great challenge for future investigation.

References

1. Donabedian A (1988) The quality of care. How can it be assessed? JAMA 260:1743–1748
2. Rubenfeld GD, Angus DC, Pinsky MR, Curtis JR, Connors AF Jr, Bernard GR (1999) Outcomes research in critical care: results of the American Thoracic Society Critical Care Assembly Workshop on Outcomes Research. The Members of the Outcomes Research Workshop. Am J Respir Crit Care Med 160:358–367
3. Sirio CA, Angus DC, Rosenthal GE (1994) Cleveland Health Quality Choice (CHQC) – an ongoing collaborative, community-based outcomes assessment program. New Horiz 2:321–325
4. Teres D, Lemeshow S (1993) Using severity measures to describe high performance intensive care units. Crit Care Clin 9:543–554
5. Knaus WA, Draper EA, Wagner DP (1983) Toward quality review in intensive care: the APACHE system. QRB Qual Rev Bull. 9:196–204
6. Mant J, Hicks N (1995). Detecting differences in quality of care: the sensitivity of measures of process and outcome in treating acute myocardial infarction. Br Med J 311:793–796
7. Baggs JG, Ryan SA, Phelps CE, Richeson JF, Johnson JE (1992) The association between interdisciplinary collaboration and patient outcomes in a medical intensive care unit. Heart Lung 21:18–24
8. Shortell SM, Zimmerman JE, Rousseau DM, et al (1994) The performance of intensive care units: does good management make a difference? Med Care 32:508–525
9. Mitchell PH, Shannon SE, Cain KC, Hegyvary ST (1996) Critical care outcomes: linking structures, processes, and organizational and clinical outcomes. Am J Crit Care. 5:353–363
10. Zimmerman JE, Shortell SM, Rousseau DM, et al (1993) Improving intensive care: observations based on organizational case studies in nine intensive care units: a prospective, multicenter study. Crit Care Med 21:1443–1451
11. Zimmerman JE, Rousseau DM, Duffy J, et al (1994) Intensive care at two teaching hospitals: an organizational case study. Am J Crit Care 3:129–138
12. Groeger JS, Strosberg MA, Halpern NA, et al (1992) Descriptive analysis of critical care units in the United States. Crit Care Med 20:846–863
13. Anonymous (1998) Future workforce needs in pulmonary and critical care medicine. Abt Associates, Cambridge
14. Vincent JL, Suter P, Bihari D, Bruining H (1997) Organization of intensive care units in Europe: lessons from the EPIC study. Intensive Care Med 23:1181–1184
15. American College of Critical Care Medicine of the Society of Critical Care Medicine (1999) Critical care services and personnel: recommendations based on a system of categorization into two levels of care. Crit Care Med 27:422–426

16. Guidelines/Practice Parameters Committee of the American College of Critical Care Medicine, Society of Critical Care Medicine (1995) Guidelines for intensive care unit design. Crit Care Med 23:582–588
17. American College of Surgeons. Committee on Trauma (1999) Resources for optimal care of the injured patient. The American College of Surgeons, Chicago
18. Calvin JE, Habet K, Parrillo JE. Critical care in the United States (1997) Who are we and how did we get here? Crit Care Clin 13:363–376
19. Task Force on Guidelines. Society of Critical Care Medicine (1988) Recommendations for critical care unit design. Crit Care Med 16:796–806
20. Anonymous (1991) Principles of design of burns units: report of a Working Group of the British Burn Association and Hospital Infection Society. J Hosp Infect 19:63–66
21. Gelsomino VV Jr (1980) Open design facilitates ICU monitoring. Hospitals. 54:121–124
22. Graven SN (1997) Clinical research data illuminating the relationship between the physical environment & patient medical outcomes. J Healthc Des 9:15–19
23. Hall B, Grossman J, Peterson FH (1992) Designing a critical care unit: description of a multidisciplinary process. Nurs Clin North Am 27:129–139
24. Harvey MA (1998) Critical-care-unit bedside design and furnishing: impact on nosocomial infections. Infect Control Hosp Epidemiol 19:597–601
25. Koay CK, Fock KM (1998) Planning and design of a surgical intensive care unit in a new regional hospital. Ann Acad Med Singapore 27:448–452
26. Krieger BP, Ershowsky P, Spivack D, Thorstenson J, Sackner MA (1988) Initial experience with a central respiratory monitoring unit as a cost- saving alternative to the intensive care unit for Medicare patients who require long-term ventilator support. Chest 93:395–397
27. Krieger BP, Ershowsky P, Spivack D (1990) One year's experience with a noninvasively monitored intermediate care unit for pulmonary patients. JAMA 264:1143–1146
28. Elpern EH, Silver MR, Rosen RL, Bone RC (1991) The noninvasive respiratory care unit. Patterns of use and financial implications. Chest 99:205–208
29. Robin ED (1985) The cult of the Swan-Ganz catheter. Overuse and abuse of pulmonary flow catheters. Ann Intern Med 103:445–449
30. Robin ED (1987) Death by pulmonary artery flow-directed catheter. Time for a moratorium? Chest 92:727–731
31. Connors AF Jr, Speroff T, Dawson NV, et al (1996) The effectiveness of right heart catheterization in the initial care of critically ill patients. SUPPORT Investigators. JAMA 276:889–897
32. Cowen JS, Matchett SC (1999) The clinical management database. Crit Care Clin 15:481–497
33. Sado AS (1999) Electronic medical record in the intensive care unit. Crit Care Clin 15:499–522
34. Anonymous (1999) Project Impact provides answers. Healthc Benchmarks. 6:91–92
35. Rubenfeld GD (1999) Workforce and organizational change: Implications for cost containment. Sem Respir Crit Care Med 20:245–251
36. Seifer SD, Troupin B, Rubenfeld GD (1996) Changes in marketplace demand for physicians: a study of medical journal recruitment advertisements. JAMA 276:695–699
37. Jollis JG, DeLong ER, Peterson ED, et al (1996) Outcome of acute myocardial infarction according to the specialty of the admitting physician. N Engl J Med 335:1880–1887
38. Kitahata MM, Koepsell TD, Deyo RA, Maxwell CL, Dodge WT, Wagner EH (1996) Physicians' experience with the acquired immunodeficiency syndrome as a factor in patients' survival. N Engl J Med 334:701–706
39. Redshaw ME, Harris A, Ingram JC (1993) Nursing and medical staffing in neonatal units. J Nurs Manag 1:221–228
40. Endacott R (1996) Staffing intensive care units: a consideration of contemporary issues. Intensive Crit Care Nurs 12:193–199
41. Reis Miranda D, Moreno R, Iapichino G (1997) Nine equivalents of nursing manpower use score (NEMS). Intensive Care Med 23:760–765
42. Cullen DJ, Civetta JM, Briggs BA, Ferrara LC (1974) Therapeutic intervention scoring system: a method for quantitative comparison of patient care. Crit Care Med 2:57–60

43. Maule WF (1994) Screening for colorectal cancer by nurse endoscopists. N Engl J Med 330:183–187
44. Mitchell-DiCenso A, Guyatt G, Marrin M, et al (1996) A controlled trial of nurse practitioners in neonatal intensive care. Pediatrics 98:1143–1148
45. Dubaybo BA, Samson MK, Carlson RW (1991) The role of physician-assistants in critical care units. Chest 99:89–91
46. Pawloski SJ, Kersh PL (1992) Therapeutic heparin monitoring service in a small community hospital. Hosp Pharm 27:703–706, 723
47. Dasgupta A, Rice R, Mascha E, Litaker D, Stoller JK (1999) Four-year experience with a unit for long-term ventilation (respiratory special care unit) at the Cleveland Clinic Foundation. Chest 116:447–455
48. Stoller JK, Skibinski CI, Giles DK, Kester EL, Haney DJ (1996) Physician-ordered respiratory care vs physician-ordered use of a respiratory therapy consult service. Results of a prospective observational study. Chest 110:422–429
49. Keenan SP, Montgomery J, Chen LM, Esmail R, Inman KJ, Sibbald WJ (1998) Ventilatory care in a selection of Ontario hospitals: bigger is not necessarily better! Critical Care Research Network (CCR-Net). Intensive Care Med 24:946–952
50. Kohn L, Corrigan J, Donaldson M (1999) To err is human: Building a safer health system. National Academy Press, Washington
51. Leape LL, Cullen DJ, Clapp MD, et al (1999) Pharmacist participation on physician rounds and adverse drug events in the intensive care unit. JAMA 282:267–270
52. Kilroy RA, Iafrate RP (1993) Provision of pharmaceutical care in the intensive care unit. Crit Care Nurs Clin North Am 5:221–225
53. Hassan Y, Aziz NA, Awang J, Aminuldin AG (1992) An analysis of clinical pharmacist interventions in an intensive care unit. J Clin Pharm Ther 17:347–351
54. Devlin JW, Holbrook AM, Fuller HD (1997) The effect of ICU sedation guidelines and pharmacist interventions on clinical outcomes and drug cost. Ann Pharmacother 31:689–695
55. Cullen DJ, Sweitzer BJ, Bates DW, Burdick E, Edmondson A, Leape LL (1997) Preventable adverse drug events in hospitalized patients: a comparative study of intensive care and general care units. Crit Care Med 25:1289–1297
56. Chuang LC, Sutton JD, Henderson GT (1994) Impact of a clinical pharmacist on cost saving and cost avoidance in drug therapy in an intensive care unit. Hosp Pharm 29:215–218, 221
57. Bates DW, Leape LL, Cullen DJ, et al (1998) Effect of computerized physician order entry and a team intervention on prevention of serious medication errors. JAMA 280:1311–1316
58. Sibbald WJ, Massaro TA, McLeod DM (1996) The business of critical care: a textbook for clinicians who manage special care units. Futura Publishing Co, Armonk
59. Fein IA, Strosberg MA (1987) Managing the critical care unit. Aspen Publishers, Rockville
60. Divine GW, Brown JT, Frazier LM (1992) The unit of analysis error in studies about physicians' patient care behavior. J Gen Intern Med 7:623–629
61. Bryk AS, Raudenbush SW (1992) Hierarchical linear models: applications and data analysis methods. Sage Publications, Newbury Park
62. Carlson RW, Weiland DE, Srivathsan K (1996) Does a full-time, 24-hour intensivist improve care and efficiency? Crit Care Clin 12:525–551
63. Hall JB (1999) Advertisements for ourselves – let's be cautious about interpreting outcome studies of critical care services. Crit Care Med 27:229–230
64. Pronovost PJ, Jenckes MW, Dorman T, et al (1999) Organizational characteristics of intensive care units related to outcomes of abdominal aortic surgery. JAMA 281:1310–1317
65. Pew Health Professions Commission. (1995) Critical challenges: revitalizing the health professions for the twenty-first century. The Commission, San Francisco
66. Baggs JG, Schmitt MH, Mushlin AI, et al (1999) Association between nurse-physician collaboration and patient outcomes in three intensive care units. Crit Care Med 27:1991–1998
67. Daly BJ, Phelps C, Rudy EB (1991) A nurse-managed special care unit. J Nurs Adm 21:31–38
68. Daly BJ, Rudy EB, Thompson KS, Happ MB (1991) Development of a special care unit for chronically critically ill patients. Heart Lung 20:45–51

69. Hughes RG, Hunt SS, Luft HS (1987) Effects of surgeon volume and hospital volume on quality of care in hospitals. Med Care 25:489–503
70. Edwards EB, Roberts JP, McBride MA, Schulak JA, Hunsicker LG (1999) The effect of the volume of procedures at transplantation centers on mortality after liver transplantation. N Engl J Med 341:2049–2053
71. Hosenpud JD, Breen TJ, Edwards EB, Daily OP, Hunsicker LG (1994) The effect of transplant center volume on cardiac transplant outcome. A report of the United Network for Organ Sharing Scientific Registry. JAMA 271:1844–1849
72. Hannan EL, Racz M, Ryan TJ, et al (1997) Coronary angioplasty volume-outcome relationships for hospitals and cardiologists. JAMA 277:892–898
73. Showstack JA, Rosenfeld KE, Garnick DW, Luft HS, Schaffarzick RW, Fowles J (1987) Association of volume with outcome of coronary artery bypass graft surgery. Scheduled vs nonscheduled operations. JAMA 257:785–789
74. Miller FG, Fins JJ (1996) A proposal to restructure hospital care for dying patients. N Engl J Med 334:1740–1742
75. Cohen IL (1993) Establishing and justifying specialized teams in intensive care units for nutrition, ventilator management, and palliative care. Crit Care Clin 9:511–520
76. Cohen IL, Bari N, Strosberg MA, et al (1991) Reduction of duration and cost of mechanical ventilation in an intensive care unit by use of a ventilatory management team. Crit Care Med 19:1278–1284
77. Maxwell G, Marion L (1997) Flexible monitoring. Bringing technology to the patient. Nurs Manage 28:48B, 48F–48G, 48I
78. Grundy BL, Jones PK, Lovitt A (1982) Telemedicine in critical care: problems in design, implementation, and assessment. Crit Care Med 10:471–475
79. Kendall J, Reeves B, Clancy M (1998) Point of care testing: randomised controlled trial of clinical outcome. Br Med J 316:1052–1057
80. Wachter RM, Goldman L (1996) The emerging role of "hospitalists" in the American health care system. N Engl J Med 335:514–517
81. Teres D, Brown RB, Lemeshow S, Parsells JL (1983) A comparison of mortality and charges in two differently staffed intensive care units. Inquiry 20:282–289
82. Li TC, Phillips MC, Shaw L, Cook EF, Natanson C, Goldman L (1984) On-site physician staffing in a community hospital intensive care unit. Impact on test and procedure use and on patient outcome. JAMA 252:2023–2027
83. Pollack MM, Katz RW, Ruttimann UE, Getson PR (1988) Improving the outcome and efficiency of intensive care: the impact of an intensivist. Crit Care Med 16:11–17
84. Reynolds HN, Haupt MT, Thill-Baharozian MC, Carlson RW (1988) Impact of critical care physician staffing on patients with septic shock in a university hospital medical intensive care unit. JAMA 260:3446–3450
85. Brown JJ, Sullivan G (1989) Effect on ICU mortality of a full-time critical care specialist. Chest 96:127–129
86. Marshall MF, Schwenzer KJ, Orsina M, Fletcher JC, Durbin CG Jr (1992) Influence of political power, medical provincialism, and economic incentives on the rationing of surgical intensive care unit beds. Crit Care Med 20:387–394
87. Pollack MM, Cuerdon TT, Patel KM, Ruttimann UE, Getson PR, Levetown M (1994) Impact of quality-of-care factors on pediatric intensive care unit mortality. JAMA 272:941–946
88. Mallick R, Strosberg M, Lambrinos J, Groeger JS (1995) The intensive care unit medical director as manager. Impact on performance. Med Care 33:611–624
89. Carson SS, Stocking C, Podsadecki T, et al (1996) Effects of organizational change in the medical intensive care unit of a teaching hospital: a comparison of 'open' and 'closed' formats. JAMA 276:322–328
90. Kollef MH, Ward S (1999) The influence of access to a private attending physician on the withdrawal of life-sustaining therapies in the intensive care unit. Crit Care Med. 27:2125–2132
91. Kollef MH (1996) Private attending physician status and the withdrawal of life-sustaining interventions in a medical intensive care unit population. Crit Care Med 24:968–975

92. Manthous CA, Amoateng-Adjepong Y, al-Kharrat T, et al (1997) Effects of a medical intensivist on patient care in a community teaching hospital. Mayo Clin Proc 72:391–399
93. Multz AS, Chalfin DB, Samson IM, et al (1998) A "closed" medical intensive care unit (MICU) improves resource utilization when compared with an "open" MICU. Am J Respir Crit Care Med 157:1468–1473
94. Tai DY, Goh SK, Eng PC, Wang YT (1998) Impact on quality of patient care and procedure use in the medical intensive care unit (MICU) following reorganisation. Ann Acad Med Singapore 27:309–313
95. Hanson CW 3rd, Deutschman CS, Anderson HL 3rd, et al (1999) Effects of an organized critical care service on outcomes and resource utilization: a cohort study. Crit Care Med 27:270–274
96. Ghorra S, Reinert SE, Cioffi W, Buczko G, Simms HH (1999) Analysis of the effect of conversion from open to closed surgical intensive care unit. Ann Surg 229:163–171

Process of Care Assessment and the Evaluation of Outcome from Intensive Care

W. A. Knaus

Introduction

Process assessment has a short and not terribly impressive record within medical science. Nevertheless there are lessons to be learned from its history that could be useful for the future direction and emphasis of clinical and health services research within intensive care medicine. More importantly, recent evidence suggests that intensive care may be very well suited to the evaluation of specific processes since these are so well defined and their impact on short term patient outcomes are remarkably large.

In this brief chapter, I will first review the modern history of process assessment, then discuss the current state of knowledge of process assessment within intensive care, and conclude with a few examples of process assessment within acute care medicine that might serve as role models for future efforts.

Brief Review of Process Assessment in Medicine

Modern attention to process assessment in medicine began when Deming [1] introduced industrial quality assurance techniques to US industries, and Donabedian [2] adapted these techniques for medical practice.

Process assessment refers to the explicit definition, measurement, and recording of the activities of health care professionals and institutions undertaken during care. Process assessment is distinct from the organization and structure of medical services or the credentials of practitioners (see Figure 2, page 163). The theory is that there are specific practices or processes that practitioners can apply to patients that will improve outcomes. Identifying and encouraging compliance to these optimal practices therefore would improve patient outcomes.

Process assessment in medicine received its first wide scale introduction through the Professional Standards and Review Organizations (PSRO) program in the US [3]. The PSRO program was a federally mandated and funded effort to measure and track process compliance with a set of utilization criteria. Every state in the United States was required to have a professionally directed PSRO that reviewed the utilization and services provided to government-funded patients, Medicare and Medicaid. This resulted in an elaborate bureaucracy and infrastructure that developed explicit criteria for the admission and treatment of hospitalized patients. Virtually all of the criteria used by the PSRO program were based on the expert judgement of practicing clinicians and, as such, represented explicit but largely unverified assumptions of the most efficient and efficacious clinical processes. There was also an ongoing controversy that, while the PSRO program was intended to improve the quality of care, its real intent was to control and limit costs. As a result it is generally accepted that the PSRO program, which is still in operation, has been a well meaning but marginally effective attempt to introduce industrial quality assurance techniques into medical services.

From a policy perspective, however, the importance of the PSRO program was substantial. It represented a very large wide scale attempt to orient the process of medical care decision making toward objective as opposed to personal criteria. These efforts continue in other forms today as well as in existing peer-review organizations.

Specifically, an effort to make medicine more objective continues within the current emphasis on outcome assessment. It has now been widely recognized and accepted that there are large variations in the process of medical care that do not appear connected to patient outcomes [4]. These variations in medical processes, while once accepted as part of the art of medical practice, are now increasingly viewed as undesirable. They are thought to increase the cost of medical care while not providing optimal care. In essence, as the scientific underpinnings of medical practice have become more secure there is less tolerance of individual variation in practice styles based on personal practitioner preferences or beliefs. One of the main differences between the outcomes assessment movement and the earlier peer review process movement is that the objective is now on measuring and improving patient outcomes. Knowledge of and adherence to specific process measures are only valuable if they have been connected to these superior outcomes. This is obviously a more difficult but ultimately more meaningful and potentially useful approach to quality assessment.

With this introduction, what do we know about the processes/outcome relationship within intensive care medicine and what tools do we have with which to measure?

Process Assessment within Intensive Care

For the purposes of this discussion, process assessment can be further defined as;

- What is done?
- When is it done?
- How is it done?

What is done?

With the introduction of the Therapeutic Intervention Scoring System (TISS) in 1974, intensive care gained a very specific and useful tool for documenting specific processes of care [5]. Within the original TISS system and its more recent refinements and derivations, there is the capability to objectively and reproducibly record a wide variety of monitoring, diagnostic, and therapeutic processes of intensive care [6]. As such, the TISS system has proved to be an invaluable resource providing a uniform standard approach to process assessment for intensive care units (ICUs).

When is it done?

Because intensive care is practiced in a designated and well-defined physical location, determining when ICU services begin would appear to be straightforward. Since many of the specific practices enumerated within the TISS system can be begun in other settings, however, there has been some confusion in regard to when it is appropriate to designate the start of intensive care. Some of the confusion of this timing issue relates to when patients are treated within emergency rooms prior to ICU admission [7]. Because emergency rooms are capable of providing many of the life support services of intensive care, it can be argued that intensive care should begin at that time. Since the subsequent admission of the patient to the ICU is not established at the time of initial emergency room admission and treatment, however, and since criteria for ICU admission are not uniform and standardized, greater uniformity in the consistency of data collection will be achieved if the actual admission of the patient to the unit is used as the operating definition (lead time bias definition) When the patient is admitted to the ICU from another hospital ward or as a transfer from another hospital, recording the hospital stay prior to ICU admission provides an important measure of time course and can assist in adjusting for the stage of illness when ICU treatment began.

How is it done?

This refers to either the technical component of intensive care processes or the manner in which the care is administered. Unlike the actual type of therapy or timing, measurement of the conduct of the process of care is more controversial and difficult. For example, it is widely believed that individuals vary in their technical competence based on their training and experience. Information describing these characteristics, however, can as easily be designated as being part of the structure or organization of the unit rather than part of the actual process of care. Other less tangible components such as the co-ordination of care, the communication among care givers, conflict resolution, etc., that are also believed to have a role in outcomes have been studied. There are specific instruments, in this case, standardized questionnaires that can be used to measure these aspects of the process of care. These have been used in ICUs and have been found to be reliable [8, 9].

What do we know about the Impact of ICU Processes on Patient Outcome?

What is done?

Our information about the impact of specific ICU processes on patient outcomes comes from applying the above tools and concepts within three major types of studies, randomized controlled trials (RCTs), meta-analysis of randomized trials, and prospective observational studies. The overall conclusion from these studies is that specific components of ICU processes appear to be closely associated with patient outcomes. In most cases, however, they have not demonstrated patient benefit but have suggested and, in some cases, concluded that there is patient harm.

Within the last decade there have been four uncoordinated but conceptually related lines of investigation that examined core components of ICU life supporting care: transfusion; colloid administration; use of vasopressors to achieve above normal hemodynamic measurements; and artificial ventilation. In three of the four cases, the process evaluation was whether an aggressive or maximal approach to use of the process improved hospital and short term mortality rates. In the fourth case, the use of colloids was contrasted with use of crystalloid solutions.

The most extensive evaluation of process in intensive care occurred in the case of using vasopressor drugs, volume loading, and other processes to attempt to achieve supernormal or above normal physiologic, specifically hemodynamic performance measurements and to increase the delivery of oxygen to vital organs. There is a long and detailed history to these proposed processes that will not be repeated here [10]. The current evidence as summarized in the review article by Heyland et al. [11] is that process interventions designed to achieve superphysiologic goals of cardiac index, and to maximize oxygen delivery do not significantly reduce mortality. This review also concluded that methodological limitations in the manner in which trials and other comparisons were conducted limited the value and implications of the evidence.

Another long-standing controversy within critical care practice concerns the process of fluid resuscitation: crystalloid versus colloids. Two recent review articles that compiled evidence from 67 RCTs concluded that there was no evidence to recommend the use of colloids over crystalloids and that, especially for the use of human albumin, the risk of death was actually higher [12, 13]. Indeed the use of crystalloid was associated with an absolute increase in mortality risk of 4% (95% confidence interval 0% to 8%). For albumin the increased risk was 6% (95% confidence intervals 3% to 9%). The latter conclusion would mean that for every 17 critically ill patients treated with albumin there is one additional death.

Closely related to the above is the recent multicenter clinical trial of transfusion requirements as conducted by the Canadian Critical Care Trials Group [14]. This trial established that a restrictive strategy of red-cell transfusion is at least as effective and may be superior to one that attempts to maintain higher hemoglobin concentrations. This finding was true for all patients with the possible exception of patients with acute myocardial infarction and unstable angina.

Finally, there was the recent and, as yet, unpublished results of the comparison of high to low volume ventilation in patients with acute respiratory distress syndrome (ARDS). That trial clearly indicated a detrimental effect when using higher volume tidal volumes for mechanical ventilation, with a significant difference in mortality [15].

Another more controversial study of ICU process involved the monitoring and diagnostic technology of right heart or Swan-Ganz catheterization. Within a retrospective observational study that went to elaborate lengths to control for confounding by selection bias, Connors and associates suggested that the use of this invasive monitoring device was associated with an increased short-term mortality rate [16]. These observations, while far from definitive, were sufficiently compelling to prompt the National Heart Blood and Lung Institute to fund a RCT of this widely used and accepted technology. Whether this effort will, like the trials that addressed the hemodynamic question, confirm or refute the results from the observational study remains to be seen.

Important lessons from these experiences, however, include the need to take into account all aspects of the process intervention especially its timing, as well as adherence to either rigorous randomization protocols or comprehensive attempts to adjust for selection bias if randomization is not possible. Some of the confusion and perhaps concern over the widescale dissemination of an aggressive approach to hemodynamic support may have been avoided if these principles had been acknowledged. This experience demonstrates how easy it is in observational studies to attribute effects to a particular process intervention that may be associated more with the characteristics of patients with superior outcomes rather than any specific therapeutic approach.

This collective experience also provides a clear if stark reminder of the dangers of relying on expert judgement to create process guidelines in the absence of objective evidence of effects on outcomes. All of the above processes were recommended and strongly endorsed by experienced and well-intentioned ICU clinicians and professional societies. Colloid administration remains a widely used process in critical care. Colloids are recommended in a number of resuscitation guidelines and intensive care management algorithms [17, 18]. The American hospital consortium guidelines recommend that colloids be used in hemorrhagic shock until blood products become available and in non-hemorrhagic shock after an initial infusion with crystalloid. A 1995 survey of American health centers found that their actual use clearly exceeds these recommendations [19]. It is not known when, if ever, this expensive and potentially dangerous approach will be altered. A process, once established, becomes very difficult to change.

When is it done?

As the above review discussion, timing of a process is critical in its proper evaluation. There is still some controversy regarding whether an aggressive approach to hemodynamic management if implemented pre-operatively for selected high-risk patients is beneficial. The fact that the implementation of protocols for maximizing oxygen delivery were applied without adequate consideration of their timing confounded interpretation of their impact.

The extensive experience within intensive care for developing and refining scoring systems for case mix adjustment has also highlighted the need to carefully document when in the course of the illness the particular process is being applied. One of the latest revisions to the APACHE classification system, APACHE III, contains an explicit variable that attempts to control for the timing of the onset of ICU process care. This variable consists of either the treatment location and/or the number of days of hospitalization that preceded ICU admission [20]. The functional form of this variable indicates that patients admitted directly from the emergency room have the lowest baseline risk of death and patients admitted after prolonged hospital stays the highest. One implication of this is that the earlier intensive care therapy is initiated the better the outcome. It certainly mandates the explicit recording of timing within any evaluation of process.

How is it done?

Because intensive care involves both technical processes and substantial human interaction there has been an interest in attempting to document whether variations in the type and quality of the human ICU team influence outcome. Interest in this area was stimulated, in part, by a study we published in 1986 suggesting that the ICU with the poorest human interactions (the doctors and nurses unable to sit together within the same room to discuss care processes) also had the lowest risk adjusted performance ranking [21]. Since this was a retrospective analysis within a relatively limited data set of 13 hospitals, we conducted a more carefully controlled prospective evaluation. That study involved 40 institutions with independent and prospective hypothesis testing that variations in the process of coordination, communication, and conflict resolution within the ICU teams would result in superior short term patient outcomes [8]. The results from that study did demonstrate some weak but unconvincing associations. Similar results were also obtained from the EURICUS-1 study [9].

One possible criticism of both of these studies is that the effect size of these human as opposed to medical and technical interventions is small and the outcome endpoint used in these studies, risk adjusted hospital mortality and length of ICU stay, would not have been affected. Also important was that these were observational studies, focusing on variations in these human interactions that were naturally occurring and that, while they achieved statistical significance, were small in overall magnitude. Contrast these results with that from a recent interventional study of outcomes from trauma care that included changing compliance with trauma team activation and consultation protocols, addressing delays for operating room transfer and other critical aspects of trauma process. This before and after study demonstrated small but significant improvements in length of stay and risk adjusted mortality [22].

The lessons from these efforts indicate that instruments developed in other non-medical settings to measure the type and quality of human interaction can be used within the intensive care setting. The association of superior team coordination with patient outcome, however, remains to be established and perhaps can be best approached within interventional as compared to observational studies.

A Descending Limb of the ICU Process-Benefit Curve?

One overall conclusion from this brief but concentrated review of the tools of measuring ICU process is that there appears to be evidence for a descending limb to the treatment benefit curve within intensive care (Fig. 1). The past three decades or so of investigations and especially evidence from the most recent ten-year period appear to suggest that too much intensive care may be harmful. Specifically the aggressive use of vasopressors, red cell transfusions, colloid administration, and large volume mechanical ventilation all increase the observed short-term death rates. I believe this is an important observation not only for its implications for patient care but also for the future of research into the value of specific ICU processes. These findings suggest that specific ICU processes are sufficiently powerful that, with the appropriate study design, their impact can be detected with logistically feasible sample sizes.

For example, the study that demonstrated the impact of a more restrictive approach to red cell transfusion enrolled 838 patients [14]. The trial that demonstrated the advantage of lower volume tidal volumes had a similar sample size [15]. These experiences suggest that a reasonably sized study with a clear operational definition of a specific process that takes into account the timing of the intervention stands a reasonable chance of detecting a clinically significant impact. Most importantly, these results suggest that fear of encountering Type II

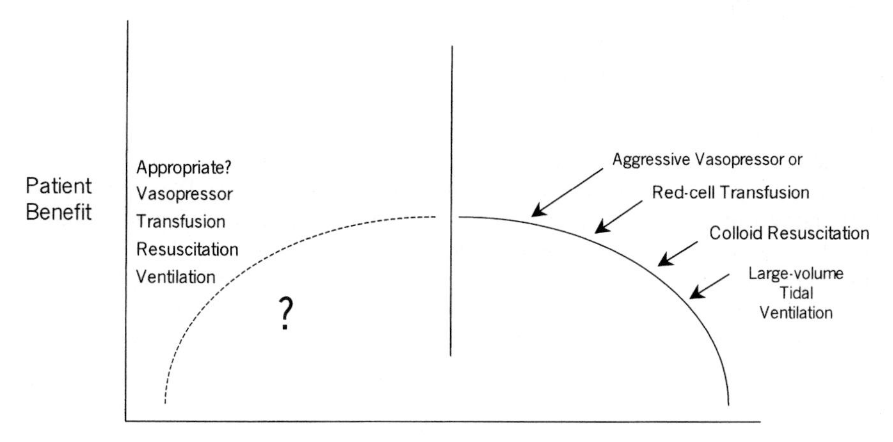

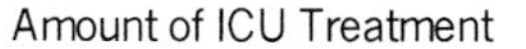

Fig. 1. The descending limb of the ICU benefit curve

errors, due to low power from either a small sample size or minimal treatment effect of the process, while still an important consideration, should not deter investigators from examining controversial, expensive, or potentially dangerous ICU processes.

Future Efforts: Two Examples of Clinically Useful Process Evaluation Efforts

This final section describes two approaches that could serve as role models for future efforts to use health services research approaches to study process with the aim of improving patient outcomes from intensive care. The first approach involves selecting a condition with associated processes that are hypothesized to have an important impact on patient outcomes but are not uniformly applied. The association between these specific processes and outcome are then analyzed within a retrospective cohort study using pre-existing information sources. An example of this approach is the process of administration of IV antibiotics for either treatment of patients hospitalized for pneumonia or as prophylaxis for postoperative infections.

The pneumonia study involved 3,555 acute care hospitals throughout the United States and 14,069 Medicare patients hospitalized with pneumonia [23]. By using a combination of routinely collected medical information and selected medical record review it demonstrated that lower 30-day mortality was associated with antibiotic administration within eight hours of hospital arrival (odds ratio 0.85; 95% CI, 0.75–0.96) and blood culture collection within 24 hours of arrival (odds ratio 0.90; 95% CI, 0.81–1.00). This study also demonstrated marked variation both by hospital and by location of the country in how well these processes were followed.

The second study that examined IV antibiotic administration was from Salt Lake and took advantage of the computerized HELP information system [24]. It examined 2,847 patients given pre-operative IV antibiotics and found that there was a significant association between the administration of antibiotics within two hours of surgery and a lower incidence of post-operative infections.

The other approach to process assessment involves selecting a procedure or diagnosis and then prospectively studying the process and outcome from care. One of the longest running and most successful such undertakings is the Northern New England Cardiovascular Disease Study Group (NNECDSG) [25]. This regional voluntary consortium was founded in 1987 to provide information about the management of cardiovascular disease in Maine, New Hampshire, Vermont, and Massachusetts. This consortium is an inter-institutional model for the improvement of medical and surgical care. Members include cardiothoracic surgeons, interventional cardiologists, administrators, operating room and cardiac nurses, anesthesiologists, perfusionists and scientists associated with six New England institutions.

The NNECDSG maintains registries for all patients receiving coronary artery bypass grafting, percutaneous coronary interventions, and heart valve surgery. During the last 12 years, data on more than 88,000 procedures have been collected and analyzed. This group adopted a uniform approach to data collection and case mix adjustment. They then scrutinized the risk-adjusted outcomes from specific procedures and related these to specific processes of care. The results have been insights into specific aspects of the per-operative and operative period with specific process interventions being associated with superior patient outcomes. The NNECDSG has also developed tools to risk adjust and provide electronic decision support for therapeutic decisions. Another result has been a dramatic improvement in the risk-adjusted outcome from coronary bypass surgery following a regional intervention to standardize care based on best processes [26]. Although some of these impressive results are due to the concentration of attention within a limited number of high volume procedures, the approach taken and the willingness of this effort to both scrutinize and then alter their clinical practices based on the results is a model worth considering for intensive care. Many of the tools necessary for the type of in depth investigation conducted by the Northern New England Group are available to intensive care practitioners.

Conclusion

This chapter has demonstrated that the field of intensive care has a variety of tools and instruments validated and ready for use in scrutiny of many aspects of its process of care. It has also concluded that the treatment effects of many specific ICU processes appears to be large enough to be detected with reasonable sample sizes. Decisions as to whether to conduct these evaluations using RCTs, retrospective record reviews, or prospective observational registries will depend on the nature of the specific process being scrutinized, the hypothesized impact on patient outcomes, and the willingness of the clinicians to consider the results as evidence for re-examining their practice style choices.

References

1. Deming WE (1986) Out of the crisis. Massachusetts Institute of Technology, Cambridge
2. Donabedian A (1966) Evaluating the quality of medical care. Milbank Memorial Fund Quarterly. 44: 166–206
3. Knaus WA (1976) Implementation versus experimentation: The federal financing question in PSRO. Proceedings of the Boston University Conference, Quality Assurance in Hospitals. November 21–22, 1975. Aspen System Press
4. Wennberg JE, Barry MJ (1994) Outcomes research. Science. 264:758–759
5. Cullen DJ, Civetta JM, Briggs BA, Ferrara LC (1974) Therapeutic intervention scoring system: a method for quantitative comparison of patient care. Crit Care Med 2: 57–60
6. Cullen DJ, Keene R, Waternaux C, Kunsman JM, Caldera DL, Peterson H (1984) Results, charges, and benefits of intensive care for critically ill patients: update 1983. Crit Care Med 12: 102–106
7. Dragsted L, Jorgensen J, Jensen NH, et al (1989) Interhospital comparisons of patient outcome from intensive care: importance of lead-time bias. Crit Care Med 17: 418–422
8. Shortell SM, Zimmerman JE, Rousseau DM, et al (1994) The performance of intensive care units: does good management make a difference? Med Care 32: 508–525
9. Miranda DR, Ryan DW, Schaufeli WB, Fider E (1998) Organization and management of intensive care. Springer, Berlin

10. Shoemaker WC, Appel PL, Kram HB (1993) Hemodynamic and oxygen transport responses in survivors and nonsurvivors of high-risk surgery. Crit Care Med 21: 977–990
11. Heyland DK, Cook DJ, King D, Kernerman P, Brun-Buisson C (1996) Maximizing oxygen delivery in critically ill patients: a methodologic appraisal of the evidence. Crit Care Med 24:517–524
12. Schierhout G, Roberts I (1998) Fluid resuscitation with colloid or crystalloid solutions in critically ill patients: a systematic review of randomised trials. Br Med J 316: 961–964
13. Anonymous (1998). Human albumin administration in critically ill patients: systematic review of randomised controlled trials. Cochrane Injuries Group Albumin Reviewers. Br Med J 317: 235–240
14. Hebert PC, Wells G, Blajchman MA, et al (1999) A multicenter, randomized, controlled clinical trial of transfusion requirements in critical care. Transfusion Requirements in Critical Care Investigators, Canadian Critical Care Trials Group. N Engl J Med 340:409–417
15. Meade MO, Cook DJ, Kernerman P, Bernard G (1997) How to use articles about harm: the relationship between high tidal volumes, ventilating pressures, and ventilator-induced lung injury. Crit Care Med 25: 1915–1922
16. Connors AF Jr, Speroff T, Dawson NV, et al (1996) The effectiveness of right heart catheterization in the initial care of critically ill patients. SUPPORT Investigators. JAMA. 276: 889–897
17. Vermeulen LC Jr, Ratko TA, Erstad BL, Brecher ME, Matuszewski KA (1995) A paradigm for consensus. The University Hospital Consortium guidelines for the use of albumin, nonprotein colloid, and crystalloid solutions. Arch Intern Med 155:373–379
18. Armstrong RF, Ballen C, Cohen SH, Webb AR (1994). Critical care algorithms. Oxford Medical Publications, Oxford
19. Yim JM, Vermeulen LC, Erstad BL, Matuszewski KA, Burnett DA, Vlasses PH (1995) Albumin and nonprotein colloid solution use in US academic health centers. Arch Intern Med 155: 2450–2455
20. Knaus WA, Wagner DP, Draper EA, et al (1991) The APACHE III prognostic system. Risk prediction of hospital mortality for critically ill hospitalized adults. Chest. 100: 1619–1636
21. Knaus WA, Draper EA, Wagner DP, Zimmerman JE (1986) An evaluation of outcome from intensive care in major medical centers. Ann Intern Med 104: 410–418
22. Simons R, Eliopoulos V, Laflamme D, Brown DR (1999) Impact on process of trauma care delivery 1 year after the introduction of a trauma program in a provincial trauma center. J Trauma 46: 811–815
23. Meehan TP, Fine MJ, Krumholz HM, Scinto JD, Galusha DH, Mockalis JT (1997) Quality of care, process, and outcomes in elderly patients with pneumonia. JAMA 278: 2080–2084
24. Classen DC, Evans RS, Pestotnik SL, Horn SD, Menlove RL, Burke JP (1992) The timing of prophylactic administration of antibiotics and the risk of surgical-wound infection. N Engl J Med 326: 281–286
25. O'Connor GT, Plume SK, Olmstead EM, et al (1991) A regional prospective study of in-hospital mortality associated with coronary artery bypass grafting. The Northern New England Cardiovascular Disease Study Group. JAMA. 266: 803–809
26. O'Connor GT, Plume SK, Olmstead EM, et al (1996) A regional intervention to improve the hospital mortality associated with coronary artery bypass graft surgery. The Northern New England Cardiovascular Disease Study Group. JAMA. 275: 841–846

Severity of Illness

R. Moreno

Introduction

As a direct result of the polio epidemics of the 1950s, critical care medicine developed in the Western world. This new field of medical practice was supported over the following decades by rapid developments in monitoring and therapeutic technologies, by a growing body of knowledge about the physiopathological alterations of the critically ill patient, and by the appearance of new therapeutic strategies. Soon, the intensive care unit (ICU) transformed itself from a small and marginal place in the hospital, where critically ill patients were monitored and treated, to a full hospital department, responsible for the consumption of a growing proportion of the health care budget.

These changes resulted in economical and political pressure to evaluate the effectiveness in the use of the intensive care facilities. From the 1960s, when patients where generally considered so sick that any survival was viewed as a miracle, to the 1990s, when governments, regulatory agencies, and consumers are evaluating in detail the cost-effectiveness of almost all the aspects of medical practice, the situation has undergone a dramatic change. Part of this process involves the precise quantification of the prognostic determinants of the critically ill patient.

Although early attempts of severity evaluation and severity quantification in some populations began in the 1950s [1], it was not until 1974 that intensivists began to use objective methods for severity stratification, applicable to the majority of patients. The publication in 1974 by David Cullen et al. of the therapeutic intervention scoring system (TISS)[2] represented a major breakthrough in this process. Hypothesizing that therapeutic intensity equates severity, these authors created a scale of 76 nursing tasks (in its last version), assigning between 1 and 4 points to each nursing task, according to their complexity. For the first time, clinicians and managers had an instrument that allowed a more precise description of the severity of illness of the critically ill patient and the quantification of the resources used in their treatment. The cumbersome nature of the instrument and its sensitivity to the intra-institution availability of specific therapeutic options were recognized at that time, and TISS never gained widespread popularity as a prognostic indicator in the critically ill patient. It is currently used mainly as a proxy for costs and as a management instrument in the planning and evaluation of the nursing workload resources used in the ICU.

William Knaus and co-workers made a second major breakthrough in 1981 with the publication of a physiologically based classification system, the acute physiology, age and chronic health evaluation (APACHE) score [3]. This instrument was soon used in multi-institutional comparisons [4] and was followed in 1985 by a revised version, the APACHE II [5]. For the first time, the use of sophisticated statistical methods, based on data collected at patient level during the first 24 hours in the ICU, allowed the prediction of mortality for groups of patients. Simplifications of the original method and competitive models appeared in the following years, such as the simplified acute physiology score (SAPS) [6]and the mortality prediction models (MPM) [7].

Now in their second or third versions [8–10], these instruments represent the state of the art in the fields of risk adjustment and severity quantification, and will be analyzed in detail below, together with their main uses and limitations.

What Are The Available Instruments?

Several instruments are available for severity evaluation and outcome prediction in intensive care. Most of them are generic, designed to be applied to all (or almost all) critically ill patients, and some are specific, that is, they can only be applied to patients with a particular condition (e.g., trauma, pancreatitis or myocardial infarction).

The instruments can be divided also according to their aim: to measure severity, assigning points according to the severity of the evaluated patient; and to predict an outcome, providing the user with a numeric estimate of the probabilities of an outcome (e.g., hospital mortality) for that patient or group of patients.

The most frequently used are described in more detail below.

APACHE II

The APACHE II was developed based on data collected from 1979 to 1982 in 13 hospitals in the US [5]. The choice of variables and their weights was made by a panel of experts, based on clinical judgment and on the relationships between the degree of physiological derangement and outcome documented in the literature. The rationale on which its construction is based is that the derangement of homeostasis has an adverse effect on mortality and that the magnitude of change from normal values for physiological and laboratory variables is proportional to their effects on outcome.

The model uses the worst value during the first 24 hours in the ICU for 12 physiologic variables (weighted from 0 to 4 points according to the degree of change from normal values), age, surgical status (non-operative, emergency surgery and elective surgery) and chronic health status. The APACHE II score varies between 0 and 71 points; up to 60 for physiological variables, up to 6 for age, and up to 5 for chronic health status.

Further information on the main diagnosis on ICU admission (chosen from a list of 50 diagnoses) allows the user to estimate the probability of hospital death using a multiple logistic regression equation.

APACHE III

The APACHE III was developed by William Knaus and co-workers between 1988 and 1989 in a sample of 40 hospitals, though to be representative of US hospitals with more than 200 beds [8].

This model comprises the APACHE III score, based on 17 acute physiological variables, age, chronic health status, and the predictive equation APACHE III. The equation uses reference data on 78 major diagnostic categories, surgical status and location before ICU admission, to provide the user with an estimate of the probability of intra-hospital death.

The APACHE III score varies between 0 and 299 points, including up to 252 for 17 physiologic variables, up to 24 for age, and up to 23 for chronic health status. All the physiological variables are registered as the worst values during the first 24 hours in the ICU. APACHE III is a commercial system; the equations are not in the public domain and must be purchased from APACHE Medical Systems, Washington.

SAPS II

SAPS II was described in 1993 by Jean-Roger Le Gall and co-workers, based on a European/North American study [9]. It was developed and validated in a large sample of patient data from 110 European hospitals and 27 North American hospitals.

This model comprises 17 variables: 12 physiological variables, age, type of admission (non-operative, emergency surgery and elective surgery) and three prior diagnoses (AIDS, metastatic cancer and hematological cancer). The SAPS II score varies between 0 and 163 points (up to 116 for the physiological variables, up to 17 for age, and up to 30 for prior diagnosis). All the physiological variables are registered as the worst values during the first 24 hours in the ICU.

The computation of the risk of death does not require an admission diagnosis or further information on chronic health status.

MPM II

The MPM II models were described in 1993–1994 by Stanley Lemeshow and co-workers [10, 11], based on the same data used for the development of SAPS II plus additional data from six ICUs in the US. In these models, the final result is expressed only as a probability of death and not as a score. MPM consists in fact of four different models:

1) The MPM II admission model (MPM II_0), computed within one hour of ICU admission
2) The MPM II 24 hour model (MPM II_{24}), computed after 24 hours in the ICU
3) The MPM II 48 hour model (MPM II_{48}), computed after 48 hours in the ICU
4) The MPM II 72 hour model (MPM II_{72}), computed after 72 hours in the ICU.

The MPM II_0 model comprises 15 variables: age, three physiological variables, three chronic diseases, five acute diagnosis, type of admission, mechanical ventilation and cardio-pulmonary resuscitation prior to ICU admission. It is the only general model that is independent from the treatment provided in the ICU and can be used for patient stratification at the time they are admitted to the ICU.

The MPM II_{24} model comprises 13 variables: age, six physiological variables, three variables evaluated at ICU admission, type of admission, mechanical ventilation and the use of vasoactive drugs. All the physiological variables are evaluated based on the worst values during the first 24 hours in the ICU.

The MPM II_{48} and MPM II_{72} models use the same variables as the MPM II_{24} model, with different weights for the computation of the risk of death. Both are based on the worst values presented by the patient during the previous 24 hours.

Organ Dysfunction/Failure Scores

The Organ Failure Score was described by William Knaus et al. [12] in 1985, to quantify organ failure in critically ill patients. Initially very simple, evaluating organ failure as an on/off phenomenon, this type of score has been replaced in recent years by more complex systems, such as the Brussels score, the multiple organ dysfunction score (MODS) [14], the logistic organ dysfunction score (LODS) [15], and the sequential organ failure assessment score (SOFA) [16]. All of these systems are built on common assumptions, being able to describe the increasing dysfunction of individual organs and evaluate multiple organ dysfunction/failure as a continuous spectrum from normality through dysfunction to failure.

All the organ failure scores aim at patient description and not at outcome prediction, except for LODS, which incorporates an equation to predict hospital mortality based on the amount of organ dysfunction/failure present at 24 hours in the ICU.

Disease Specific Models

Several models have been proposed for severity evaluation in specific groups of patients, such as patients with trauma or with pancreatitis.

In trauma, the most used system is the injury severity score (ISS) that assigns points at time of death or discharge according to the severity of injury for six anatomical areas [17]. Evaluated together with the revised trauma score (rTS), that evaluates the physiology impact of trauma for the Glasgow Coma Scale, for blood pressure and for respiratory rate [18], the ISS constitutes the basis for the TRISS methodology [19], which has been used in several studies. Other systems have been proposed, such as the ASCOT (a severity characterization of trauma) method [20], but have not gained widespread acceptance.

Another field where specific instruments have been developed and gained some popularity is acute pancreatitis, where several disease-specific systems have been described [21], based on clinical and physiological variables [21–28] or on computed tomography (CT) scan findings [29]. Their use is still controversial, since several studies have not shown a clear superiority of these instruments over general severity scores [30–35] or even versus organ dysfunction/failure scores [36].

What are the Prognostic Determinants in the Critically Ill Patient?

All the general outcome prediction models aim at predicting a result (vital status on hospital discharge) based on a given set of variables, evaluated and registered on admission or at 24 hours in the ICU. In other words, they predict what the outcome of a patient, with a certain background and acute clinical condition (defined by the values of the predictive variables), will be if the patient was treated in a reference (theoretical) ICU, used to develop the model.

As presented above, the existing models differ greatly in the number and type of variables used, as well as in the timeframe for data collection (Table 1). In almost all of them, physiologic data are evaluated and registered during the first 24 hours after ICU admission, the exception being the admission component of the MPM (MPM II_0), which uses only data registered within one hour of ICU admission. The predictive variables can be divided into two groups:

1) Those that evaluate the chronic health status and the degree of physiological reserve of the patient (age, chronic diagnosis)
2) Those that evaluate the acute health status of the patient (acute diagnosis, and the presence and degree of physiological dysfunction such as heart rate, blood pressure, or leukocyte count).

Location before ICU admission also seems to be of prognostic significance [37–39]. The most important of these variables are those that evaluate the degree of physiological derangement presented by the patient during the first 24 hours in the ICU. It has been found that acute physiological derangement is uniquely responsible for almost 50% of the explanatory power of the models. This fact is illustrated in Figure 1, using data from the APACHE III model [8].

Table 1. Variables used in general outcome prediction models

Model	Number of variables	Time frame for data collection	Age	Origin of the patient	Surgical status	Chronic health status	Physiology	Acute diagnosis
APACHE [3]	34	24 hours	No	No	No	Yes	Yes	No
SAPS [6]	14	24 hours	Yes	No	No	No	Yes	No
APACHE II [5]	17	24 hours	Yes	No	Yes	Yes	Yes	Yes
MPM [133]	11	Within one hour and 24 hours	Yes	No	Yes	Yes	Yes	No
APACHE III [8]	26	24 hours	Yes	Yes	Yes	Yes	Yes	Yes
SAPS II [9]	17	24 hours	Yes	No	Yes	Yes	Yes	No
MPM II_0 [10]	15	Within one hour	Yes	No	Yes	Yes	Yes	Yes
MPM II_{24} [10]	13	24 hours	Yes	No	Yes	Yes	Yes	Yes
MPM II_{48} [11]	13	24 hours	Yes	No	Yes	Yes	Yes	Yes
MPM II_{72} [11]	13	24 hours	Yes	No	Yes	Yes	Yes	Yes

Depending on the degree of departure from normal values, points are assigned to each variable. The impact on mortality of the variations in the values of the variable can occur in just one direction (e.g., low values for the Glasgow Coma score, Fig. 2) or in both directions (e.g., lower and higher values for leucocytes, Fig. 3). An aggregated score is then computed, summing the values for all the variables.

Once computed, a logistic regression equation converts the score (or the variables directly, as in the case of MPM II) into a probability of hospital death. In this technique, the dependent variable or hospital mortality, Y is related to a series of independent or predictive variables through the equation

$$Y = b_0 + b_1x_1 + b_2x_2 \ldots b_kx_k$$

b_0 being the intercept of the model, x_1 to x_k the predictive variables, and b_1 to b_k the estimated regression coefficients. Then, a logistic transformation is applied, with the probability of death computed according to the equation:

$$\text{Probability of death} = \frac{e^{\text{logit}}}{1 + e^{\text{logit}}}$$

with *logit* = Y as described before. Using this curve, at the extremes of the score (very low or very high values), the associated changes in the probabilities of death are small. For intermediate values even small changes in the score are associated with large changes in the probability of death.

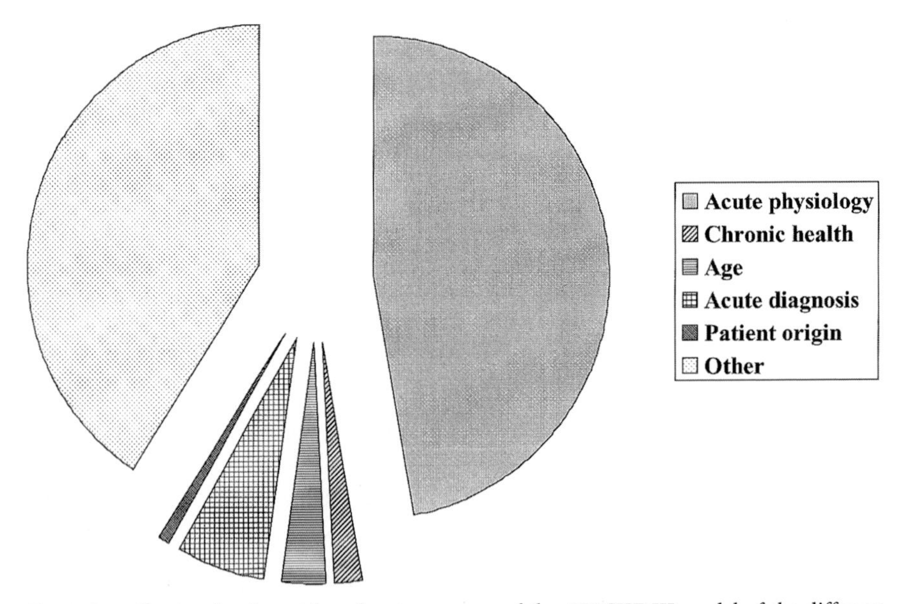

Fig. 1. Contribution for the total explanatory power of the APACHE III model of the different variables. Other, refers to the interaction among all other explanatory variables together. Adapted from Knaus et al. [8]

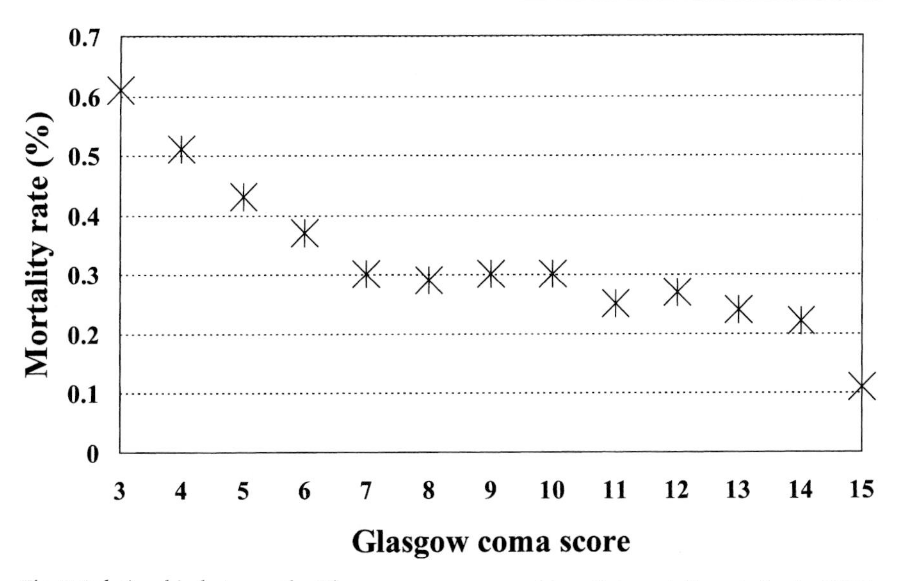

Fig. 2. Relationship between the Glasgow coma score and hospital mortality rate in the EURICUS-I database. With decreasing values in the score we can observe an increase in the mortality rate

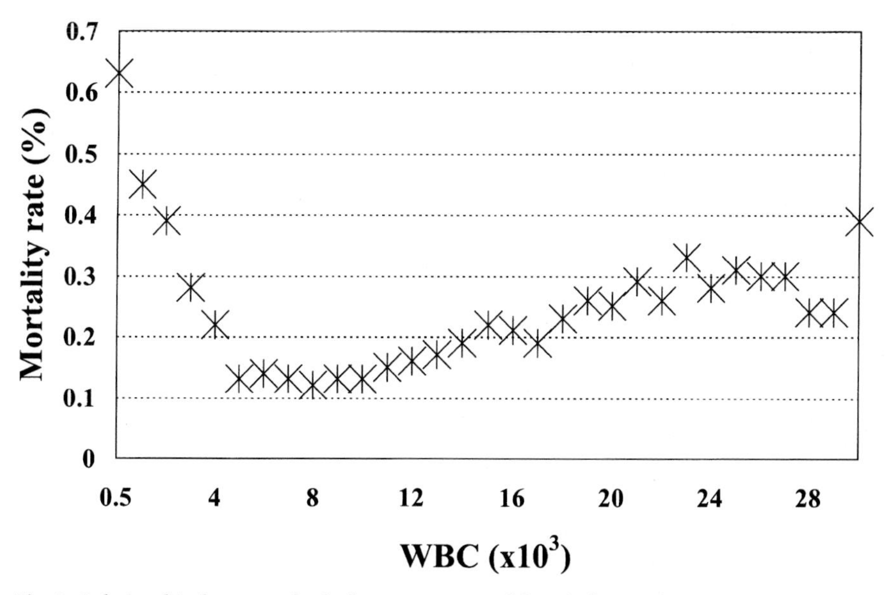

Fig. 3. Relationship between the leukocyte count and hospital mortality rate in EURICUS-I database. With very low or very high leukocyte counts, an increase in the mortality rate can be observed

When necessary, the model can be adapted to local situations through the computation of new coefficients for the logistic regression equation in a process termed customization [40–42].

It should be noted that the variables must be collected with great care. Several authors have analyzed this problem and found a great variation in the literature in the definitions used for the application of the models [43–45]. The errors most frequently noted are:

1) differences in definitions of the variables
2) differences in the time frame for data collection
3) very large variations in the exclusion criteria used for data collection and/or data analysis

In addition, the escalating use of information systems for data collection and management in the ICU can alter outcome prediction [46]. As a result, although in the original datasets reliability in data collection is described as high [9, 10, 47], several authors present a much darker picture of the use of outcome prediction models when applied out of the experimental context [48]. Two such studies, published in 1999, deserve a comment.

The first was published by Kess Polderman and co-workers [49], who assessed the inter-observer variation in the application of the APACHE II score in one Dutch ICU. They found a very large inter-observer variability between the scores (mean 14, standard deviation 6), similar in residents and in trained intensivists.

The second was published by Liddy Chen and co-workers [50], who assessed the inter–observer variation in the application of the APACHE II model in a network database. These authors did not find significant inter-observer differences in the mean global scores or in the mean predicted risks of death but described an agreement rate as low as 66.1% in the choice of the admission diagnosis.

These findings urge all researchers and clinicians who want to use these instruments to compare patient groups or ICUs, to be very careful in the definition of the variables and in the training of data abstractors. Up to now, intensivists have been more prone to check carefully the application of new drugs or the use of new monitoring devices. It is time to afford the same careful attention to this type of instrument.

Why I Need to Measure the Severity of Illness in the Critically Ill Patient?

Several reasons support the use of severity scores and general outcome prediction models in critically ill patients:

1) at the patient level, to describe the severity of illness of the individual patient and as an aid in the process of clinical decision making and in the allocation of resources
2) at the ICU level, for purposes of auditing, benchmarking, multi-institutional comparisons and intra-institutional comparisons.

Patient Level

Severity scores can be used to describe, in a language that everybody can understand, the severity of illness of individual patients. This information can then be used, for example, as a criterion for inclusion in clinical studies [51, 52]. This utilization is not controversial, but often requires the use of repetitive evaluations to capture and describe the evolution of the pathological process. Up to now, given the work involved in data collection, general severity scores have not been used routinely for this task, although some preliminary results support their use [53, 54]. The scores have also been used to predict which patients are going to die [55]. This utilization, which raises several ethical problems, is still very controversial and should not be routinely employed [56].

As an aid to the process of clinical decision-making, evidence suggests that outcome prediction models perform better than clinicians in prognostic prediction [57–65], or that they are helpful in this process [66–68]. This opinion is not supported by all [69–71], especially in the process of therapeutic limitation [72]. Moreover, the application of different models to the same patient often results in very different predictions [73]. As a result, the routine application of outcome prediction models to individual patients is still far from being incorporated into routine clinical practice and current recommendations do not allow their use in prognosis prediction in individual patients [74].

Moreover, we should not forget the probabilistic nature of the predictions given by existing instruments. A very well calibrated model can only, when applied to an individual patient, say that there exists a 46% probability of death; it can never say if that individual patient is one of the 54 of the 100 that will survive or one of the 46 in each 100 who will die. This fact makes such systems almost useless in the process of withholding or withdrawing therapy. They can, however, be useful in discussions with relatives, if they are well calibrated in that particular ICU. Some authors have demonstrated that the knowledge by the clinician of the predictions did not have a negative influence in quality of care but allowed a reduction in costs [75]. However, not all studies have confirmed this positive effect of clinician knowledge of prognosis in individual patients [76, 77].

Several studies exist in the literature describing methods for the identification and characterization of patients with a very low risk of developing complications [78–82]. These patients, who require only general care and basic monitoring, could eventually be transferred to other areas in the hospital [68, 83]. It can however be argued that the low mortality of these patients is explained by the fact that they are treated in the ICU, with transfer to other areas in the hospital resulting in a more frequent deterioration in their clinical status and in a higher mortality rate [84]. Moreover, the cost of a patient in intensive care depends mainly on the amount of nursing workload used. The clinical characteristics of the patient (diagnosis, severity of disease) are not the only determinants of this process, the practices and policies in each ICU playing an important role. To focus only on patient characteristics at ICU admission or at 24 hours ignores all the subsequent process of care. Consequently, we should focus on the balance between the required and the supplied nursing workload and in the appropriateness of their use [85]. This strategy seems preferable to approaches based on the condition of the patient or on the relationship between predicted and actual length of stay [86–88].

On the other hand, outcome prediction models have been used to identify the patient who potentially uses more resources [89], and in whom care is potentially ineffective [90, 91]. Examples of such use are the evaluation of the appropriateness of total parenteral nutrition [92], the identification of futile treatment in intensive care [93] or the prediction of prolonged support after coronary revascularization [94]. Unfortunately, this kind of patient can rarely be identified on ICU admission, since their degree of physiological derangement, although very variable, is usually not very high [95–97]. And, if one day we could identify such patients in a cost-effective way [98], what would we do with the information? Withdraw or withhold therapy from potentially expensive patients?

ICU Level

At the ICU level, general outcome prediction models have been used in auditing, benchmarking, multi-institutional comparisons and intra-institutional comparisons [99].

Several researchers have suggested the use of the ratio between actual and predicted death, the standard mortality ratio (SMR), in this process, assuming that the models can take into account the main prognostic determinants of the critically ill patient (e.g., age, previous health status, admission diagnosis, degree of physiologic derangement) [100]. The ratio is computed by dividing the actual mortality by the predicted mortality (summing up the individual probabilities of mortality) in the sample under analysis. Additional computations can be made for the estimation of the confidence interval of the SMR [101]. The interpretation of the SMR is easy: a ratio less than 1 implies that the performance is better than in the reference group, and a ratio greater than 1 that the performance is worse than in the reference group. An example of the application of this methodology can be found in Figure 4, using SAPS II to predict mortality, in the Portuguese Multicenter Study.

This methodology has been used in international comparisons of ICUs [102–107], comparisons of hospitals [4, 86, 87, 100, 108–113], evaluation of ICUs [114–118], and in the evaluation of the effects of organization and management on ICU performance [111, 119–121]. This approach has been subject to severe criticism and a few points should always be addressed before conclusions can be made [122]:

1) were valid methods used to compared the ICUs?
   - are the outcome measures accurate and comprehensive?
   - do the compared ICUs serve similar patients?
   - was the sample of patients sufficient and unbiased?
   - was appropriate risk adjustment undertaken?
   - do the comparisons really focus on care in the ICU?
2) how do we interpret these performance results?
   - what was the difference in outcome?
   - how confident are we in the results?

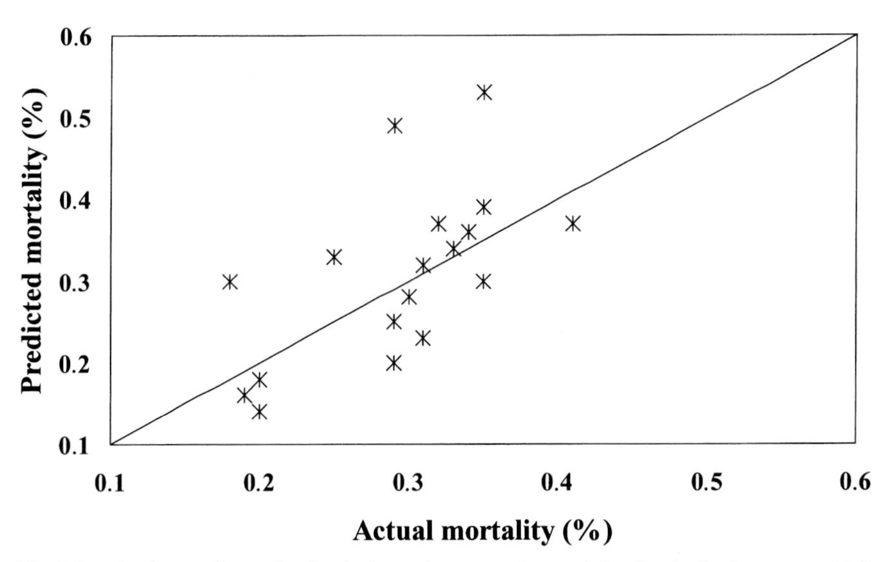

Fig. 4. Standard mortality ratios for the intensive care units participating in the Portuguese Multicenter Study, using SAPS II to compute the predicted mortality. Adapted from Moreno and Morais [109]

Moreover, to be meaningful, this comparison should be undertaken separately in low-, medium- and high-risk patients, as discussed before [123]. Only then could possible league tables or other benchmarking processes be done with confidence, as in other fields [124].

What are the Limitations of the Instruments?

Several examples can be found in the literature of an inadequate predictive capability of existing outcome prediction models, when applied in independent populations [41, 42, 103, 104, 108, 109, 125–127]. This feature was already recognized back in 1993 in a RAND Consensus Conference that stated "Mortality prediction models are almost always overspecific for the patient samples upon which they were developed, and thus performance usually deteriorates when models are applied to different population samples..." and recommended that "mortality prediction models should always be tested in patient samples distinct from those in which the models were developed".

Several explanations have been proposed for this problem [107], with previous research from our group demonstrating clearly that the performance of the models presents very large differences among relevant patient subgroups, varying from excellent to almost random predictive accuracy [129]. These differences can explain some of the difficulties the models show in accurately predicting mortality when applied to different populations with distinct patient baseline characteristics.

Conclusion: What the Future Holds

Over recent years, we have witnessed the transformation of prognostic science into a full scientific discipline. The amount of information about the prognostic determinants of the critically ill patient is today greater than ever and new statistical methods, aided by developments in medical informatics, are appearing in the ICU [130, 131].

It is time to step forwards, providing the clinician, in real time, with relevant prognostic information about their patients. To achieve this, we must complement the existing static models with dynamic scoring, which can be adapted to new information as it becomes available. Similarly, the benchmarking process should be refined. Increasingly, regulatory agencies and the general public are demanding that clinicians demonstrate the adequacy and quality of their practices [132]. New ways are needed to evaluate ICU performance, taking into account not only mortality but also other outcomes, such as quality of life, quality of death, and the appropriateness of the use of resources. The scope of our performance evaluation should also change, moving from the ICU to the health system as a whole, studying the interactions and the appropriateness of the use of all components of the system, starting with the general practitioner and finishing with post-hospital, long-term rehabilitation care. The ICU, which is part of this continuum of care, can and should be evaluated, not only in the short-term results it produces but also in its interactions with the global health care system.

As clinicians, we have the duty to provide the best and most human care to all our patients, employing to the best of our knowledge the resources we have to those who will survive, and allowing those who will die to do so with respect and dignity. For this, we need new and better instruments, properly tested and validated, that can be used to review and improve our practice. These are the challenges of the next decade.

References

1. Apgar V (1953) A proposal for a new method of evaluation of the newborn infant. Anaesth Analg 32:260–267
2. Cullen DJ, Civetta JM, Briggs BA, Ferrara LC (1974) Therapeutic intervention scoring system: a method for quantitative comparison of patient care. Crit Care Med 2:57–60
3. Knaus WA, Zimmerman JE, Wagner DP, Draper EA, Lawrence DE (1981) APACHE – acute physiology and chronic health evaluation: a physiologically based classification system. Crit Care Med 9:591–597
4. Knaus WA, Draper EA, Wagner DP, et al (1982) Evaluating outcome from intensive care: A preliminary multihospital comparison. Crit Care Med 10:491–496
5. Knaus WA, Draper EA, Wagner DP, Zimmerman JE (1985) APACHE II: a severity of disease classification system. Crit Care Med 13:818–829
6. Le Gall JR, Loirat P, Alperovitch A, et al (1984) A simplified acute physiologic score for ICU patients. Crit Care Med 12:975–977
7. Lemeshow S, Teres D, Pastides H, et al (1985) A method for predicting survival and mortality of ICU patients using objectively derived weights. Crit Care Med 13:519–525
8. Knaus WA, Wagner DP, Draper EA, et al (1991) The APACHE III prognostic system. Risk prediction of hospital mortality for critically ill hospitalized adults. Chest 100:1619–1636

9. Le Gall JR, Lemeshow S, Saulnier F (1993) A new simplified acute physiology score (SAPS II) based on a European/North American multicenter study. JAMA 270:2957–2963
10. Lemeshow S, Teres D, Klar J, Avrunin JS, Gehlbach SH, Rapoport J (1993) Mortality Probability Models (MPM II) based on an international cohort of intensive care unit patients. JAMA 270:2478–2486
11. Lemeshow S, Klar J, Teres D, et al (1994) Mortality probability models for patients in the intensive care unit for 48 or 72 hours: a prospective, multicenter study. Crit Care Med 22:1351–1358
12. Knaus WA, Draper EA, Wagner DP, Zimmerman JE (1985) Prognosis in acute organ-system failure. Ann Surg 202:685–693
13. Bernard G (1997) The Brussels score. Sepsis 1:43–44
14. Marshall JC, Cook DA, Christou NV, Bernard GR, Sprung CL, Sibbald WJ (1995) Multiple organ dysfunction score: a reliable descriptor of a complex clinical outcome. Crit Care Med 23:1638–1652
15. Le Gall JR, Klar J, Lemeshow S, et al (1996) The logistic organ dysfunction system. A new way to assess organ dysfunction in the intensive care unit. JAMA 276:802–810
16. Vincent J-L, Moreno R, Takala J, et al (1996) The SOFA (Sepsis-related organ failure assessment) score to describe organ dysfunction/failure. Intensive Care Med 22:707–710
17. Baker SP, O'Neill B, Haddon W Jr, Long WB (1974) The injury severity score: a method for describing patients with multiple injuries and evaluating emergency care. J Trauma 14:187–196
18. Chamion HR, Sacco WJ, Copes WS, Gann DS, Gennarelli TA, Flanagan ME (1989) A revision of the trauma score. J Trauma 29:623–629
19. Boyd C, Tolson M, Copes W (1987) Evaluating trauma care: the TRISS method. J Trauma 27:370–378
20. Champion HR, Copes WS, Sacco WJ, et al (1996) Improved predictions from a severity characterization of trauma (ASCOT) over trauma and injury severity score (TRISS): results of an independent evaluation. J Trauma 40:42–49
21. Agarwal N, Pitchumoni CS (1991) Assessment of severity in acute pancreatitis. Am J Gastroenterol 86:1385–1391
22. Ranson JHC, Rifkind KM, Roses DF, et al (1974) Prognostic signs and the role of operative management in acute pancreatitis. Surg Gynecol Obstet 139:69–81
23. Osborne DH, Imrie CW, Carter DC (1981) Biliary surgery in the same admission for gallstone-associated acute pancreatitis. Br J Surg 68:758–761
24. Fan ST, Choi TK, Wong J (1989) Prediction of severity of acute pancreatitis: an alternative approach. Gut 30:1591–1595
25. Tran DD, Cuesta MA (1992) Evaluation of severity in patients with acute pancreatitis. Am J Gastroenterol 87:604–608
26. Bradley EL (1993) A clinically based classification system for acute pancreatitis. Arch Surg 128:586–590
27. Niederau C, Luthen R, Heise JW, Becker H (1993) Prognosis of acute pancreatitis. In: Beger HG, Buchler M, Malfertheiner P (eds) Standards in Pancreatic Surgery. Springer-Verlag, Berlin pp76–91
28. Tran DD, Cuesta MA, Schneider AJ, Wesdorp RI (1993) Prevalence and prediction of multiple organ system failure and mortality in acute pancreatitis. J Crit Care 8:145–153
29. Balthazar EJ, Ranson JHC, Naidich DP, Megibaw AJ, Caccavale R, Cooper MM (1985) Acute pancreatitis: prognostic value of CT. Radiology 156:767–772
30. Larvin M, McMahon MJ (1989) APACHE-II score for assessment and monitoring of acute pancreatitis. Lancet 2:201–205
31. Wilson C, Heath DI, Imrie CW (1990) Prediction of outcome in acute pancreatitis: a comparative study of APACHE II, clinical assessment and multiple factor scoring systems. Br J Surg 77:1260–1264
32. Arnell TD, de Virgilio C, Chang L, Bongard F, Stabile BE (1996) Admission factors can predict the need for ICU monitoring in gallstone pancreatitis. Dig Surg 14283–14298

33. Brisinda G, Maria G, Ferrante A, Civello IM (1999) Evaluation of prognostic factors in patients with acute pancreatitis. Hepatogastroenterology 46:1990–1997
34. Armengol-Carrasco M, Oller B, Escudero LE, et al (1999) Specific prognostic factors for secondary pancreatic infection in severe acute pancreatitis. Dig Surg 16:125–129
35. Williams M, Simms H (1999) Prognostic usefulness of scoring systems in critically ill patients with severe acute pancreatitis. Crit Care Med 27:901–907
36. Matos R, Moreno R, Fevereiro T (2000) Severity evaluation in acute pancreatitis: the role of SOFA score and general severity scores. Crit Care 4:S138 (abst)
37. Dragsted L, Jorgensen J, Jensen NH, et al (1989) Interhospital comparisons of patient outcome from intensive care: importance of lead-time bias. Crit Care Med 17:418–422
38. Tunnell RD, Millar BW, Smith GB (1998) The effect of lead time bias on severity of illness scoring, mortality prediction and standardised mortality ratio in intensive care – a pilot study. Anaesthesia 53:1045–1053
39. Lundberg JS, Perl TM, Wiblin T, et al (1998) Septic shock: an analysis of outcomes for patients with onset on hospital wards versus intensive care units. Crit Care Med 26:1020–1024
40. Moreno R, Apolone G (1997) The impact of different customization strategies in the performance of a general severity score. Crit Care Med 25:2001–2008
41. Metnitz PG, Valentin A, Vesely H, et al (1999) Prognostic performance and customization of the SAPS II: results of a multicenter Austrian study. Intensive Care Med 25:192–197
42. Rivera-Fernandez R, Vazquez-Mata G, Bravo M, et al (1998) The Apache III prognostic system: customized mortality predictions for Spanish ICU patients. Intensive Care Med 24:574–581
43. Abizanda Campos R, Balerdi B, Lopez J, et al (1994) Fallos de prediccion de resultados mediante APACHE II. Analisis de los errores de prediction de mortalidad en pacientes criticos. Med Clin Barc 102:527–531
44. Fery-Lemmonier E, Landais P, Kleinknecht D, Brivet F (1995) Evaluation of severity scoring systems in the ICUs: translation, conversion and definitions ambiguities as a source of interobserver variability in APACHE II, SAPS, and OSF. Intensive Care Med 21:356–360
45. Rowan K (1996) The reliability of case mix measurements in intensive care. Curr Opin Crit Care 2:209–213
46. Bosman RJ, Oudemane van Straaten HM, Zandstra DF (1998) The use of intensive care information systems alters outcome prediction. Intensive Care Med 24:953–958
47. Damiano AM, Bergner M, Draper EA, Knaus WA, Wagner DP (1992) Reliability of a measure of severity of illness: acute physiology and chronic health evaluation -II. J Clin Epidemiol 45:93–101
48. Goldhill DR, Sumner A (1998) APACHE II, data accuracy and outcome prediction. Anaesthesia 53:937–943
49. Polderman KH, Thijs LG, Girbes AR (1999) Interobserver variability in the use of APACHE II scores. Lancet 353:380
50. Chen LM, Martin CM, Morrison TL, Sibbald WJ (1999) Interobserver variability in data collection of the APACHE II score in teaching and community hospitals. Crit Care Med 27:1999–2004
51. Gattinoni L, Brazzi L, Pelosi P, et al (1995) A trial of goal orientated hemodynamic therapy in critically ill patients. N Engl J Med 333:1025–1032
52. Galbán C, Montejo JC, Masejo A, et al (2000) An immune-enhancing enteral diet reduces mortality rate and episodes of bacteremia in septic intensive care unit patients. Crit Care Med 28:643–648
53. Moreno R, Estrada H, Miranda I, Massa L (1994) SAPS II over time: a preliminary study. Clin Intensive Care 5:S122 (abst)
54. Wagner DP, Knaus WA, Harrel Jr. FE, Zimmerman JE, Watts C (1994) Daily prognostic estimates for critically ill adults in intensive care units: results from a prospective, multicenter, inception cohort analysis. Crit Care Med 22:1359–1372
55. Chang RW (1989) Individual outcome prediction models for intensive care units. Lancet i: 143–146

56. Jacobs S, Arnold A, Clyburn PA, Willis BA (1992) The Riyadh intensive care program applied to a mortality analysis of a teaching hospital intensive care unit. Anaesthesia 47:775–780
57. Perkins HS, Jonsen AR, Epstein WV (1986) Providers as predictors: using outcome predictions in intensive care. Crit Care Med 14:105–110
58. Silverstein MD (1988) Predicting instruments and clinical judgement in critical care. JAMA 260:1758–1759
59. Dawes RM, Faust D, Mechl PE (1989) Clinical versus actuarial judgement. Science 243:1668–74.
60. Kleinmuntz B (1990) Why we still use our heads instead of formulas: toward an integrative approach. Psychol Bull 107:296–310
61. McClish DK, Powell SH (1989) How well can physicians estimate mortality in a medical intensive care unit? Med Decis Making 9:125–132
62. Poses RM, Bekes C, Winkler RL, Scott WE, Copare FJ (1990) Are two (inexperienced) heads better than one (experienced) head? Averaging house officers prognostic judgement for critically ill patients. Arch Intern Med 150:1874–1878
63. Poses RM, Bekes C, Copare FJ, et al (1989) The answer to "what are my chances, doctor?" depends on whom is asked: prognostic disagreement and inaccuracy for critically ill patients. Crit Care Med 17:827–833
64. Winkler RL, Poses RM (1993) Evaluating and combining physicians' probabilities of survival in an intensive care unit. Manag Sci 39:1526–1543
65. Marcin JP, Pollack MM, Patel KM, Ruttimann UE (1998) Decision support issues using a physiology based score. Intensive Care Med 24:1299–1304
66. Chang RWS, Lee B, Jacobs S, Lee B (1989) Accuracy of decisions to withdraw therapy in critically ill patients: clinical judgement versus a computer model. Crit Care Med 17:1091–1097
67. Knaus WA, Rauss A, Alperovitch A, et al (1990) Do objective estimates of chances for survival influence decisions to withhold or withdraw treatment? Med Decis Making 10:163–171
68. Zimmerman JE, Wagner DP, Draper EA, Knaus WA (1994) Improving intensive care unit discharge decisions: supplementary physician judgment with predictions of next day risk for life support. Crit Care Med 22:1373–1384
69. Branner AL, Godfrey LJ, Goetter WE (1989) Prediction of outcome from critical illness: a comparison of clinical judgement with a prediction rule. Arch Intern Med 149:1083–1086
70. Kruse JA, Thill–Baharozin MC, Carlson RW (1988) Comparison of clinical assessment with APACHE II for predicting mortality risk in patients admitted to a medical intensive care unit. JAMA 260:1739–1742
71. Marks RJ, Simons RS, Blizzard RA, et al (1991) Predicting outcome in intensive therapy units – a comparison of APACHE II with subjective assessments. Intensive Care Med 17:159–163
72. Knaus WA, Wagner DP, Lynn J (1991) Short-term mortality predictions for critically ill hospitalized adults: science and ethics. Science 254:389–394
73. Lemeshow S, Klar J, Teres D (1995) Outcome prediction for individual intensive care patients: useful, misused, or abused ? Intensive Care Med 21:770–776
74. Suter P, Armagandis A, Beaufils F, et al (1994) Predicting outcome in ICU patients: consensus conference organized by the ESICM and the SRLF. Intensive Care Med 20:390–397
75. Murray LS, Teasdale GM, Murray GD, et al (1993) Does prediction of outcome alter patient management ? Lancet 341:1487–1491
76. Knaus WA, Harrell FE, Lynn J, et al (1995) The SUPPORT prognostic model. Objective estimates for seriously ill hospitalized adults. Study to understand prognoses and preferences for outcomes and risks of treatments. Ann Intern Med 122:191–203
77. Bellamy PE (1997) Why did prognosis presentation not work in the SUPPORT study? Curr Opin Crit Care 3:188–191
78. Henning RJ, McClish D, Daly B, et al (1987) Clinical characteristics and resource utilization of ICU patients: implementation for organization of intensive care. Crit Care Med 15:264–269
79. Wagner DP, Knaus WA, Draper EA (1987) Identification of low-risk monitor admissions to medical–surgical ICUs. Chest 92:423–428

80. Wagner DP, Knaus WA, Draper EA, et al (1983) Identification of low-risk monitor patients within a medical-surgical ICU. Med Care 21:425–433
81. Zimmerman JE, Wagner DP, Knaus WA, Williams JF, Kolakowski D, Draper EA (1995) The use of risk predictors to identify candidates for intermediate care units. Implications for intensive care unit utilization. Chest 108:490–499
82. Zimmerman JE, Wagner DP, Sun X, Knaus WA, Draper EA (1996) Planning patient services for intermediate care units: insights based on care for intensive care unit low-risk monitor admissions. Crit Care Med 24:1626–1632
83. Strauss MJ, LoGerfo JP, Yeltatzie JA, Temkin N, Hudson LD (1986) Rationing of intensive care unit services. An everyday occurrence. JAMA 255:1143–1146
84. Civetta JM, Hudson-Civetta JA, Nelson LD (1990) Evaluation of APACHE II for cost containment and quality assurance. Ann Surg 212:266–276
85. Moreno R, Reis Miranda D (1998) Nursing staff in intensive care in Europe. The mismatch between planning and practice. Chest 113:752–758
86. Knaus WA, Wagner DP, Zimmerman JE, Draper EA (1993) Variations in mortality and length of stay in Intensive Care Units. Ann Intern Med 118:753–761
87. Zimmerman JE, Shortell SM, Knaus WA, et al (1993) Value and cost of teaching hospitals: a prospective, multicenter, inception cohort study. Crit Care Med 21:1432–1442
88. Rapoport J, Teres D, Lemeshow S, Gehlbach S (1994) A method for assessing the clinical performance and cost-effectiveness of intensive care units: a multicenter inception cohort study. Crit Care Med 22:1385–1391
89. Teres D, Rapoport J (1991) Identifying patients with high risk of high cost. Chest 99:530–531
90. Esserman L, Belkora J, Lenert L (1995) Potentially ineffective care. A new outcome to assess the limits of critical care. JAMA 274:1544–1551
91. Rapoport J, Teres D, Lemeshow S (1998) Can futility be defined numerically? Crit Care Med 26:1781–1782.
92. Chang RW, Jacobs S, Lee B (1986) Use of APACHE II severity of disease classification to identify intensive-care-unit patients who would not benefit from total parenteral nutrition. Lancet i:1483–1486
93. Atkinson S, Bihari D, Smithies M, Daly K, Mason R, McColl I (1994) Identification of futility in intensive care. Lancet 344:1203–1206
94. Shaughnessy TE, Mickler TA (1995) Does acute physiology and chronic health evaluation (APACHE II) scoring predict need for prolonged support after coronary revascularization? Anaesth Analg 81:24–29
95. Cerra FB, Negro F, Abrams J (1990) APACHE II score does not predict multiple organ failure or mortality in post-operative surgical patients. Arch Surg 125:519–522
96. Rapoport J, Teres D, Lemeshow S, Avrunin JS, Haber R (1990) Explaining variability of cost using a severity of illness measure for ICU patients. Med Care 28:338–348
97. Oye RK, Bellamy PF (1991) Patterns of resource consumption in medical intensive care. Chest 99:695–689
98. Glance LG, Osler T, SWhinozaki T (1998) Intensive care unit prognostic scoring systems to predict death: a cost-effectiveness analysis. Crit Care Med 26:1842–1849
99. Patel PA, Grant BJ (1999) Application of mortality prediction systems to individual intensive care units. Intensive Care Med 25:977–982
100. Knaus WA, Draper EA, Wagner DP, Zimmerman JE (1986) An evaluation of outcome from intensive care in major medical centers. Ann Intern Med 104:410–418
101. Hosmer DW, Lemeshow S (1995) Confidence interval estimates of an index of quality performance based on logistic regression estimates. Stat Med 14:2161–2172
102. Knaus WA, Le Gall JR, Wagner DP, et al (1982) A comparison of intensive care in the U.S.A. and France. Lancet i:642–646
103. Sirio CA, Tajimi K, Tase C, et al (1992) An initial comparison of intensive care in Japan and United States. Crit Care Med 20:1207–1215
104. Rowan KM, Kerr JH, Major E, McPherson K, Short A, Vessey MP (1993) Intensive Care Society's APACHE II study in Britain and Ireland – II: Outcome comparisons of intensive care

units after adjustment for case mix by the American APACHE II method. Br Med J 307:977–981
105. Rapoport J, Teres D, Barnett R, et al (1995) A comparison of intensive care unit utilization in Alberta and western Massachusetts. Crit Care Med 23:1336–1346
106. Wong DT, Crofts SL, Gomez M, McGuire GP, Byrick RJ (1995) Evaluation of predictive ability of APACHE II system and hospital outcome in Canadian intensive care unit patients. Crit Care Med 23:1177–1183
107. Moreno R, Reis Miranda D, Fidler V, Van Schilfgaarde R (1998) Evaluation of two outcome predictors on an independent database. Crit Care Med 26:50–61
108. Bastos PG, Sun X, Wagner DP, Knaus WA, Zimmerman JE, The Brazil APACHE III Study Group (1996) Application of the APACHE III prognostic system in Brazilian intensive care units: a prospective multicenter study. Intensive Care Med 22:564–570
109. Moreno R, Morais P (1997) Outcome prediction in intensive care: results of a prospective, multicentre, Portuguese study. Intensive Care Med 23:177–186
110. Le Gall JR, Loirat P, Nicolas F, et al (1983) Utilisation d'un indice de gravité dans huit services de réanimation multidisciplinaire. Presse Médicale 12:1757–1761
111. Zimmerman JE, Rousseau DM, Duffy J, et al (1994) Intensive care at two teaching hospitals: an organizational case study. Am J Crit Care 3:129–138
112. Goldhill DR, Sumner A (1998) Outcome of intensive care patients in a group of British intensive care units. Crit Care Med 26:1337–1345
113. Zimmerman JE, Wagner DP, Draper EA, Wright L, Alzola C, Knaus WA (1998) Evaluation of acute physiology and chronic health evaluation III predictions of hospital mortality in an independent database. Crit Care Med 26:1317–1326
114. Chisakuta AM, Alexander JP (1990) Audit in Intensive Care. The APACHE II classification of severity of disease. Ulster Med J 59:161–167
115. Marsh HM, Krishan I, Naessens JM, et al (1990) Assessment of prediction of mortality by using the APACHE II scoring system in intensive care units. Mayo Clin Proc 65:1549–1557
116. Turner JS, Mudaliar YM, Chang RW, Morgan CJ (1991) Acute physiology and chronic health evaluation (APACHE II) scoring in a cardiothoracic intensive care unit. Crit Care Med 19:1266–1269
117. Oh TE, Hutchinson R, Short S, Buckley T, Lin E, Leung D (1993) Verification of the acute physiology and chronic health evaluation scoring system in a Hong Kong intensive care unit. Crit Care Med 21:698–705
118. Parikh CR, Karnad DR (1999) Quality, cost, and outcome of intensive care in a public hospital in Bombay, India. Crit Care Med 27:1754–1759
119. Zimmerman JE, Shortell SM, Rousseau DM, et al (1993) Improving intensive care: observations based on organizational case studies in nine intensive care units: a prospective, multicenter study. Crit Care Med 21:1443–1451
120. Shortell SM, Zimmerman JE, Rousseau DM, et al (1994) The performance of intensive care units: does good management make a difference? Med Care 32:508–525
121. Reis Miranda D, Ryan DW, Schaufeli WB, Fidler V (1997) Organization and management of intensive care: a prospective study in 12 European countries. Springer–Verlag, Heidelberg.
122. Randolph AG, Guyatt GH, Carlet J, for the Evidence Based Medicine in Critical Care Group (1998) Understanding articles comparing outcomes among intensive care units to rate quality of care. Crit Care Med 26:773–781
123. Teres D, Lemeshow S (1993) Using severity measures to describe high performance intensive care units. Crit Care Clin 9:543–554
124. Goldstein H, Spiegelhalter DJ (1996) League tables and their limitations: statistical issues in comparisons of institutional performance. J R Stat Soc A 159:385–443
125. Castella X, Gilabert J, Torner F, Torres C (1991) Mortality prediction models in intensive care: Acute Physiology and Chronic Health Evaluation II and Mortality Prediction Model compared. Crit Care Med 19:191–197

126. Apolone G, D'Amico R, Bertolini G, et al (1996) The performance of SAPS II in a cohort of patients admitted in 99 Italian ICUs: results from the GiViTI. Intensive Care Med 22:1368–1378
127. Nouira S, Belghith M, Elatrous S, et al (1998) Predictive value of severity scoring systems: comparison of four models in Tunisian adult intensive care units. Crit Care Med 26:852–859
128. Hadorn DC, Keeler EB, Rogers WH, Brook RH (1993) Assessing the performance of mortality prediction models. RAND/UCLA/Harvard Center for Health Care Financing Policy Research, Santa Monica
129. Moreno R, Apolone G, Reis Miranda D (1998) Evaluation of the uniformity of fit of general outcome prediction models. Intensive Care Med 24:40–47
130. Dybowski R, Weller P, Chang R (1996) Prediction of outcome in critically ill patients using artificial neural network, synthesised by genetic algorithm. Lancet 347:1146–1150
131. Wong LS, Young JD (1999) A comparison of ICU mortality prediction using the APACHE II scoring system and artificial neural networks. Anaesthesia 54:1048–1054
132. Green J, Wintfeld N (1995) Report cards on cardiac surgeons: assessing New York State's approach. N Engl J Med 332:1229–1232
133. Lemeshow S, Teres D, Avrunin JS, Pastides H (1987) A comparison of methods to predict mortality of intensive care unit patients. Crit Care Med 15:715–722

Measuring Treatment Outcomes in Intensive Care: Mortality, Morbidity, and Organ Dysfunction

J.C. Marshall

Learning Points

- Survival is no longer the only, nor even the most important, outcome for patients admitted to an intensive care unit (ICU)
- Although methodologies for developing and validating outcome measures reflecting quality of life are becoming well-established, these have not been extensively applied to the evaluation of ICU care
- The construct of the multiple organ dysfunction syndrome reflects the process of ICU care, and so can serve as a measure of ICU-related quality of life
- Approaches for modeling organ dysfunction as an ICU outcome are underdeveloped, but evolving

A previously healthy 93 year old man was admitted to the ICU in septic shock, four days following an elective sigmoid colectomy for resolving diverticulitis. He was anuric and ventilator-dependent. Following resuscitation, he was taken to the operating room for a laparotomy that revealed diffuse fecal peritonitis; the peritoneal cavity was irrigated, and the dehisced anastomosis converted to a sigmoid end colostomy. The patient was transferred back to the ICU in stable condition.

Discussions with the patient and his family prior to his initial operation revealed that he wanted to avoid a colostomy or prolonged hospitalization at all costs. Following this complication, the family requested a brief course of aggressive ICU care, but asked that supportive care not be prolonged. He was weaned from mechanical ventilation in 24 hours, and his acute renal failure resolved without dialysis. He was discharged from hospital 2 weeks later, and had his colostomy reversed 3 months later, in time for his 70th wedding anniversary.

It is increasingly evident that survival per se is not necessarily the most important outcome for patients admitted to an ICU, but rather quality of life, reflected in minimizing the time spent in the ICU, and returning to a pre-morbid level of physical and mental functioning. Yet survival has been the touchstone for assessing ICU care, or for evaluating the utility of new therapies. What are the alternatives?

Introduction

The ability to effect change presupposes an ability to measure, describe, and predict. In the greater world outside the boundaries of the ICU, measurement and behavior are inextricably linked. I change my socks because I have worn them for a day, and carry an umbrella when it threatens to rain. The government changes when a rival party gains more votes than the party in power, and the melange of attitudes that create a culture change through the interplay of the events and perceptions that comprise our daily existence. The ability to measure, and to make a decision based on an awareness of the value of that measure, is fundamental to survival. I fight because my intuitive measurements tell me I am likely to win, and flee when they suggest that victory is improbable.

Within the ICU, a particularly intense microcosm of the world of health care delivery, measurement forms the basis for clinical decision-making, for the evaluation of therapies, for the establishment of prognosis, and for the ethical allocation of resources [1]. As the discipline of intensive care acquires sophistication, its measurement tools must do likewise.

Effective measurement tools must reflect the objectives of the measuring exercise. In a democracy, the objective is the equal exercise of decision-making ability in a non-coercive fashion: the appropriate measurement tool is the secret ballot. In other areas, the connection between the measurement tool and the objective is indirect, a result of an ability to predict the consequences of a decision that is made. I do not want my feet to smell, therefore I change my socks every day. Time is used as a predictor, or as a surrogate measure of a subthreshold process that I do not wish to become manifest. It is equally important that the measurement tools employed in the ICU reflect the events or processes that they purport to measure: the proper interpretation of the significance of the resulting data depends on an explicit understanding of the nature of the tool employed.

ICU Outcome Measures: A Taxonomy

For the purposes of this chapter, an outcome is defined as a quantifiable measure of a physiologic state. The clinician records and analyzes outcomes for a variety of different purposes (Table 1); the optimal characteristics of a given outcome measure depend on the purpose it is designed to serve.

The ICU has evolved over less than half a century as a geographic locale for the monitoring and support of otherwise lethal, physiologic, organ system insufficiency during a time of acute, and potentially reversible derangement [2]. The objective of critical care is not so much to treat diseases, as it is to sustain vital functions that have been compromised as a complication of a broad spectrum of disorders. The decision-making process in optimizing mechanical ventilation is similar, whether the need for that ventilation results from pneumonia, pancreatitis, or fluid overload in a patient with end stage chronic lung disease, while the decision to transfuse red blood cells is largely independent of the particular circumstances that caused the hemoglobin to fall. The assumption that we make is that by optimizing physiologic function we can maximize the clinical benefit for the patient, although our notions of optimizing deranged physiology may include not only trying to restore normal physiologic parameters, but also accepting subnormal values [3–5] or striving to achieve supraphysiologic values [6]. The consequences of the application of that body of knowledge – its outcome – can be evaluated from at least four different perspectives: that of the patient, of his or her family or relatives, of the ICU health care team, and of the larger society (Table 2). These are of necessity interrelated, and usually, although not always, congruent.

Table 1. Important outcomes in intensive care medicine

Focus	Characteristics
Diagnosis	Specific to the process of interest; maximize positive and negative predictive value
Titration of therapy	Sensitive to physiologically relevant change
Evaluation of response to therapy	Sensitive to clinically important changes in morbidity or mortality
Prognostication	Calibrated to maximize association with dependent variable, e.g., mortality
Evaluation of process of care	Comprehensive reflection of relevant manifestations of ICU morbidity
Evaluation of costs and utilization or need for resources	Reflective of events or processes that generate costs or need for personnel or equipment

Table 2. Outcome perspectives in intensive care medicine

Outcome Perspective	Focus of Interest
Patient-centered	Survival
	Quality of life: *Short term* – freedom from pain, frustration, helplessness *Long term* – independence; freedom from physical or mental debility
Family-centered	Survival Freedom from uncertainty Rapidity of resolution
Treatment-centered	Survival Identification of treatable disease or correctable physiologic derangement Organ dysfunction – the rationale and need for ICU intervention Potential to do more good than harm: The ability to predict that a given treatment plan will help the patient and not simply prolong his or her suffering
Society-centered	Costs Appropriate use of resources Ethical and legal appropriateness

Patient-Centered Outcomes

From the perspective of the patient, there are two important outcomes: survival and quality of life. Yet critically ill patients rarely recall the time spent in the ICU, and to speak of ICU quality of life is almost a contradiction in terms. Pain or agitation are inferred by the medical and nursing staff, and treated with analgesics and sedatives. Beyond this, however, we have no means of defining what comprises a preferable quality of life for a critically ill patient, poised on the brink of death, and sustained, albeit transiently by multiple lines, tubes, and interventions. Quality of life beyond the ICU is easier to define, although the ICU-related factors that predict post-ICU quality of life are not well-defined. Quality of life as an ICU outcome is discussed in greater detail elsewhere in this volume.

Family-Centered Outcomes

The survival of a loved one is clearly an important concern of the family, relatives, and friends of a critically ill patient. However the experience of witnessing prolonged illness, with its attendant uncertainties, gives rise to a new spectrum of concerns. On the one hand, they seek freedom from pain, fear, and therapeutic indignity for their loved one, and assume a role as patient advocate. On the other hand, for those who are waiting, freedom from uncertainty or ambiguity, and a rapid resolution of the process are important and desirable outcomes. Indeed discussions regarding the withdrawal of life support frequently hinge not only on the improbability of long term survival, but also on the concern that a patient would not want prolonged life support. Moreover, the economic and emotional demands on the family of a protracted illness can be substantial.

Treatment-Centered Outcomes

Treatment-centered outcomes are the focus of the health care team looking after the critically ill patient. Survival is one measure of success, but, as discussed later, it is not the only, and perhaps not even the primary, objective of therapy for the majority of critically ill patients. Rather, physicians, nurses, and other ICU health care staff are concerned with doing more good than harm for a particular patient. This objective presupposes an ability to evaluate care as being both medically and ethically appropriate, and to discriminate interventions that can be successful from those that are ultimately futile. Since the focus of medical care is the identification and management of treatable disease or correctable physiologic derangement, outcomes of relevance to the physician include the individual or aggregate results of diagnostic tests, and other parameters that delineate a need for an intervention that may benefit the patient [7].

Society-Centered Outcomes

ICU care is costly. In Canada, ICU costs account for approximately 8% of all in patient hospital costs, and 0.2% of the Gross National Product (GNP) [8]. From a social perspective, therefore, interest lies in assuring that resources are adequate, but that costs are controlled, and the use of ICU resources is appropriate. Society is also concerned with ensuring that the use of ICU resources is ethically and legally appropriate.

The particular perspective and priorities of each of the above stakeholders will be reflected in differing outcome measures, and even in different interpretations of the same outcome measure. For example, ICU survival may be a measure of therapeutic success to the clinician, but not for the patient who dies shortly after ICU discharge, or who must be institutionalized for chronic irreversible disability. The focus of this chapter is treatment-centered outcomes – those of primary interest to the health care team.

Treatment-Centered Outcomes in Intensive Care

The evaluation of a therapeutic intervention – whether a discrete treatment such as the administration of a drug, or the entire process of care – centers on two distinct, but related questions:
1) Does the treatment work? Is it producing a biologic effect?
2) Does the treatment help? Is it resulting in net benefit to the patient?

These questions correspond roughly to the epidemiologic concepts of efficacy and effectiveness, respectively. For example, a new antimicrobial agent will show evidence that it works by demonstrating an ability to kill micro-organisms *in vitro*, and to result in sterilization of sites of infection *in vivo*; that it helps will be reflected in the clinical resolution of infection. Similarly, the efficacy of an anti-arrhythmic agent will be reflected in its ability to reverse arrhythmias, its effectiveness in its ability to prevent the complications of these arrhythmias, including death. The ability to produce a biologic effect does not guarantee that the agent will be beneficial to a patient. The anti-arrhythmic agents flecainide and encainide prevented arrhythmias following myocardial infarction, but were associated with an increased risk of mortality [9]. Similarly vasoactive agents such as dobutamine [10] or the nitric oxide synthase inhibitor, L-NMMA [11] proved capable of achieving a physiologic target, but did so at the cost of increased mortality. In general, an intervention that produces clinical benefit will show some evidence of a biologic effect, although the reverse is not necessarily true.

What is the Treatment Objective of Intensive Care?

The focus of intensive care is not the management of any distinct disease process, but rather the support of patients with a broad spectrum of diseases whose complications pose an immediate threat to life, yet are potentially reversible. As a result, the outcomes of interest to the intensivist are not those that reflect the cure of a disease, but rather those that mirror successful support or reversal of its complications. At first blush, the primary objective of the aggregate of interventions that comprise ICU care is saving the lives of desperately ill patients who, in the absence of these interventions, would die. By virtue of their need for ICU admission, critically ill patients are at very high risk of death, and the decision to admit to an ICU implies a therapeutic desire to reduce or eliminate that risk. This goal, however, is neither absolute or immutable. Even if we are able to preserve a life in the present, we recognize that the ultimate measure of success will not be immortality, but simply a process of procrastination, a delay in the inevitable.

Perhaps the objective of intensive care is the treatment of disease and the restoration of a state of normal health. However for many of the most complex patients in an ICU, therapy is not directed at the disease *per se*, but rather at its complications. And for many of the patients we attempt to treat, the primary disease itself may be incurable, for example, in the patient with disseminated fungemia following a bone marrow transplant, or the patient with end-stage chronic obstructive pulmonary disease who becomes ventilator-dependent following an acute exacerbation.

If survival is not the only, nor even the predominant, objective of therapy for the intensivist managing a critically ill patient in an ICU, then what other outcomes are important? The process of intensive care involves three elements:

1) Resuscitation and physiologic stabilization
2) Diagnostic assessment and initiation of therapy
3) Evaluation of the response to therapy, and determination of potential for reversibility.

During the first stage of resuscitation we focus on those measures of acute life-threatening instability: respiratory parameters such as tachypnea, hypoxemia, cyanosis; hemodynamic measures such as tachycardia, hypotension, urine output or lactate levels; and other clinical or biological parameters that suggest the need for emergent intervention. The measures employed are physiologic variables that must, by virtue of their role in resuscitation, be reproducible, readily and rapidly measured, and responsive to the institution of resuscitative measures. The ability of these measures in aggregate to predict short and long term outcome is underscored by their inclusion in the physiologic domain of composite severity of illness scoring systems such as SAPS (simplified acute physiology score) [12] and APACHE (acute physiology and chronic health evaluation [13].

During the diagnostic phase of ICU care, our focus is on measures that will provide information about pathologic derangements that are amenable to therapy. Attention is turned, for example, to the diagnosis of infection with appropriate cultures or radiologic investigations, the detection of altered myocardial function with invasive hemodynamic monitoring or markers of myocardial injury, or the optimization of ventilatory support through blood gas determinations and measures of pulmonary physiology. The outcome measures of interest are diagnostic tests, and emphasis is placed on their accuracy, reflected in positive and negative predictive values, and likelihood ratios.

The evaluation of the response to therapy involves both measures that reflect the immediate success or failure of the intervention employed (blood pressure in the case of a vasopressor, or urine output following the administration of a diuretic) and more generic measures of global physiologic status. These latter typically include individual or aggregate measures reflecting normalization of the physiologic state; for example, her temperature is back to normal and she is beginning to wake up, or his ventilator requirements are increasing, and the platelet count is falling. Intensivists select those variables that best reflect the clinical gestalt of improvement or deterioration, choosing not to comment on the fact, for example, that the white count has gone up in the former case, or that the dose of inotropes has been reduced to half in the latter. Indeed a significant step in the maturation of a critical care physician is the ability to interpret an enormous body of variable and often contradictory data in a selective and coherent fashion that leads to clinical decisions that will help the patient.

However, this process is inherently subjective and non-reproducible. More objective methods of integrating important, yet contradictory data in a quantitative and reproducible manner are needed: this need has been the stimulus for organ dysfunction scales. Their evolution as clinically useful measurement tools is in its infancy.

Mortality as a Clinical Outcome

Despite its limitations, discussed in greater detail below, survival remains the *sine qua non* for the measurement of a successful outcome in critical care [14]. Admission to an ICU carries an implicit acceptance of a desire to intervene using heroic measures to subvert a potentially lethal process. Even if this objective is abandoned early because survival is improbable, the transition from hope for survival to acceptance of its impossibility reflects a failure of the global intervention to produce the possible modification of clinical course. Survival is an intuitively sensible outcome measure for any process that carries a risk of death. Moreover, as an outcome measure it is simple, definitive, and dichotomous.

Survival, however, is not absolute, and an evaluative process must indicate the time interval over which survival is deemed to indicate therapeutic success. In practice, this is a trade-off between a shorter interval, during which the outcome is more likely to be directly linked to the therapeutic process of interest, and a longer interval that is more clinically relevant, but that is confounded by intercurrent events that may be entirely unrelated to that therapy. A survival time measured in hours may provide evidence of effectiveness during cardiopulmonary resuscitation, but if it is followed by death over the next few days, it is difficult to view the effect as clinically valuable. On the other hand, survival status at six months would be expected to reflect the restoration of most patients to a stable, post-illness state. However multiple intercurrent events may have occurred that can impact on survival during this time interval.

The use of 28 or 30 day all-cause mortality as an endpoint in ICU-based clinical trials reflects a compromise between these two extremes. Survival to ICU discharge is an alternative that reflects the ability of the patient to survive, for however briefly, independent of a need for ICU technology; thus it has been used as an endpoint for calibrating organ dysfunction scales as measures of ICU-based morbidity [15]. Conversely hospital survival reflects a presumed ability to live independent of hospital care.

The benefits of survival to a landmark timepoint occur when the patient is free of the burden of disease for at least a portion of that time. An increase in survival from cancer of two years would not represent a desirable clinical outcome if those two years were spent in severe pain and debility. Yet prolongation of ICU survival represents precisely such an outcome, unless that survival also results in resolution of the process that led to ICU admission, and a return to a premorbid state of health.

From the perspective of the patient, however, survival alone may well not be the most important objective of care in the ICU [16]. Prolonged intensive care is associated with a significant diminution in quality of life, often of a degree sufficient to preclude a return to an independent existence; this loss of independence is, for many patients, worse than the prospect of death. An Australian study, for example, found that 80% of women over the age of 75 would rather die than sustain a hip fracture that necessitated their admission to a nursing home [17]. Yet an intervention that improves survival could decrease mean quality of life by salvaging patients whose illness was the most severe. Indeed a reduction in quality of life is almost an expected consequence of an advance that improves survival; the increased life expectancy that has resulted from improvements in public health and social policy has resulted in an aging population that has survived to become afflicted with the degenerative conditions of advancing age. The ICU cares for a significant number of patients who are justifiably considered to be nearing the end of their natural life expectancy, and evaluation of ICU outcomes will need to focus increasingly on quality as well as quantity of life.

Mortality in critical illness is heavily influenced by factors beyond the scope of ICU care, with the result that the potentially modifiable component of mortality risk may be relatively small. The ability of physiologic severity scales such as APACHE and SAPS to produce reliable estimates of the probability of survival at the time the patient is admitted to the ICU speaks to the fact that a significant component of mortality risk, perhaps as much as 75%, is established prior to the onset of ICU care, and hence will not be altered by interventions occurring subsequently. Pre-morbid diseases exert a significant, but unquantified impact on the likelihood of ICU survival. Impaired ability to walk or perform normal activities of daily living, for example, is associated with a net 20% increment in hospital mortality above that predicted by the APACHE II score [18]. Finally patient preferences, as reflected in advanced directives or religious beliefs can exert an important influence on therapeutic decisions that in turn influence survival.

Finally the use of landmark (fixed timepoint) measures of mortality can influence the determination of whether a particular patient is a survivor or non-survivor. The time course to death for non-survivors is quite variable, and 30 day mortality will fail to capture patients who die after a longer ICU stay. ICU survival may reflect a decision by the caregivers to transfer a patient who can no longer benefit from ICU care to a private room where he or she will be allowed to die in privacy. The need to establish an arbitrary point for the determination of mortality status runs the risk of overestimating the rate of resolution of the morbid conditions that led to ICU admission, while increasing the impact of unrelated events that may result in patient mortality. Moreover the time interval between ICU admission and death is a costly, emotionally demanding, and complex interval that mortality measures alone are incapable of describing.

Organ Dysfunction as a Clinical Outcome

The majority, perhaps as many as 80%, of patient deaths in a contemporary ICU are a consequence of a deliberate decision to terminate life-sustaining interventions because of a failure to respond to therapy [19, 20]. In a very real sense, mortality is a surrogate for the clinically important outcome – reversal of the life-threatening process that triggered ICU admission. The development of scales to measure organ dysfunction as an ICU outcome reflects an evolving attempt to quantify clinical improvement or deterioration.

The attraction of such scales is obvious. ICU care is primarily directed to the support of organs whose dysfunction would otherwise be lethal. The response to organ dysfunction reflects the concerns and capabilities of ICU care; it is what we do as intensivists. At another level, altered organ system function is an important sequel of the activation of a systemic inflammatory response, and a measure of the morbidity that results from important physiologic threats managed in the ICU, including infection, ischemia, and injury.

The first descriptions of what has come to be called the multiple organ dysfunction syndrome [21] emphasized the concept that the failure of vital organ system function in critically ill patients both predicted a high probability of subsequent death [22–24], and served as a harbinger of occult and untreated infection [25–27]. Goris et al. [28] developed the first organ dysfunction scale in 1985, and transformed the concept of organ failure from a syndrome of multiple failed (and presumably irretrievable) organs to one of organ dysfunction, in which the degree of severity of a potentially reversible process was the measure of interest. We published a similar score in 1988 [29], and a revised version of that score, the Multiple Organ Dysfunction (MOD) score, in 1995 [15]. Three other scales were developed almost simultaneously: the Sequential Organ Failure Assessment (SOFA) score [30]; the Logistic Organ Dysfunction (LOD) Score [31]; and the Brussels Score [32].

The development of organ dysfunction scales is a relatively recent phenomenon, and the methodologic principles guiding their development are still in their infancy. Some general observations, however, can be made.

Organ Dysfunction Scales: Methodologic Considerations

I. Selection of Variables

The construction of a scale to quantify organ dysfunction requires that explicit decisions be made about which systems will be included in the scale, and what variables will be used to describe their dysfunction. Unlike a prognostic score, in which the developer selects component variables primarily on the basis of their ability to predict the outcome of interest, an organ dysfunction scale emphasizes face or construct validity; it must look like the entity of organ dysfunction as seen by the clinician. Two approaches have been used to accomplish this, with similar results. To select the organ systems that are included in the MOD score, we undertook a systematic review of published reports of multiple organ failure or the multiple organ dysfunction syndrome. Thirty reports were identified that presented specific definitions for organ failure. Although the systems and criteria used were variable, seven organ systems – the respiratory, renal, cardiovascular, gastrointestinal, neurologic, hepatic and hematologic systems – were included in more than half of the reports, and were therefore selected as the appropriate systems for inclusion in the MOD score, based on their demonstration of construct validity [33]. The SOFA score used a process of expert consensus involving members of the European Society of Intensive Care Medicine (ESICM), and identified the same seven systems [30]. Because a satisfactory variable to describe gastrointestinal dysfunction could not be found, this system was dropped from both scores. The same six systems appear in the Brussels and LOD scores, confirming that there is a general consensus on the systems whose dysfunction comprises the multiple organ dysfunction syndrome.

The selection of variables to describe dysfunction within a given system requires consideration of both construct and content validity; the variable must not only look on organ dysfunction as the clinician sees it, but it should also incorporate the entire spectrum of dysfunction within the system of interest. The SOFA score used the same process of expert consensus to select variables, while the MOD score evaluated candidate variables against a series of criteria for the ideal descriptor of organ dysfunction [33]. Moreover, it is apparent that organ dysfunction can be described from several differing perspectives:

1) as the physiologic derangement of the organ system in question – for example, using measures of oxygenation such as the PO_2/FiO_2 ratio for the respiratory system, or the creatinine level or urine output for the renal system
2) as the therapeutic response to deranged physiology – for example, using the institution of mechanical ventilation for the respiratory system, or the use of diuretics or dialysis for the renal system
3) as a syndrome of organ dysfunction within each system, using several variables to establish its presence – for example, acute respiratory distress syndrome (ARDS) defined as a PO_2/FiO_2 ratio of less than 200, bilateral fluffy infiltrates on chest X-ray, and a pulmonary capillary wedge pressure of less than 18, or acute renal failure defined as anuria, an elevated creatinine level, and the institution of dialysis.

The latter approach maximizes content validity, but at a cost of creating a complex variable that is categorical (yes or no), rather than continuous. The use of physiologic variables addresses the question – "Does it work?", while the use of therapeutic variables addresses that of "Does it help?". The MOD sore was deliberately constructed using physiologic variables alone, without reference to the therapeutic intervention, while the other organ dysfunction scales use a combination of physiologic and therapeutic variables.

II. Weighting of Variables

Weights for variables in a prognostic score are developed based on their ability to predict mortality, using techniques of logistic regression; hospital mortality is used as the dependent variable. In contrast, an organ dysfunction scale that is concerned with maximizing construct validity uses alternate approaches. The MOD score weights each of the six component systems equally, on a scale that ranges from 0 to 4, even though logistic regression analysis showed that the impact of neurologic dysfunction on survival was much greater than that of hepatic dysfunction [15]. Within each system, variables are weighted so that a score of 0 describes essentially normal physiologic function, and is associated independently with a mortality of less than 5%, while a score of 4 represents marked dysfunction, and is associated with a mortality in excess of 50%; intervening intervals are selected so that they are roughly equal in size, with sensible, whole-number boundaries. ICU mortality, rather than hospital mortality is selected as the dependent variable, since organ dysfunction is conceptualized as the need for ICU care.

An organ dysfunction scale that emphasizes construct validity should, by definition, be less powerful than a prognostic scale in discriminating survivors and non-survivors. Indeed an organ dysfunction scale should record a low score for a patient who dies without organ dysfunction of a process such as a myocardial infarction, pulmonary embolism, or exsanguinating hemorrhage.

III. Timing of Variable Measurement

Each of the available organ dysfunction scales records its component variables on a daily basis. Three select the worst value for a given day, while the MOD score records a representative value – the first recorded on that day. This approach is taken to emphasize a concept of organ dysfunction as stable, post-resuscitation physiologic derangement, and to reduce the potential for bias that might result from sampling frequency. In practice, the impact of these differences is relatively modest, for the intervals in each scale are broad.

The features of the four most widely-used organ dysfunction scales are summarized in Table 3; their differences reflect areas for debate, development, and ultimately, it is hoped, consensus.

Uses of Organ Dysfunction Scales

Organ dysfunction scales can serve a variety of uses as validated measures of ICU morbidity (Table 4).

Quantification of Baseline Severity of Illness

The score calculated on the day of admission to the ICU or at some other discrete timepoint (for example, immediately prior to an experimental intervention in a

Table 3. Organ dysfunction scales

	Multiple Organ Dysfunction (MOD) Score [15]	Sequential Organ Failure Assessment (SOFA) Score [30]	Brussels Score [32]	Logistic Organ Dysfunction (LOD) Score [31]
Variable Selection	Systematic literature review	Expert consensus	Expert consensus	SAPS database
Timing of measurement	Representative daily value (first AM value)	Worst daily value	Worst daily value	Worst daily value
Variables	Physiologic	Physiologic and therapeutic	Physiologic and therapeutic	Physiologic
Cardiovascular variable	Pressure-adjusted heart rate (Heart rate X MAP/CVP)	Dosage of vaso-active agents	pH, fluid requirements, inotropes	Hyper- or hypo-tension, heart rate (bradycardia or tachycardia)

MAP: mean arterial pressure; CVP: central venous pressure.

Table 4. Models for the description of the outcome of critical illness using the construct of organ dysfunction (from [40] with permission).

Objective	Approach	Uses
To quantify the baseline severity of organ dysfunction	Calculate organ dysfunction score on day of admission (Admission MODS)	To establish baseline severity, eg for entry criteria for a clinical trial, or to ensure comparability of study groups
To quantify severity of organ dysfunction at a point in time	Calculate score on a particular ICU day (Daily MODS)	To determine the intensity of resource utilization, or the evolution or resolution of organ dysfunction at a discrete point in time
To measure aggregate severity of organ dysfunction over ICU stay	Sum the individual worst scores for each organ system over a defined time interval (Aggregate MODS)	To determine severity of physiologic derangement over a defined time interval (e.g., ICU stay)
To quantify new organ dysfunction arising following ICU admission	Calculate difference between aggregate and admission scores (Delta MODS)	To measure organ dysfunction attributable to events occurring following ICU admission
To provide a combined measure of morbidity and mortality	Adjust aggregate score so that all patients dying receive maximal number of points (Mortality-adjusted MODS)	To create a single measure that integrates impact of morbidity in survivors, and mortality for non–survivors
	Organ failure-free days = days alive and free of organ failure	

clinical trial) provides an objective baseline assessment of severity of organ dysfunction at the start of therapy. Baseline severity of illness is strongly associated with the ultimate risk of ICU death (Fig. 1). More importantly, however, it represents physiologic derangement that cannot be modified by changes in practice. Admission or baseline scores permit objective quantification of the acuity of illness (and therefore the need for medical and nursing intervention) in a given ICU, and can be used to evaluate baseline comparability of patient populations in a clinical trial [5].

Quantification of Daily Severity of Illness

Daily organ dysfunction scores can be used to track the aggregate clinical course of a patient or population of patients; in the context of a clinical trial, divergence of scores between the two study groups suggests a therapeutic effect (Fig. 2). Daily scores can also be considered as a measure of the serial acuity of illness, and hence as a measure of the intensity of care, analogous to scales such as the Therapeutic Intervention Scoring System (TISS) [34]. An improvement in scores over time correlates with ICU survival, while deterioration is associated with mortality [35–37].

Aggregate Scores

Organ dysfunction can be quantified as an outcome over time using one of several approaches. The simplest is the compilation of an aggregate or cumulative score, calculated by summing the worst scores for each organ system over a defined period of time. Thus, if the worst respiratory score is obtained on day 1,

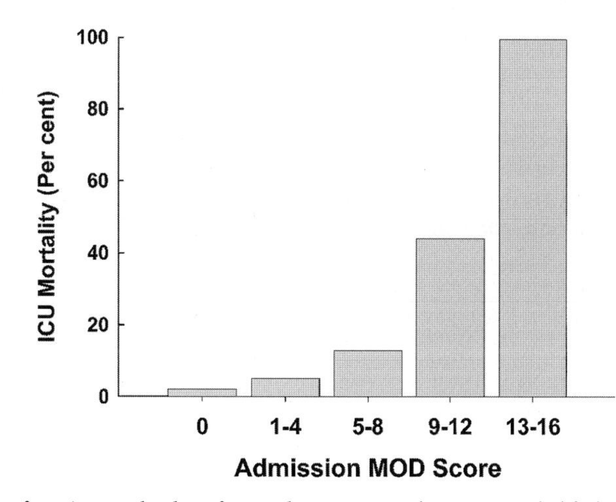

Fig. 1. The severity of organ dysfunction on the day of ICU admission correlates in a graded fashion with the ultimate risk of ICU mortality (from [15] with permission)

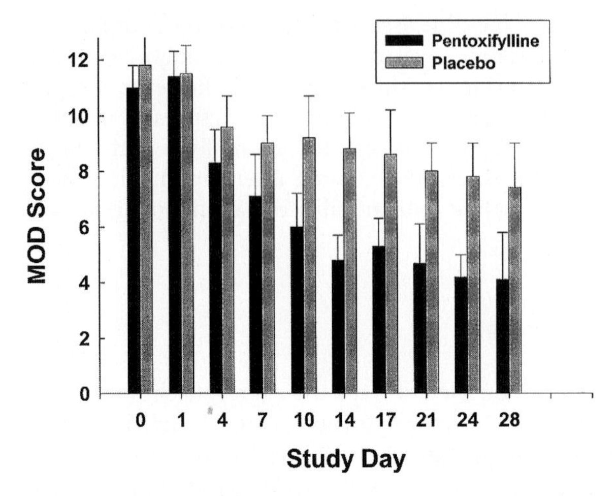

Fig. 2. Daily organ dysfunction scores comparing a population of patients receiving adjuvant pentoxifylline with placebo controls. Reduction in organ dysfunction scores in the treated group suggests a treatment effect (from [41] with permission)

and the worst renal score on day 7, these are summed to produce an aggregate score. An alternative approach is to sum the scores from each day over a defined period of time.

Delta Scores

Computation of an aggregate score allows the quantification of organ dysfunction arising following ICU admission as a delta score – the difference between the aggregate and admission scores. The delta score reflects morbidity that is potentially reversible by interventions undertaken in the ICU, and thus of potential use as an outcome measure for clinical trials. The delta score, too, correlates with outcome [15,38] (Fig. 3), confirming that despite the impact of illness severity at the time of ICU admission, clinical management in the ICU affects outcome. It has been shown, for example, that a restrictive transfusion strategy improves ICU outcome, measured as a smaller increase in delta MODS [5].

Combined Measures of Mortality and Morbidity

In practice, the most useful ICU outcome measures are those that can evaluate not only ICU morbidity, but also ICU mortality. It is entirely conceivable, for example, that an intervention that improves organ dysfunction does so because it hastens the deaths of the sickest patients, and prevents their developing organ dysfunction. Conversely an effective ICU therapy may be associated with worsening of organ dysfunction scores by virtue of salvaging desperately ill patients

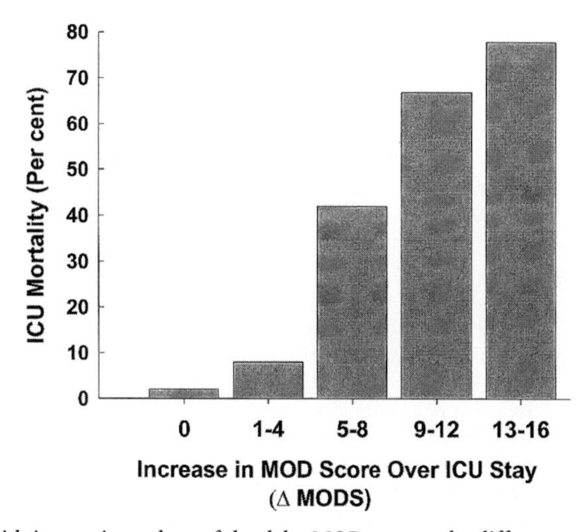

Fig.3. ICU mortality is increased with increasing values of the delta MOD score – the difference between aggregate scores and those present on admission, and a measure of morbidity that arises following ICU admission. (from [15] with permission)

who otherwise would have died. There are two methods of combining morbidity and mortality into a single, continuous measure.

Bernard and colleagues introduced the concept of 'organ failure-free' days to integrate mortality and morbidity measures. Organ failure-free days are defined as the number of days over a fixed time interval (for example, the 28 days of an interventional study) that the patient is both alive and free of organ failure by predetermined criteria [39].

An alternate approach to integrate mortality and morbidity is to calculate mortality-adjusted scores, in which survivors are assigned the measured number of organ dysfunction points (either aggregate or delta), and non-survivors are assigned a maximal number of points. Such an approach was used in a recently published clinical trial that demonstrated the clinical superiority of a restrictive transfusion strategy in anemic, critically ill patients [5].

Conclusion

It is common for the contemporary intensivist to be confronted with a patient who indicates that he or she wants aggressive therapy, but does not want prolonged life support. Death, for this individual, is not failure; prolonged support or persistent debility is. We do not know at the time that therapy is instituted whether the patient will improve quickly, deteriorate quickly and die, improve slowly and die, or improve slowly and live. Prognostic scales are highly influenced by patients in the first two groups – the majority of critically ill patients admitted to an ICU. Costs and morbidity are driven by the latter two – the population of patients who develop the multiple organ dysfunction syndrome. The tools for describing such a complex group of critically ill patients are still in their infancy. As ICUs care for an increasingly aged population of patients whose underlying medical disorders are complex or even irreversible, and as ICU care providers and patients and their families become more realistic about the limitations of ICU care, the concept of critical care as compassionate care gains greater sway, and the need for robust and validated measures of morbidity becomes more pressing.

References

1. Knaus WA, Wagner DP, Lynn J (1991) Short-term mortality predictions for critically ill hospitalized adults: science and ethics. Science 254:389–394
2. Safar P, DeKornfeld T, Pearson J, Redding JS (1961) The intensive care unit. A three year experience at Baltimore city hospitals. Anesthesia 16:275–284
3. Hickling KG, Walsh J, Henderson S, Jackson R (1994) Low mortality rate in adult respiratory distress syndrome using low-volume, pressure-limited ventilation with permissive hypercapnia: A prospective study. Crit Care Med 22:1568–1578
4. Zaloga GP, Roberts P (1994) Permissive underfeeding. New Horiz 2:257–263
5. Hebert PC, Wells G, Blajchman MA, et al (1999) A multicentre randomized controlled clinical trial of transfusion requirements in critical care. N Engl J Med 340:409–417
6. Shoemaker WC, Appel PL, Kram HB, Waxman K, Lee TS (1988) Prospective trial of supranormal values of survivors as therapeutic goals in high risk surgical patients. Chest 94:1176–1186
7. Cook DJ, Brun-Buisson C, Guyatt GH, Sibbald WJ (1994) Evaluation of new diagnostic technologies: Bronchoalveolar lavage and the diagnosis of ventilator-associated pneumonia. Crit Care Med 22:1314–1322
8. Jacobs P, Noseworthy TW (1990) National estimates of intensive care utilization and costs: Canada and the United States. Crit Care Med 18:1282–1286
9. Echt DS, Liebson PR, Mitchell LB, et al (1991) Mortality and morbidity in patients receiving encainide, flecainide, or placebo. The Cardiac Arrhythmia Suppression Trial. N Engl J Med 324:781–788
10. Hayes MA, Timmins AC, Yau EHS, Palazzo M, Hinds CJ, Watson D (1994) Elevation of systemic oxygen delivery in the treatment of critically ill patients. N Engl J Med 330:1717–1722
11. Grover R, Lopez A, Lorente J, et al (1999) Multicenter, randomized, placebo-controlled, double blind study of the nitric oxide synthase inhibitor 546C88: Effect on survival in patients with septic shock. Crit Care Med 27:A33 (Abst)
12. Le Gall J-R, Lemeshow S, Saulnier F (1993) A new simplified acute physiology score (SAPS II) based on a European/North American multicenter study. JAMA 270:2957–2963
13. Knaus WA, Draper EA, Wagner DP, Zimmerman JE (1985) APACHE II: a severity of disease classification system. Crit Care Med 13:818–829
14. Hebert PC (1997) Mortality as an outcome in sepsis trials. Sepsis 1:35–40
15. Marshall JC, Cook DJ, Christou NV, Bernard GR, Sprung CL, Sibbald WJ (1995) Multiple organ dysfunction score: A reliable descriptor of a complex clinical outcome. Crit Care Med 23:1638–1652
16. Petros AJ, Marshall JC, van Saene HKF (1995) Is mortality an appropriate endpoint for clinical trials in critical illness? Lancet 345:369–371
17. Salkeld G, Cameron ID, Cumming RG, et al (2000) Quality of life related to fear of falling and hip fracture in older women: A time trade off study. Br Med J 320:341–346
18. Gurman GM, Roy-Shapira A, Weksler N, Fisher A, Almog Y (1999) Prior functional status is a predictor of outcome in critically ill patients. Crit Care Med 27:A27 (Abst)
19. Deitch EA (1992) Multiple organ failure. Pathophysiology and potential future therapy. Ann Surg 216:117–134
20. Beal AL, Cerra FB (1994) Multiple organ failure syndrome in the 1990s. Systemic inflammatory response and organ dysfunction. JAMA 271:226–233

21. Bone RC, Balk RA, Cerra FB, et al (1992) ACCP/SCCM Consensus Conference. Definitions for sepsis and organ failure and guidelines for the use of innovative therapies in sepsis. Chest 101:1644–1655
22. Skillman JJ, Bushnell LS, Goldman H, Silen W (1969) Respiratory failure, hypotension, sepsis, and jaundice. A clinical syndrome associated with lethal hemorrhage and acute stress ulceration in the stomach. Am J Surg 117:523–530
23. Tilney NL, Bailey GL, Morgan AP (1973) Sequential system failure after rupture of abdominal aortic aneurysms: an unsolved problem in postoperative care. Ann Surg 178:117–122
24. Baue AE (1975) Multiple, progressive, or sequential systems failure. A syndrome of the 1970s. Arch Surg 110:779–781
25. Polk HC, Shields CL (1977) Remote organ failure: a valid sign of occult intraabdominal infection. Surgery 81:310–313
26. Fry DE, Pearlstein L, Fulton RL, Polk HC (1980) Multiple system organ failure. The role of uncontrolled infection. Arch Surg 115:136–140
27. Meakins JL, Wicklund B, Forse RA, Mclean APH (1980) The surgical intensive care unit: current concepts in infection. Surg Clin North Am 60:117–132
28. Goris RJA, te Boekhorst TPA, Nuytinck JKS, Gimbrere JSF (1985) Multiple organ failure. Generalized autodestructive inflammation? Arch Surg 120:1109–1115
29. Marshall JC, Christou NV, Horn R, Meakins JL (1988) The microbiology of multiple organ failure. The proximal GI tract as an occult reservoir of pathogens. Arch Surg 123:309–315
30. Vincent JL, Moreno R, Takala J, et al (1996) The sepsis-related organ failure assessment (SOFA) score to describe organ dysfunction/failure. Intensive Care Med 22:707–710
31. Le Gall JR, Klar J, Lemeshow S, et al (1996) The logistic organ dysfunction system – A new way to assess organ dysfunction in the intensive care unit. JAMA 276:802–810
32. Marshall JC, Bernard G, Le Gall J–R, Vincent J-L (1997) The measurement of organ dysfunction/failure as an ICU outcome. Sepsis 1:41–57
33. Marshall JC (1995) Multiple organ dysfunction syndrome (MODS). In: Sibbald WJ, Vincent JL (eds) Clinical Trials for the Treatment of Sepsis. Springer–Verlag, Berlin, pp 122–138
34. Keene AR, Cullen DJ (1983) Therapeutic intervention scoring system: Update 1983. Crit Care Med 11:1–3
35. Barie PS, Hydo LJ (1996) Influence of multiple organ dysfunction syndrome on duration of critical illness and hospitalization. Arch Surg 131:1318–1324
36. Vincent JL, De Mendonca A, Cantraine F, et al (1998) Use of the SOFA score to assess the incidence of organ dysfunction/failure in intensive care units: results of a multicenter, prospective study. Crit Care Med 26:1793–1800
37. Maziak DE, Lindsay TF, Marshall JC, Walker PM (1998) The impact of multiple organ dysfunction on mortality following ruptured abdominal aortic aneurysm repair. Ann Vasc Surg 12:93–100
38. Moreno R, Vincent JL, Matos R, et al (1999) The use of maximum SOFA score to quantify organ dysfunction/failure in intensive care. Results of a prospective, multicentre study. Intensive Care Med 25:686–696
39. Bernard GR, Wheeler AP, Russell JA, et al (1997) The effects of ibuprofen on the physiology and survival of patients with sepsis. N Engl J Med 336:912–918
40. Marshall JC (1999) Charting the course of critical illness: Prognostication and outcome description in the intensive care unit. Crit Care Med 27:676–678
41. Staubach KH, Schröder J, Stüber F, Gehrke K, Traumann E, Zabel P (1998) Effect of pentoxifylline in severe sepsis. Results of a randomized, double-blind, placebo-controlled study. Arch Surg 133:94–100

Health-Related Quality of Life: During and Following Critical Care

D. J. Kutsogiannis and T. Noseworthy

Learning Points

- Both the extent and nature of survival are fundamentally important; accordingly, outcomes of critical care should include measures of health-related quality of life (HRQL), as well as survival
- HRQL is multidimensional, with each dimension having many components; instruments for measuring it may be generic or specific, and used in a cross-sectional or longitudinal evaluation
- Which instrument(s) is chosen to measure HRQL, depends on the purpose of measurement, and should be chosen on the basis of the strengths and weaknesses taking into account reliability, validity, responsiveness, relevance and perceived interpretability of the test results
- HRQL during ICU stay is largely a measure of the extent and effect of the acute illness and the associated interventions; measurement should include physical, psychological, interpersonal and environmental factors
- A single, ICU-specific, universal HRQL instrument to measure outcomes following critical care is unrealistic

"As a pedestrian, I was severely injured by an automobile; entered into the trauma system in severe pain and dependent upon others for everything; intubated emergently for acute upper airway obstruction; underwent several major surgeries; entered an intensive care unit, still intubated; unable to work for months; and became depressed and lonely. ..... There is not a day that passes that I am not reminded of my critical illness by the patients I care for and that I don't apply the lessons from my experience. Hopefully, the personal experiences I am sharing here will help readers understand what I perceive as the important issues to patients who are critically ill. (Hayden WR. Pediatric Critical Care Program, Rush Medical College/Cook County Children's Hospital, Chicago, 1994).

Introduction

A philosopher's writings of 1843 conveyed the thought, "life can only be understood backwards, but it must be lived forwards" (Søren Kierkegaard). With this context applied to intensive care units (ICUs), we need to better understand the impact of critical care on patients who have lived through the experience and have survived. The nature and extent of that survival is, of course, of fundamental importance.

With better knowledge about the quality of life experienced during the ICU stay, clinicians and the ICU team would be better able to triage, treat or ameliorate pain and suffering, and address a variety of physical, mental, emotional and perhaps spiritual needs of patients during the care process. Correspondingly, following discharge and beyond the ICU stay, the concepts of benefit and the value of critical care encompass measures, and compel a better understanding, of quantity, and quality of life.

Not surprisingly, there has been a good deal of interest in quality of life assessments and from multiple perspectives. These have been intended to better inform or understand clinical management, health outcomes, resource allocation, or policy, to name but a few. Despite such apparent interest, there remains insufficient literature bearing on these subjects, and an undeniable argument for a unified approach to more and better research [1]. The following two chapters deal with quality of life and long-term outcomes.

The first briefly reviews the measures and studies used in quality of life assessment, during and after the ICU stay; what we have learned, thus far, with particular attention to the elderly, long-stay and other particular types of patients; and, suggests further direction for analysis and evaluation in quality of life, following critical care.

The second chapter by Dr Ridley points to the importance of choosing tools for outcome measurement based on the question being asked and how the result will be applied. Long-term survival analysis is discussed, together with non-mortality measures, indicating quality of life.

Health-Related Quality of Life (HRQL): What is it?

Measuring health status is central to understanding clinical care and its value. From a broader context, it is fundamental to analyzing differences in health, predicting the need for care, and assessing the value and outcome of therapies and interventions [2,3].

Health and wellbeing is multidimensional. Its dimensions encompass consequences for individuals' daily lives, how they perceive and are able to live them. Accordingly, measurement of health and wellbeing embraces HRQL and broadly includes values, preferences and perceptions related to health, as well as functionality, and symptoms [4–6].

Why Measure HRQL in and Beyond the ICU?

In the face of illness which threatens life and requires admission to an ICU, measuring health and quality of life during critical illness in effect becomes an exercise in measuring the nature and degree of illness and, secondarily, the short- and long-term effects and responses to care and treatment that is administered.

Assuming that care and, correspondingly, quality of life can be maintained or improved during the ICU stay, measurement is central to managing improvements.

Within the broader, long-term context, measuring HRQL takes on particular importance as issues such as total and societal cost, and the benefit and value of critical care, justifiably receive continuing attention.

Characteristics of HRQL Measurements

Domains

While research and understanding of HRQL associated with critical care may be limited, in broader terms and for many specific illnesses, it is better measured and understood [7–10]. In determining the aspects of life that must be included in such measures, classification by health-related domain has been widely adopted. At least five specific domains have been categorized, including pain and impairment, functional status and mobility, social role, satisfaction and perceptions, and death. All measures of HRQL include one or more such domains. This clearly points to the need for designing and using instruments that incorporate elements at varying degrees of detail to be used for general, or more specific purposes.

Generic or Specific Instruments

Generic instruments attempt to capture a broad range of elements and are more widely applicable across the case mix. However, generic instruments are not as responsive to changes over time in specific illnesses, as are disease-specific instruments. In contrast, specific instruments focus on diseases, individuals, or indicators. While they provide tangible and relevant information, they may not provide comprehensive or unexpected information. Whether generic or specific instruments are used largely depends on the goals of measurement and the availability of necessary information. Clearly, more can be accomplished by using a combination of generic and specific measures, though the cost and effort is greater.

Cross-Sectional or Longitudinal Measures

Assessment of HRQL may be used to choose between alternatives. This can be evaluated with a discriminative instrument at a point in time, using a cross-sectional method. Alternatively, the purpose of evaluation may be to assess changing quality of life over time, requiring a longitudinal method. Both discriminative and evaluative instruments must be reproducible (test-retest reliability) and must accurately measure what they are intended to measure (validity) [4,6,11]. Additionally, tools used to measure HRQL over time must be responsive to change over time (responsiveness) [12].

The measures chosen for a given analysis must align to the purposes of the evaluation and be selected on the basis of strengths and weaknesses (content validity). This should take into account reliability, validity, responsiveness and perceived interpretability, as well as the relevance of the test results derived from such instruments.

What is Known About Quality of Life During the ICU Stay?

Reviews and Studies

From the English language literature indexed in Medline, Cinhal and Health Star from 1990–1999, we reviewed 18 journal articles pertaining to quality of life during the ICU stay. Seven of these were descriptive in nature, or represented personal experiences or perspectives [13–19]. Of the remaining 11 studies, seven used qualitative methods, mostly interviews, aimed at recalling or recollecting the ICU experience [20–26], and one was a cross-sectional study of patients evaluated during the ICU stay [27]. An additional three articles focused on pain during critical care, two using recollection techniques, and one a controlled study of pain management [28–30]. Six of the studies included quality of life considered from broad dimensions. The remaining focused on specific dimensions or components such as pain, noise, and dyspnea.

Instruments and Component Measures

Of the studies focusing on quality of life during the ICU stay, semi-structured or focused interviews were the primary source of data collection. Four instruments, two generic and two specific, were used, including:
- Environmental stressor scale [31,32]
- Short form McGill [33]
- Brief pain inventory [34]
- Visual analog scale for pain [30]

The component measures covered different aspects of quality of life, broadly categorized into physical, psychological, interpersonal, and environmental factors. Physical factors included the impact of pain and lack of sufficient sedation, altered cognitive function, difficulty in recall, physical discomfort due to tubes in the mouth or nose, and impact of procedures such as mechanical ventilation, arterial and venous access procedures, and tracheal suctioning. Psychological factors included fear, loss of control, dependency, anxiety, and serious or advanced states of delirium and psychosis. Interpersonal factors included relationships with ICU staff, particularly physicians and nurses, and the impact on patients' personal relationships. Environmental measures included impact of noise and the physical environment in general.

Current Understanding

In addition to whatever additional burden critical illness brings, patients in the ICU feel pain, countless discomforts, loss of control, loss of role, and unfulfilled commitments and expectations. As previously categorized, the quality of life experienced during the ICU stay is influenced, if not determined, by physical, psychological, interpersonal, and environmental factors.

By far, the best-studied physical factor is pain, while sleep disorders, anxiety and altered states of consciousness, such as delirium, are the most frequently evaluated psychological impacts. Less understood, but of particular importance, are the interpersonal factors between patients and their nurses, physicians and family. Such factors, combined with the sense of loss of control of one's immediate environment, form a complex interplay. At the same time, the patient may be feeling the loss of participation in normal roles and activities. In the surrounding environment, factors best studied include noise and temperature, but minimal if any attention has been directed at countless interventions, disturbances, and discomforts, all of which are factors of varying importance to the individual patient's quality of life during the ICU stay. Powerful personal experiences related by former ICU patients, some of which have been physicians, have drawn attention, for example, to the extent of pain and discomfort, such as comes from tracheal suction, as well as the overwhelming sense of loss of control in the ICU [14, 19].

There have been at least seven studies in the last decade in the area of recollection, recall, or perceptions of the ICU experience. The broad intent of these has been to gather information from those with a recent ICU experience, as a means of getting as close as possible to the perspective of the critically ill patient. Accordingly, five papers have evaluated recall within 48 hours of discharge from the ICU [20–24], though an additional two collected recall data for periods of up to 6–12 months after discharge [25, 26].

One recent cross-sectional study used the Intensive Care Unit Environmental Stressor Scale in 50 patients and showed that pain and sleep disturbance, noise and interventions were important physical stressors [27]. These were complemented by loss of self-control and lack of understanding about the attitudes and procedures as major psychological stressors. All of the recollection studies point to the same factors: pain, noise, sleeplessness, loss of control, as the principal sources of stress, and factors which negatively impact the quality of life during the ICU stay.

Notwithstanding that recall of ICU pain and its treatment may be altered by the medications themselves, all evaluations of pain in the ICU confirm frequent painful experiences in patients [28–30]. Despite advances in pain management, patients frequently report that pain relief is incomplete and, furthermore, that communications about pain and its treatment are often frustrating and ineffective, in part because of endotracheal intubation.

As for environmental factors, research on hospital noise has suggested that adverse behavioral changes in the critically ill may be potentiated by noise [16, 35, 36]. A number of studies have recorded hospital noise at greater than 45 decibels (dBA) [35–38]. In the ICU, noise has been recorded by audiometers at 58–72 dBA.

Loud noises over 70 dBA are especially common in the ICU, and may occur, on average, every 9 minutes [35]. Such noise levels are of sufficient intensity to interfere with rest and sleep. Countless other factors, of course, contribute to sleep disturbances in the ICU, which may evolve to full manifestations of the ICU syndrome, a severe, reversible, confusional state secondary to prolonged hospitalization in the ICU [39, 40]. Lesser states of confusion, anxiety, or delirium are, unquestionably, of major significance. Anxious patients are less cooperative with respiratory management and toilet, while delirious patients may be completely non-cooperative, if not combative.

It appears clear that quality of life during the ICU is seriously impacted by physical, psychological, interpersonal and environmental factors, all of which require better knowledge. There is, nonetheless, at this point, no common understanding as to the instruments, component measures, or dimensions to be included in quality of life measurement during the ICU stay. The development of better instruments to measure the components of HRQL in the ICU would permit us to better understand the relationship between external stimuli and a patient's health status while in the ICU, which may influence HRQL following critical care. By doing so, changes in these stimuli or new therapies could be more objectively evaluated in an effort to improve the patient's HRQL.

What is Known About Quality of Life Following the ICU Stay

Reviews and Studies to Date

From the English language literature indexed in Medline, Cinhal and Health Star from 1990–1999, we reviewed 21 journal articles pertaining to quality of life following the ICU stay, a subgroup of which provided longitudinal evaluation of HRQL. The studies were subdivided into four general groups: three articles provided a qualitative or methodological review and recommendations about the existing literature [1, 41, 42], two articles were of a descriptive nature [43, 44], seven articles evaluated either validated or non-validated original instruments developed specifically for assessing quality of life after ICU admission [45–51], and 10 articles utilized one or more previously validated instruments developed to measure both global domains and disease-specific quality of life [52–61].

There is a requirement for better instruments which move beyond simple mortality prediction models and encompass the assessment of morbidity, disability, and quality of life following critical care. This has been recognized and recommended by a consensus conference of the European Society of Intensive Care Medicine [41], as well as by a prominent review [42]. Moreover, the lack of a unified measure of HRQL after critical care has been emphasized. In a methodological review of 1073 articles relevant to the practice of adult intensive care, only 1.7% included quality of life measures [1]. Of the few studies which include some form of measurement of quality of life after ICU discharge, there are few comparisons of quality of life between study populations, in part, because of the heterogeneous nature of the instruments utilized in the studies.

Instruments and Component Measures

The seven studies which utilized a newly developed instrument for assessing quality of life after critical care, were published within the past 12 years, but only three of the seven provided some form of validation for the developed instruments. Ten studies utilized a previously validated instrument for measuring global and/or specific domains of HRQL, or modified previously validated tools for their intended purposes. These instruments were not initially developed with the intent of using them to study critically ill patients. Table 1 shows the instruments used solely or simultaneously within these studies.

The domains in these instruments included: physical and physiological measures; activities of daily living; degree of dependence; employment; emotional status; social functioning; and perceived quality of life.

The physical and physiological domain included mobility, weakness, measures of oral communication, ability to think and remember, ability to drive a vehicle, regular medication usage, readmission to hospital, disturbance of sleep, pain perception and intensity, and sphincter control.

The activities of daily living domain included activities such as bathing, dressing and preparing meals. The place of residence (e.g., nursing home) and degree of physical dependence comprised the dependence domain. Items within the employment domain included the capacity to work, and satisfaction with current income. Emotional status encompassed a broad array of measures including happiness and energy, strength of relationships with family and friends, self-respect and respect by others, meaning/purpose in life, anxiety/depression, sexual relationships, personal appearance, spiritual satisfaction, somatic symptoms, self-worth, control over life, and elements embodying the stress following a traumatic life event, similar to that documented with post-traumatic stress disorder.

Contribution to the community, leisure activities, social appearance, social relationships and isolation, hobbies, holidays were characteristic of the social domain. Finally, general questions pertaining to overall perceived quality of life were included as a separate domain.

Table 1. Validated instruments for measuring global/specific health-related quality of life (HRQL)

Short Form (SF-36) [62]
Sickness Impact Profile (SIP) [63]
Rosser's Disability Categories [64]
Katz's Activities of Daily Living [65]
General Health Questionnaire 28-Item Version
Rosenberg Self–Esteem Scale [67]
The Impact of Event Scale [68]
The Psychological General Well-Being Schedule [69]
Nottingham Health Profile [70]
Spitzer's Quality of Life Index [71]

Current Understanding

One validated instrument for measuring HRQL following critical care is comprised of an 11-item measure of need satisfaction, namely, the Perceived Quality of Life Scale (PQOL) [45]. This instrument has demonstrated internal consistency and reliability (Cronbach's alpha coefficient = 0.88). However, criterion validity against various social characteristics was limited (R = 0.18 to 0.50). Likewise, criterion validity as evidenced by the correlation between the PQOL and other global measures was limited (Sickness Impact Score [R = –0.49]; the Psychological General Well–Being Schedule [R=0.54]). In the original description of the PQOL scale, the mean score, out of a total of 100 points for maximum satisfaction, at a median of 19 months following ICU discharge was 75. This compared favorably to a mean score of 79 in a group of healthy, elderly patients living in the community. The PQOL scale has also been incorporated into a larger instrument by other investigators who have demonstrated that patients who are admitted with a good pre-admission quality of life suffered a significant decrease in quality of life, whereas those with a lower pre-admission quality of life did not experience a significant change [59].

A second validated HRQL instrument originally described in Spanish and specific to the ICU, the Quality of Life Score (QLS), focuses mainly on functional status, including questions pertaining to oral communication, sphincter control, movement and exercise, physical dependence, requirement for regular medications, and capacity to work [72]. A subsequent study of 606 patients utilizing this QLS, demonstrated a general worsening of quality of life from the time of ICU admission to 12 months post ICU discharge, with the exception of the subgroup with the worst initial QLS, who demonstrated an overall improvement in quality of life at 12 months [46]. Although a poor association was demonstrated between the APACHE II and the QLS, only the initial QLS and age were predictive of the 12 month QLS, after adjustment in a multivariate model. The QLS was subsequently expanded into a 15-item validated instrument developed specifically for critical care, within the Spanish 'Project for the Epidemiological Analysis of Critical Care Patients'. Hence this third instrument was comprised of three subscales including basic physiological measures, normal daily activities, and emotional state. This has proven to have good internal consistency (Cronbach's alpha coefficient = 0.85), and reproducibility (correlation > 0.90), within and between various populations. The instrument has content validity, as evidenced by the extraction of 3 distinct factors, using factor analysis techniques. These factors corresponded to the three subscales proposed *a priori* [47].

Four remaining studies have utilized non-validated, ICU-specific instruments. Of 504 ICU patients surveyed 3 months after hospital discharge, 47% indicated their health was good to very good, fair in 42% and poor/very poor in 11% [48]. Moreover, patients' activity level was found to be unchanged in 59%, worse in 33% and improved in 8% of respondents. Of 238 patients studied 16 months after ICU discharge and compared with a random community sample [49], using the ICU-specific Health-Related Quality of Life Questionnaire, critically ill patients developed more symptoms, depression and dependence, and reduced sexual activity.

In a third study, utilizing a 6-domain HRQL instrument in 160 patients 6 months after hospital discharge, physical activity decreased in 31%, social function decreased in 32% and functional limitation increased in 30% of respondents [50]. Finally, a smaller evaluation of 13 patients demonstrated mostly minor complaints related to physical condition in 54%, an increase in anxiety in 46% and a return to living at home in 100% of respondents [51].

Of the 10 studies that utilized validated instruments not initially designed for critical care, five utilized generic instruments, either the Sickness Impact Profile (SIP) or the Short Form-36 (SF-36). In a Dutch study [52] of 3655 respondents 1 year after hospital discharge, mean SIP scores ranged between 5.8 for those aged 17–29 to 10.5 for those > 70 years old (with an overall mean SIP score of 8.5). This was dominated by dysfunction in the physical dimension, with the exception of those aged 30–49 years in whom categories comprising the psychosocial dimension represented approximately 50% of the total variance [52]. More optimistic results were reported in a cohort surviving to 1 year after admission to a multidisciplinary ICU in Hong Kong. The median SIP score was found to be 5.1 [53]. In this study, age, cardiac/respiratory arrest, intracranial hemorrhage, and trauma were identified as independent predictors of a higher SIP score. Both the Dutch and the Hong Kong studies failed to identify a strong correlation between SIP score and the severity of illness as measured by APACHE II, nor was there a correlation between the SIP score, therapeutic intervention scoring system (TISS), and length of ICU stay. One caveat with using the SIP as well as other instruments is the form in which the questionnaire is distributed. Previous investigators have demonstrated that response rates after the distribution of the SIP to ex-ICU patients varied from 56% in those where the instrument was mailed, to 77% if patients were telephoned with an invitation to participate prior to distributing the questionnaire [54]. Moreover, significant differences in SIP scores were noted between these groups compared with those being personally interviewed using the SIP, although the differences in scores may have been attributed to sample characteristics.

With respect to the reliability and validity of the SF-36 after discharge from a general ICU, internal consistency and reliability as measured by Cronbach's alpha, exceeded 0.85 for all dimensions except for mental health. Construct validity was demonstrated by a difference in the distribution of scores by age and gender, and content validity was demonstrated by the broad distribution of scores throughout the range of answers [55]. In a corresponding study utilizing the same ICU population, the SF-36 was distributed to 166 patients at ICU discharge and 6 months later. Overall, the patients' premorbid scores at discharge were lower than normal for all dimensions of the SF-36, and 6 months later, there were significant increases in mental health, vitality, social functioning, and a reduction in bodily pain scores compared to baseline [56]. However, the overall mean score decreased at 6 months for those patients admitted with acute problems, as compared with patients with chronic comorbidities. This is consistent with the findings of a previous study [57].

Five additional studies utilized either individual quality of life scales [58, 59, 61], or a composite instrument made up of previously validated scales [57, 60].

Both the Nottingham Health profile (NHP) and the PQOL correlated well. However, good quality of life as measured by the NHP was present in only 38.8% of respondents and a high PQOL was observed in only 23.7% of respondents. Moreover, in a separate study assessing psychological dysfunction after an ICU admission, the General Health questionnaire 28-item version, the Rosenberg Self-esteem Scale, and the Impact of Event Scale were administered to 72 patients at 6 weeks, 6 and 12 months after ICU discharge [59]. Changes in the scores of these instruments were found to be dependent on the indication for admission to the ICU, the mode of admission (e.g., elective, post-operative vs unconscious from the ward) and the patient recall of the ICU. Hence, these factors must be considered when validating any future HRQL instruments in critical care.

One study, which utilized Spitzer's Quality of Life Index on admission to the ICU and at 6 and 12 months after the initial survey, demonstrated a reduction in activity and activities of daily living at 6 months and 12 months [61]. However, perceived health improved over the year, which was consistent with the findings utilizing the SF-36 instrument [56].

In the only study that assessed a composite quality of life measure with a cost-utility analysis, the quality of life for the majority of patients remained the same following ICU, except for survivors who previously perceived a good quality of life or were admitted with respiratory problems, in which case their quality of life diminished [60]. Furthermore, the hospital cost per quality-adjusted life year was approximately £ 7500.

Attention to Specific Groups

The Elderly

The disproportionately large effect that the elderly have on health care costs is well established. Depending on the nature and location of ICUs, utilization by the elderly may range between 26–51% of admissions. Epidemiologic trends in the burden of disease towards an increasing proportion of non-communicable diseases, twinned with the aging of the population will, no doubt, give rise to complex questions about the nature and extent of critical care benefit and to whom it should be directed, if not limited.

Interest in elderly patients being admitted to ICUs has prompted at least six studies and two review articles since 1990 dealing with the impact of age as a contributor to outcome following critical care [73–80]. This work suggests that age has little or no important impact on outcome from critical illness, which is most strongly predicted by severity of illness and, to a varying extent, prior health status and ICU length of stay.

Viewing the world as over and under 65 is, however, simplistic. What about the oldest of the old [77,78]? Two studies dealing with patients over 85 years of age similarly concluded that advanced age was an incomplete criterion for allocation of ICU resources, and was of lesser importance than acute severity of illness, as a determinant of outcome. Other information suggests that advanced age cannot be used to predict functional ability.

The ICU follow–up studies of the elderly evaluated quality of life in a variety of ways, using such defined instruments as:

- Katz and Downs Activity of Life Scale [81]
- Lawton and Brody Instrumental Activities of Daily Living [82,83]
- Geriatric Depression Scale [84]
- Mini–Mental State [85]
- Centre for Epidemiologic Studies Depression Score. [86]

Other less defined information has come from personal and telephone interviews collecting data on subjective perceptions of quality of life, as well as a variety of indicators of functional ability.

While our understanding to date suggests that age is not a major factor, in and of itself, influencing either quantity or quality of survival following critical care, this generalization requires clearer understanding in relation to many specific diseases and interventions, and changing perspectives of what is 'old age'.

Long-Stay Patients

The assumption that long-stay patients in the ICU have a diminishing probability of survival, with poor HRQL, has repeatedly raised questions about the value of prolonged critical care. Two studies addressing this topic arrive at similar conclusions [87,88]. Namely, prolonged ICU stay is not a reliable marker for survival or for quality of life. Indeed, using a novel approach to economic evaluation, the value of treating patients beyond 14 days in the ICU has been investigated [89]. Not surprisingly, a considerable proportion of patients with a prolonged length of stay in the ICU survive their critical illness. Furthermore, their HRQL at 12 months is comparable to short-stay patients, with an incremental cost-effectiveness ratio of $4350 (CND) per life-year saved.

Cardiac Patients

Quality of life following multisystem ICU support of patients after cardiac surgery has been evaluated with retrospective, cohort, and case-control methods [90–92]. Not surprisingly, the cost of severe complications in the ICU is extremely high. While not incompatible with a good long-term outcome, multiple organ failure and prolonged critical care after heart surgery has provided mixed results with respect to HRQL. However, when compared to uncomplicated controls, cardiac surgery patients with prolonged ICU stays have poorer outcomes and a significantly negative impact on activities such as housework, hobbies, and sexual practices.

Trauma

Analysis of HRQL has been prospectively evaluated in post–traumatized patients after critical care [93, 94]. Patients report significant social disability, work impairment, psychological and emotional perturbations. This is particularly marked in those suffering head injuries. Pre-trauma quality of life, injury severity, and age appear to be the best predictors of outcome.

Acute Respiratory Distress Syndrome (ARDS)

Systematic study of functional recovery in survivors of ARDS has largely focused on pulmonary function [95]. Beyond this, long-term survivors of ARDS achieve good HRQL, though with impairment in all health domains, as compared with controls and as measured by the SF-36 [96]. Moreover, for those who experience repeatedly adverse experiences during the ICU stay, there is a strong association with post–traumatic stress disorders and a negative impact on HRQL.

Other Disorders and Conditions

A variety of other disorders and conditions, such as abdominal sepsis [97], hematologic malignancy [98], and liver transplantation [99], have been evaluated with respect to HRQL following critical care. In the case of abdominal sepsis, long-term survivors were independent, ambulatory, and capable of self-care, with no patients being completely disabled. The determinants of survival did not predict subsequent quality of life.

Study of long-term HRQL following critical care for life-threatening, potentially reversible complications of hematologic malignancies is complicated by the direct impact of the malignancy on survival and outcome. Nonetheless, it appears that HRQL in the long-term survivors is good, permitting return to such activities as employment. Furthermore, when questioned more than one year following discharge, survivors appear willing to re-enter the ICU, if confronted with similar circumstances.

Survivors of liver transplantation who have required ICU admission appear to do as well in terms of post-discharge HRQL, as those not requiring ICU, and whose course was not complicated by critical illness.

Future Directions

Beyond Survival and Morbidity

Over the past decade, it has become apparent that models for predicting ICU survival are useful, yet limited in their ability to confidently predict for individual patients, and are not well correlated with current measures of HRQL after the ICU experience. This has implications for economic evaluation and resource allocations in the ICU, as well as for both individual and patient/family decision-making. This emphasizes the importance of developing a variety of instruments better suited for predicting HRQL in those patients likely to survive the ICU stay.

Future instruments specific to assessing HRQL following critical care must be developed and refined, taking into account a method of evaluating societal values and preferences. If prospective patients were informed of the likelihood of changing from one health state before their ICU admission to a different state, during and after discharge from the ICU, this would enable them to make better decisions about choosing to enter an ICU for treatment.

Comparative Studies and Economic Evaluation

Any research of critical care value and outcomes must include comparative studies of models of delivery and alternate care formats, both within and outside of the ICU. Longitudinal studies of general and specific patient cohorts are essential, with assessment of HRQL as an outcome measure or key independent variable. Furthermore, in consideration of overall benefit of critical care, economic evaluation which includes quality of life assessment is of central importance. Economic evaluation without assessment of HRQL undervalues the effectiveness or benefit. Alternatively, assessing HRQL without economic evaluation weakens tradeoff decisions and considerations involved in resource allocation.

To undertake this type of research agenda, prospective data collection is essential. While cross-sectional studies are important contributors to knowledge and hypothesis generation, better evidence is likely from patient-specific, longitudinal studies. This implies a need for data standards, data collection methods, and the information systems needed for storage, retrieval, data management, and analysis.

Towards a Universal HRQL Measure for General Intensive Care

It appears that different measurement instruments for HRQL should be applied to patients during their ICU stay, when external physical and psychological stimuli vary little from patient to patient. Instruments developed for the purposes of evaluating HRQL within the ICU must encompass the domains of sleep, pain, and loss of control, to name a few. Such instruments could be easily developed and adopted and validated against objective measures of external stimuli such as electroencephalographic measurement of rapid eye movement (REM) sleep, visual analog scales of pain, or measurements of ambient noise within the ICU.

Measurement of HRQL after ICU discharge poses more difficult problems. Given the heterogeneity of the general ICU population, the severity of the critical illness incurred by most of these patients, and the inability to accurately predict those patients destined to enter the ICU *a priori*, development of a single, universal HRQL measure in the ICU is both daunting and, arguably, unrealistic. A sounder approach would be to develop and rigorously validate a group of instruments based on the predominant diagnosis or case type (e.g., trauma, respiratory failure, hematological or other malignancies). This would permit improved responsiveness, valuable to longitudinal studies, and would avoid the possibility of floor or ceiling effects, which may be encountered with more generic instruments. With specific instruments, one must account for the presence of co-morbidities (versus a healthy pre-morbid state), as this has been consistently found to influence the transitional probabilities of moving from a specific health status prior to ICU admission to a predicted outcome after ICU discharge.

The timing of assessment using any newly developed instrument is important, as recovery from the initial illness precipitating an ICU admission may be prolonged. Hence, it is proposed that such instruments be evaluated over the course of two and perhaps three years, using methods of longitudinal data analysis. Mean recuperation times as long as 23 months may be required for severely traumatized patients [100], and regaining employment may require up to 3 years for certain individuals [101].

Given the multi-dimensional impact of ICU admission on the health status of an individual, measurement instruments for HRQL must be multi-dimensional and composed of several component measures within each domain. Each domain should be subjected to rigorous assessment for internal consistency, test-retest reliability, and content, construct, and criterion validity.

In conjunction with ICU-specific instruments, further research is essential using generic instruments of HRQL such as the SIP and the SF-36, which have demonstrated validity in this population in a small number of examples. Comparison of any proposed ICU-specific instrument with these generic tools would improve the criterion validity of the instrument. The ability to understand and use generic instruments for measuring HRQL would enable researchers to evaluate generic measures of quality of life across various diseases and populations in and outside of the ICU.

Given the limitation of recall bias in obtaining baseline measures of HRQL in patients admitted to the ICU, other epidemiological methodologies must be adopted to answer questions pertaining to the improvement or decline, and the utility of moving from one health state prior to ICU admission to a different health state after ICU discharge. Methodologies such as case-control and cohort studies may prove useful in determining the additional benefit of an ICU admission for certain populations. This would require periodic evaluation using an established HRQL instrument in a homogeneous population of patients at high risk of requiring ICU admission at some point in their lives, for example, those with advanced chronic obstructive lung disease or chronic renal failure. Should a subgroup of patients from this population subsequently require ICU care, comparisons of the change in HRQL could subsequently be made between the cases requiring ICU care and similar control patients from the original population.

Unquestionable progress has been made over the past decade in the development of mortality prediction models for critical care and there is growing interest in a broad array of HRQL issues and measures, during and after the ICU experience. Notwithstanding the need to be better informed, there exists a considerable gap in understanding and a substantial opportunity for the development and use of ICU-specific measures in the future.

Beyond this, as the next chapter points out, there are many difficulties in assessing outcomes following critical care. This has been particularly exemplified through experiences from follow-up clinics, which have identified the nature of long-term consequences in survivors of critical care.

References

1. Heyland DK, Guyatt G, Cook Deborah J (1998) Frequency and methodologic rigor of quality-of-life assessments in the critical care literature. Crit Care Med 26:592–598
2. Clancy M, Eisenberg JM (1998) Outcomes research: Measuring the end results of health care. Science 282:245–246
3. McDowell I, Newll C (1996) The theoretical and technical foundations of health measurement. In: McDowell I, Newll C (eds) Measuring health: A guide to rating scales and questionnaires, 2nd edn. Oxford University Press, New York, pp 10–46
4. Juniper EF, Guyatt GH, Jaeschke R (1996) How to develop and validate a new health-related quality of life instrument. In: Spiker B (ed) Quality of life and pharmacoeconomics in clinical trials, 2nd edn. Lippincott-Raven Publishers, Philadelphia, pp 49–56
5. Feeny DH, Torrance GW, Furlong WJ (1996) Health utilities index. In: Spiker B (ed) Quality of life and pharmacoeconomics in clinical trials, 2nd edn. Lippincott-Raven Publishers, Philadelphia, pp 239–252
6. Guyatt GH, Feeny DH, Patrick DL (1993) Measuring health-related quality of life. Ann Intern Med 118:622–629
7. Osoba D (1995) Measuring the effect of cancer on health-related quality of life. Pharmacoeconomics 7:308–319
8. Hillers TK, Guyatt GH, Oldridge N, et al (1994) Quality of life after myocardial infarction. J Clin Epidemiol 47:1287–1296
9. Feeny DH, Torrance GW (1989) Incorporating utility-based quality-of-life assessment measures in clinical trials: Two examples. Med Care 27:S190–S204
10. Guyatt G, Feeny D, Patrick D (1991) Issues in quality-of-life measurement in clinical trials. Control Clin Trials 12 (suppl 4):81S–90S
11. Hays RD, Anderson R, Revicki D (1993) Psychometric considerations in evaluating health-realted quality of life measures. Qual Life Res 2:441–449
12. Deyo RA, Diehr P, Patrick D (1991) Reproducibility and responsiveness of health status measures. Control Clin Trials 12 (suppl 4):142S–158S
13. McCartney JR, Boland RJ (1994) Anxiety and delirium in the intensive care unit. Crit Care Clin 10:673–680
14. Lloyd G (1993) Psychological problems and the intensive care unit. Br Med J 307:458–459
15. Schwab RJ (1994) Disturbances of sleep in the intensive care unit. Crit Care Clin 10:681–695
16. Griffin JP (1992) The impact of noise on critically ill people. Holistic Nurs Pract 6:53–56
17. Compton P (1991) Critical illness and intensive care: What it means to the client. Crit Care Nurs 11:50–56
18. Norrie P (1992) The intensive care experience. Nursing Times 88:40–42
19. Hayden WR (1994) Life and near-death in the intensive care unit. Crit Care Clin 10:651–657
20. Turner JS, Briggs SJ, Springhorn HE, Potgieter PD (1990) Patients' recollection of intensive care unit experience. Crit Care Med 18:966–968
21. Simpson TF, Armstrong S, Mitchell P (1989) Critical care management. Heart Lung 18: 325–332
22. Shih FJ, Chu SH (1999) Comparisons of American-Chinese and Taiwanese patients' perceptions of dyspnea and helpful nursing actions during the intensive care unit transition from cardiac surgery. Heart Lung 28:41–54
23. Helpern EH, Patterson PA, Gloskey D, Bone RC (1992) Patients' preferences for intensive care. Crit Care Med 20:43–47
24. Holland C, Cason CL, Prater LR (1997) Patients' recollections of critical care. Dimens Crit Care Nurs 16:132–141
25. Johnson MM, Sexton DL (1990) Distress during mechanical ventilation: patients' perceptions. Crit Care Med 10:48–57
26. Green A (1996) An exploratory study of patients' memory recall of their stay in an adult intensive therapy unit. Intensive Crit Care Nurs 12:131–137
27. Novaes M, Aronovich A, Ferraz MB, Knobel E (1997) Stressors in ICU: patients' evaluation. Intensive Care Med 23:1282–1285

28. Valdix SW, Puntillo KA (1995) Pain, pain relief and accuracy of their recall after cardiac surgery. Prog Cardiovasc Nurs 10:3:3–11
29. Puntillo KA (1990) Pain experiences of intensive care unit patients. Heart Lung 19:526–533
30. Tittle M, McMillan SC (1994) Pain and pain-related side effects in an ICU and on a surgical unit: Nurses' management. Am J Crit Care 3:25–30
31. Ballard KS (1981) Identification of environmental stressors for patients in a surgical intensive care unit. Issues Ment Health Nurs 1:89–108
32. Enastasy EL (1985) Identifying environmental stressors for cardiac surgery patients in a SICU. In: Proceedings of the 12th Annual National Teaching Institute of AACN. AACN, Newport Beach, p 357
33. Melzack R (1987) The short-form McGill pain questionnaire. Pain 30:191–197
34. Cleeland C (1985) Measurement and prevalence of pain in cancer. Semin Oncol Nurs 87–92
35. Falk S, Woods N (1973) Hospital noise levels and potential health hazards. N Engl J Med 289:774–781
36. King TA, Craddock J (1975) Measuring and reducing noise. Hospitals 49:85–90
37. Topf M (1985) Noise induced stress in hospital patients: coping and nonauditory health outcomes. J Human Stress 11:3:125–134
38. Hilton A (1985) Noise in acute patient areas. Res Nurs Health 8:283–291
39. Snyder-Halpern R (1985) The effect of critical care unit noise on patient sleep cycles. CCQ 7:41–51
40. Weber RJ, Soak MA, Bolender BJ, et al (1985) The intensive care unit syndrome: Causes, treatment and prevention. Drug Intell Clin Pharm 19:13–20
41. Suter P, Armaganidis A, Beaufils F, et al (1994) Predicting outcome in ICU patients. Intensive Care Med 20: 390–397
42. Brooks R, Bauman A, Daffurn K, Hillman K (1995) Post-hospital outcome following intensive care. Clin Intensive Care 6: 127–135
43. Sawdon V, Woods I, Proctor M (1995) Post-intensive care interviews: implications for future practice. Critl Care Nurs 11:329–332
44. Daffurn K, Bishop GF, Hillman KM, Bauman A (1994) Problems following discharge after intensive care. Intensive Crit Care Nurs 10:244–251
45. Patrick DL, Danis M, Southerland LI, Hong G (1988) Quality of life following intensive care. J Gen Intern Med 3:218–223
46. Vazquez Mata G, Rivera Fernandez R, Gonzalez Carmona A, Delgado-Rodriguez M, Miguel Torres Ruiz J, Raya Pugnaire A, Aguayo De Hoyos E (1992) Factors related to quality of life 12 months after discharge from an intensive care unit. Crit Care Med 20:1257–1262
47. Rivera Fernandez R, Sanchez Cruz JJ, Vazquez Mata G (1996) Validation of a quality of life questionnaire for critically ill patients. Intensive Care Med 22:1034–1042
48. Munn J, Willatts SM, Tooley MA (1995) Health and activity after intensive care. Anaesthesia 50:1017–1021
49. Brooks R, Kerridge R, Hillman K, Bauman A, Daffurn K (1997) Quality of life outcomes after intensive care: comparison with a community group. Intensive Care Med 23:581–586
50. Capuzzo M, Bianconi M, Contu P, Pavoni V, Gritti G (1996) Survival and quality of life after intensive care. Intensive Care Med 22:947–953
51. Rustom R, Daly K (1993) Quality of life after intensive care. Br J Nurs 2:316–320
52. Tian ZM, Reis Miranda D (1995) Quality of life after intensive care with the sickness impact profile. Intensive Care Med 21:422–428
53. Short TG, Buckley TA, Rowbottom MY, Wong E, Oh TE (1999) Long-term outcome and functional health status following intensive care in Hong Kong. Crit Care Med 27:51–57
54. Hulsebos RG, Beltman FW, dos Reis Miranda D, Spangenberg JFA (1991) Measuring quality of life with the sickness impact profile: a pilot study. Intensive Care Med 17:285–288
55. Chrispin PS, Scotton H, Rogers J, Lloyd D, Ridley SA (1997) Short form 36 in the intensive care unit: assessment of acceptability, reliability and validity of the questionnaire. Anaesthesia 52:15–23

56. Ridley SA, Chrispin PS, Scotton H, Rogers J, Lloyd (1997) Changes in quality of life after intensive care: comparison with normal data. Anesthesia 52: 195–202
57. Ridley SA, Wallace PGM (1990) Quality of life after intensive care. Anaesthesia 45:808–813
58. Hurel D, Loirat P, Saulnier F, Nicolas F, Brivet F (1997) Quality of life 6 months after intensive care: results of a prospective multicenter study using a generic health status scale and a satisfaction scale. Intensive Care Med 23:331–337
59. Perrins J, King N, Collings J (1998) Assessment of long-term psychological well-being following intensive care. Intensive Crit Care Nurs 14:108–116
60. Ridley S, Biggam M, Stone P (1994) A cost-utility analysis of intensive therapy. Anesthesia 49:192–196
61. Konopad E, Noseworthy TW, Johnston R, Shustack A, Grace M (1995) Quality of life measures before and one year after admission to an intensive care unit. Crit Care Med 23: 1653–1659.
62. Ware JE (1993) SF-36 Health Survey Manual and Interpretation Guide. The Medical Outcomes Trust, Boston
63. Bergner M, Bobbitt RA, Kressel S, Pollard WE, Gibson BS, Morris JR (1981) The sickness impact profile: development and final revision of a health status measure. Med Care 19: 787–805
64. Kind P, Rosser RM, Williams A (1982) Valuation of quality of life: some psychometric evidence. In: Jones-Lee MW (ed). The value of life and safety. North Holland Publishing Co, Amsterdam, pp 159–170
65. Katz S (1983) Assessing self-maintenance: activities of daily living, mobility, and instrumental activities of daily living. J Am Geriatr Soc 31:721–727
66. Goldberg DP, Hillier VF (1979) A scaled version of the General Health Questionnaire. Psychol Med 9: 139–145
67. Rosenberg M (1965) Society and the adolescent self-image. Princeton University Press, New Jersey
68. Horowitz M, Wilner N (1979) The impact of event scale: a measure of subjective stress. Psychosom Med 41: 209–218
69. Dupuy H. The Psychological General Well–being (PGWB) Index (1984) In: Wenger NK, Mattson ME, Furberg CD, Elinson (eds). Assessment of quality of life in clinical trials of cardiovascular therapies. LeJacq, New York.
70. Hunt SM, McKenna SP, McEwen J, Williams J, Rapp E (1981) The Nottingham Health Profile: subjective health status and medical consultations. Soc Sci Med 15A: 221–229
71. Spitzer WO, Dobson AJ, Hall J, et al (1981) Measuring the quality of life of cancer patients: A concise Quality of Life Index for use by physicians. J Chronic Dis 34:585–597
72. Rivera Fernandez R, Vazquez Mata G, Gonzalez Carmona A, et. al. (1991) Descripcion de una encuesta de calidad de vida en medicina intensive. Medica Intensiva 15:313–318
73. Rockwood K, Noseworthy TW, Gibney RTN, et al. (1993) One-year outcome of elderly and young patients admitted to intensive care units. Crit Care Med 21:687–691
74. Broslawski GE, Elkins M, Algus M (1995) Functional abilities of elderly survivors of intensive care. J Am Osteopath Assoc 92:12:712-717
75. Chelluri L, Pinsky MR, Donahoe MP, Grenvik A (1993) Long-term outcome of critically ill elderly patients requiring intensive care. JAMA 269:3119–3123
76. Mahul Ph, Perrot D, Tempelhoff G, et al. (1991) Short- and long-term prognosis, functional outcome following ICU for elderly. Intensive Care Med 17:7–10
77. Chelluri L, Pinsky MR, Grenvik ANA (1992) Outcomes of intensive care of the "oldest-old" critically ill patients. Crit Care Med 20:757–761
78. Kass JE, Castriotta RJ, Malakoff F (1992) Intensive care unit outcome in the very elderly. Crit Care Med 20:1666–1671
79. Chelluri L, Grenvik A (1995) Intensive care for critically ill elderly: mortality, costs, and quality of life. Arch Intern Med 155:1013–1022
80. Rubins HB (1989) Intensive care and the elderly. Hospital Practice. January 30:9–12
81. Katz S, Downs TD, Cash HR, et al. (1970) Progress in development of the index of ADL. Gerontologist 10:20–30

82. Lawton MP (1971) The functional assessment of elderly people. J Am Geriatr Soc 19:465–481
83. Lawton MP (1969) Assessment of older people: Self-maintaining and instrumental activities of daily living. Gerontologist 9:179–186
84. Sheikh JI, Yesavage JA (1986) Geriatric depression scale (GDS): Recent evidence and development of a shorter version. Clin Gerontol 4:165–173
85. Folstein MF, Folsttein SE, McHugh PR (1975) "Mini-mental state": a practical method for grading the cognitive state of patients for the clinician. J Psychiat Res 12:189–198
86. Weissman MM, Sholomskas D, Pottenger M Prusoff BA, Locke B (1977) Assessing depressive symptoms in five psychiatric populations: a validation study. Am J Epidemiol 106: 203–214
87. Fakhry SM, Kercher KW, Rutledge R (1996) Survival, quality of life, and charges in critically ill surgical patients requiring prolonged ICU stays. J Trauma 41:999–1007
88. Trouillet JL, Scheimberg A, Vuagnat A, Fagon JY, Chastre J, Gibert C (1996) Long-term outcome and quality of life of patients requiring multidisciplinary intensive care unit admission after cardiac operations. J Thorac Cardiovasc Surg 112:926–934
89. Heyland DK, Konopad E, Noseworthy TW, Johnston R, Gafni A (1998) Is it 'worthwhile' to continue treating patients with a prolonged stay (>14 days) in the ICU? An economic evaluation. Chest 114:192–198
90. Soderlind K, Rutberg H, Olin C (1997) Late outcome and quality of life after complicated heart operations. Ann Thorac Surg 63:124–128
91. McHugh GJ, Havill JH, Armistead SH, Ullal RR, Fayers TM (1997) Follow up of elderly patients after cardiac surgery and intensive care unit admission, 1991 to 1995. N Z Med J 110:432–435
92. Nielsen D, Sellgren J, Ricksten SE (1997) Quality of life after cardiac surgery complicated by multiple organ failure. Crit Care Med 25:52–57
93. Mata GV, Fernandez RR, Aragon AP, Carmona AG, Mondejar EF, Navarro PN (1996) Analysis of quality of life in polytraumatized patients two years after discharge from an Intensive Care Unit. J Trauma 41:326–332
94. Thiagarajan J, Taylor P, Hogbin E, Ridley S (1994) Quality of life after multiple trauma requiring intensive care. Anaesthesia 49:211–218
95. McHugh LG, Milberg JA, Whitcomb ME et al. (1994) Recovery of function in survivors of the acute respiratory distress syndrome. Am J Respir Crit Care Med 150:90–94
96. Schelling G, Stoll C, Haller M, et al. (1998) Health-related quality of life and posttraumatic stress disorder in survivors of the acute respiratory distress syndrome. Crit Care Med 26:651–659
97. McLauchlan GH, Anderson ID, Grant IS, Fearon KCH (1995) Outcome of patients with abdominal sepsis treated in an intensive care unit. Br J Surg 82:524–529
98. Yau E, Rohatiner AZS, Lister TA, Hinds CJ (1991) Long-term prognosis and quality of life following intensive care for life-threatening complications of haematological malignancy. Br J Cancer 64:938–942
99. Singh N, Gayowski T, Wagener MM (1997) Intensive care unit management in liver transplant recipients: beneficial effect on survival and preservation of quality of life. Clin Transplant 11:113–120
100. Kivioja AH, Myllynen PJ, Rokkanen PU (1990) Is the treatment of the most severe multiply injured patients worth the effort? J Trauma 30:480–483
101. Benzer H, Mutz N, Pauser G (1983) Psychological sequelae of intensive care. Int Anesthesiol Clin 21:1659–1678

Quality of Life and Longer Term Outcomes

S. A. Ridley

Learning Points

1. Longer-term outcome following ICU may be examined from the perspective of the patient, attendant staff or society. All of these perspectives are different and will require different measurement tools
2. Long term follow-up of critically ill patients should be extended until the gradient of their survival curves parallels that of a comparison group. This may require follow-up for up to four or more years and is probably country specific
3. The selection of a comparison group requires carefully consideration. Patients admitted to ICU are not a random selection of the normal population and so comparisons with age and sex matched normal populations may not be valid. Diagnosis on ICU admission affects long term survival and so the comparison group should be similar in this respect
4. Functional outcome measures physical and mental capacity, neuropsychological function and recovery. Functional outcome has been widely measured outside critical care but the psychometric properties of assessment tools have not been rigorously reported for use in the survivors of critical illness

Figure 1 plots two possible outcomes for a critically ill patient following rupture of an abdominal aortic aneurysm. After a protracted ICU stay involving mechanical ventilation, renal replacement therapy and a further laparotomy for an ischemic sigmoid colon, the patient is discharged to the general ward where he develops a hospital-acquired chest infection. After two months in hospital, the patient is considered well enough to return home. However, he is weak, his limbs are stiff, and he is having problems coping with his colostomy; understandably he is anxious and depressed.

At this stage his clinical course could diverge to follow one of several outcomes. For example, shortly after hospital discharge, the patient could suffer a cerebrovascular accident and develop a dense hemiparesis. Although he is re-admitted to hospital, he remains aphasic and wheelchair bound. As he cannot return to his previous employment, he loses his income and subsequently his home. On the other hand the patient could continue to make a gradual improvement and be well enough to return to his previous job. Unfortunately he dies in a road traffic accident three months later.

This clinical history usefully illustrates some of the problems when measuring the longer-term outcomes following critical illness. At present, survival is mea-

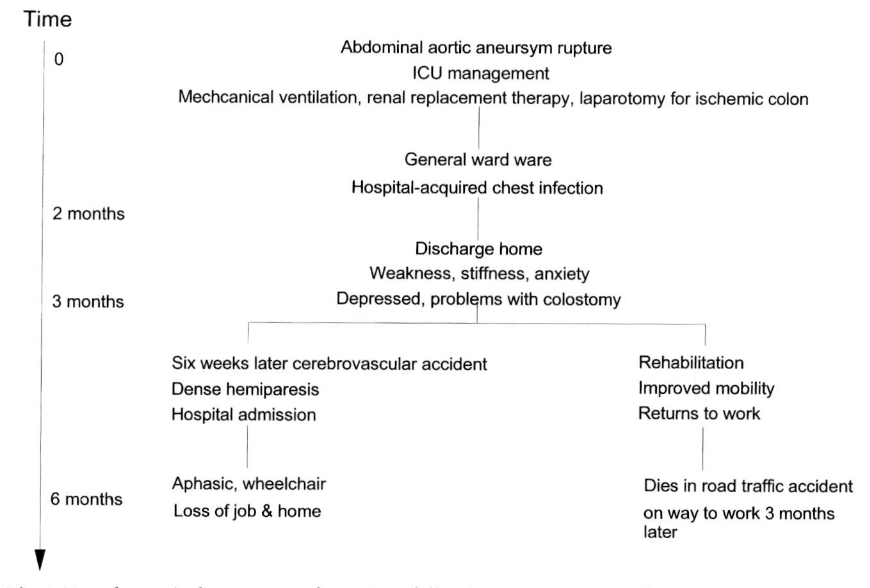

Fig. 1. Two theoretical outcomes of a patient following emergency aortic aneurysm repair

sured at arbitrary calendar periods after ICU admission. If survival was measured at six months in the above example, then the patient might have died in the road traffic accident. Unless his cause of death is known, this might be attributed to his critical illness rather than an unfortunate twist of fate. If quality of life is measured, then the patient in the wheelchair may not have too bad a quality of life because as a result of being so ill he is just grateful to be alive. Before his death, the quality of life of the patient who returned to work may not be as good as expected because he has lost his chances of promotion, enhanced salary and as a result his wife has left him. Clearly the functional outcome of this patient is much better that the patient who suffered the significant physical handicap due to the cerebrovascular accident.

From the patient's perspective, survival, quality of life and functional outcome are the most important outcome measures after critical illness. However, the timing of measurement will influence the results and it may be difficult to unravel the effects of important socio-economic influences that may not be directly related to ICU management.

Introduction

The analytical tools chosen for outcome measurement depend upon the question being asked and how the result will be applied. Outcome from intensive care can be measured from at least three different perspectives: that of the patient and their relatives, that of the staff on the intensive care unit (ICU) and finally the perspective of health managers, economists and politicians. As none of these perspectives is similar, different measurement tools will be required to investigate the areas of interest to each of the three groups.

Patient-Orientated Outcomes

The patients and their relatives will be primarily interested in long-term outcome measures. Relatives will have a keen interest in knowing whether the patient will be capable of independent living and of returning to work, or will suffer permanent disability once they have recovered from their critical illness. Patients will be interested in the duration and quality of survival; however, what defines 'adequate' survival is a personal perception varying with the individual's view of the value of life, their expectations and possibly age. For the purposes of research, a standard definition of an acceptable duration of survival will be required. Calendar periods are used but evidence that one follow-up period is more representative and useful than another is lacking. A frequently used definition of adequate survival is when the patient returns home (not necessarily back to work since there may be good reasons why the patient was not working prior to ICU admission). Leaving hospital alive could be considered a health care success but it ignores the high post-hospital mortality in some patient groups.

Patients will also be interested in outcome measures such as complications and other adverse events occurring during critical illness. Adverse events and complications may reflect the standard of care delivered on the ICU and so will also be of interest to staff. Cross infection rates may reflect professional standards of practice and in Europe, higher rates of nosocomial infection have been linked to higher ICU mortality rates [1]. Adverse events and complications may be pathology dependent (for example, amputation of peripheries because of ischemia or extensive bowel resection leading to prolonged dependence on total parenteral nutrition) or they may be treatment dependent. Treatment dependent complications may be divided into general complications such as weight loss, critical illness neuropathy and joint stiffness, or specific treatment related complications such as tracheal stenosis following tracheostomy. Unfortunately, complications occur commonly on the ICU. Giraud et al. [2] recorded 316 iatrogenic complications in 124 out of 400 admissions (31%) in two centers in France. The commonest complications involved ventilator procedures or therapeutic errors. This distribution of complications was confirmed by the Australian Incident Monitoring Study (AIMS) which analyzed 610 complications involving drugs (28%), procedures (23%), patient environment (21%), airway (20%), and ICU management (9%) [3]. Some complications may be categorized as both treatment and pathology dependent. For example, the post traumatic stress disorder following acute respiratory distress syndrome (ARDS) has a reported incidence of 27.5% [4] which is similar to the incidence of post traumatic stress disorder following road traffic and industrial accidents and terrorism. Post traumatic stress disorder following ARDS may also have a specific and severe effect on health related quality of life of patients when compared to other forms of critical illness [4].

Other areas of interest to the patient are functional outcome and quality of life. Functional outcome encompasses physical impairment, handicap or disability. Functional outcome is not the same as quality of life, although it has been used, incorrectly, as being synonymous with quality of life. Functional outcome concentrates on physical and mental capacity and does not measure well being or sense of satisfaction. Quality of life measures cover a broad range of physical and psychological attributes (domains). For example, the Short Form 36 [6] has eight domains (physical functioning, role-physical, bodily pain, general health, vitality, social functioning, role-emotional, mental health), the Nottingham Health Profile [7] has five (activity level, pain, emotional reactions, sleep, social isolation and physical abilities) while the Sickness Impact Profile [8] has twelve (sleep and rest, eating, work, home management, recreation and pastimes, ambulation, mobility, body care and movement, social interaction, alertness behavior, emotional behavior and communication).

Staff-Orientated Outcomes

The effects of disease and the consequences of new medical interventions resulting in changes in mortality are important. New therapeutic options are frequently introduced on the basis of reduced mortality. For example, the improved survival of patients with human immunodeficiency virus (HIV) following the introduction of highly active anti-retroviral therapy [9] has improved the prognosis of such patients following ICU admission [10]. Prior to the introduction of such therapy, the prognosis of critically ill patients with acquired immunodeficiency syndrome (AIDS) was so poor as to be considered almost futile.

Long-term mortality is also of interest to intensivists because, in the face of increasing ICU demand and the relative paucity of resources, ICU physicians have to carefully triage patients in order to direct resources towards patients with the best chance of long-term survival. Sprung et al. [11] have shown that the decision whether or not to admit a patient depends upon the number of ICU beds available, the admission diagnosis, the severity of disease, age and surgical status. Three of these factors (diagnosis, severity of illness and age) all influence long-term survival. Other studies have shown that while some patients may survive having been declined ICU admission, the majority suffer a higher mortality [12]. It is therefore important that physicians recognize the consequences of declining admission and be certain that the information upon which they base their decision is as robust as possible. As a large quantity of resources are expended on patients who do not survive intensive care [13], attempts to identify potentially ineffective care are being made. For example, Esserman et al. [14] have developed a model where, if the product of the APACHE III risk estimates on day 1 and day 5 is greater than 0.35, then the specificity for a prediction of death is 98%. This, and similar prognostic tools, may help physicians in their difficult task of directing ICU resources to those patients who are likely to benefit the most.

Society-Orientated Outcomes

Health managers, economists and politicians are not necessarily interested in an individual's prognosis or clinical problems. Their task involves distributive justice to maximize the good for the whole of society. They are required to make rational decisions about health care resourcing based on accurate and reliable data. They must resolve conflicts concerning areas of health care, not only within hospital but also in trying to establish the appropriate balance between primary and secondary health care. Their decision making should be based upon rigorous economic evaluation using techniques of cost-minimization, cost-effectiveness, cost-benefit and cost-utility analyses. The data required for such outcome measures will probably be of little interest to the critically ill individual presenting to the ICU. However, for the professionals involved in intensive care, one of the pressing tasks must be to produce accurate and reliable information to allow rational decision making.

Long-Term Survival

Difficulties with Survival Analysis

Theoretically, measurement of mortality should be easy, but the reliability of information concerning survival depends upon a national system that collects this data centrally. For example, the Scandinavian countries have developed an effective system for identifying deaths based upon the individual's unique social security number. In the United Kingdom, the Office for Population Census and Survey uses the patient's National Health Service (NHS) number which is not the same as their hospital number or any other nationally used identifier. If the NHS number is not available, then identifying the patients depends upon their address and date of birth. With a mobile population, patients can easily be lost. Contact with their primary care physician may be fruitless if no follow-up details are provided by the patient on moving. Therefore, unless the national system for recording deaths can easily interact with the hospital system, following patients is more difficult because of data collection inadequacies.

When performing survival analysis, either special statistical methods must be used to compensate for censored observations or all the patients must be followed for a specified minimum period of time. Statistical tests include actuarial (or life table) analysis and hazard function calculation. However, one of the most frequently used analysis tools is the Kaplan-Meier product limit method and the graphical representation of such analysis is the step-wise decreasing Kaplan-Meier curves. Ninety-five percent confidence intervals for the survival curves can be calculated for both the actuarial and Kaplan-Meier analyses. If there are no censored observations, then two survival curves may be compared with the Wilcoxon Rank Sum test, but if censored observations are included then the Gehan (otherwise known as the Breslow) test or the log rank test should be employed. Modeling survival needs advanced techniques such as Cox's proportional hazard modeling. Details of such advanced statistics for survival analysis are available [15].

As mentioned above, survival has been reported at differing times following the onset of critical illness or admission to ICU. There is no standardized time at which survival figures are consistently reported. This makes interpretation and comparison of the survival figures difficult. Furthermore, reporting survival at different times allows other influences to confound the results. Survival is most frequently reported at ICU or hospital discharge, and then at various calendar periods up to many years following admission. Each of these reported survival periods has its shortcomings.

ICU mortality is frequently quoted and, while it provides a global impression of ICU performance, it can be affected by various factors. Some of these factors are well recognized and include case-mix, severity of illness, co-morbidity, and age of patients. However, there may be more subtle effects that influence ICU mortality figures; for example, a discharge policy whereby no terminal care is given on the ICU with hopelessly ill patients being discharged to the general ward. Such practice will reduce the ICU mortality rate. Similarly, if the ICU workload has a large elective surgical component, these low risk patients should depress the overall mortality figure.

Hospital mortality is frequently quoted as an outcome measure following critical illness. However, hospital mortality is influenced by care outside the ICU physician's control and really reflects the institution's performance. Unfortunately, the in-hospital mortality rate following intensive care is surprisingly high. Goldhill [16] reported a 27% 'post-ICU but in-hospital' mortality rate in 12,762 patients. Most deaths occurred in elderly patients who had spent a short time on the ICU. In Norwich, the post-ICU discharge mortality rate of medical patients is 21% with a median survival of only 40 days after ICU admission [17]. This is alarming when many of the patients are returned to a general ward with the expectation that they will survive.

Wallis et al. [18] reviewed the causes of hospital death following ICU discharge in 1700 patients in a district hospital over a five-year period (Table 1). The main causes of death on the general wards following ICU discharge were pneumonia, hypoxic or structural brain damage, cerebrovascular accident, malignancy, myocardial infarction, renal or multiple organ failure, and sepsis. The management of four of these conditions, namely pneumonia, renal or multiple organ failure, and sepsis, are certainly within the realms of the critical care services and it is disappointing to see these conditions being responsible for patients' deaths.

Long-term survival is dependent upon a combination of the degradation of physiological reserve by critical illness and the natural progression of the underlying pathology that precipitated critical illness. With appropriate follow-up, it is possible to draw a survival curve for a group of critically ill patients. However, interpretation of the patients' survival requires comparison with an appropriate control group. Two new problems then need careful consideration. First, which individuals should make up the control group? The ICU patient population is not a representative sample of the general population because ICU patients tend to be chronically ill with pre-existing physiological derangement due to co-morbidity. Comparing their survival with that of an age and sex matched normal population may not be appropriate. Even so this comparison has been most frequently

Table 1. Causes of death on the ward following ICU discharge [18]

Cause of death	Number	%
Pneumonia (no other major precipitating factor apart from recent critical illness)	43	28.1
Hypoxic brain damage	21	13.7
Structural brain damage (trauma, surgery or cerebrovascular accident prior to ICU admission)	13	8.5
Cerebrovascular accident (occurring during or after critical illness but not the primary event)	12	7.8
Malignancy (direct cause of death)	11	7.2
Myocardial infarction	10	6.5
Renal failure	9	5.9
Multiple organ failure	8	5.2
Sepsis	8	5.2
Thrombo-embolism	5	3.3
Pulmonary aspiration	4	2.6
Hepatic failure	1	0.7
Miscellaneous	4	2.6

reported because of the relative ease of obtaining death rate data in the national population. Comparing ICU survivors with hospital patients would be a more representative comparison but there may still be real differences due to case–mix. For example, patients with advanced cancer are frequently admitted to hospital but not necessarily to the ICU. Ideally ICU survivors should be compared with a group of hospital patients with the same disease who did not develop critical illness and so did not require ICU admission (Fig. 2). Unfortunately it is difficult to identify this group of patients and even then such a comparison would determine the effect of critical illness on survival rather than the influence of ICU management.

Second, the question of how long to follow-up the patients arises. The ICU survivors should be followed until the gradient of their survival curve parallels that of the control group. However, the length of time taken for the gradients of the survival curves to become parallel depends upon the control groups chosen (Fig. 2). It will take the longest time with an age and sex matched normal population and probably the shortest time with hospital patients with the same condition. When the curves of the critically ill patients match those of a comparable population, then the effects of critical illness in combination with the underlying pathological process will have run their course. However, not all the long-term mortality observed in critically ill patients is due to the effects of the disease that precipitated their ICU admission. For example, the survival of patients following esophagogastrectomy is dependent upon their tumor histology, while their ICU admission is required for cardiorespiratory observation and monitoring after long and difficult surgery.

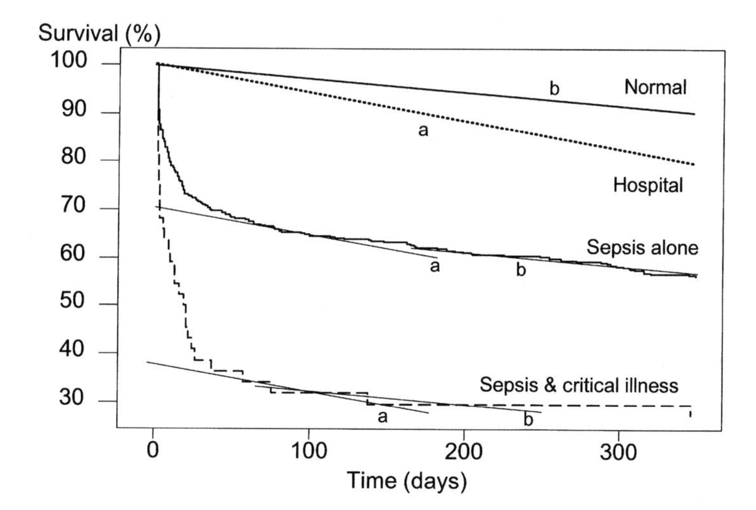

Fig. 2. The theoretical survival curves for four patient groups (normal individuals, hospital patients, patients suffering from sepsis but not ill enough to warrant ICU admission, and critically ill septic patients). Lines marked 'a' or 'b' are parallel with each other, thus represent when the survival curves of patients with sepsis parallel the other two possible control groups

Long-Term Survival

Unfortunately most of the studies that have followed critically ill patients have matched their survival to that of a normal population. There is conflicting data concerning the length of time taken for survival curves to parallel the normal population. Niskanen et al. [19] followed 12,180 Finnish patients for five years. The 5-year survival rate was 66.7% and overall the survival rate paralleled that of the general population at two years. However, the time at which this happened varied with diagnostic category. For example, the survival of trauma victims and patients with a cardiovascular diagnosis equaled that of the general population after three months (Fig. 3). If they survived the initial episode, patients admitted following cardiac arrest had a similar mortality rate to the general population after one year. In contrast, there were more deaths than expected throughout the follow up period among patients with respiratory failure and attempted suicide.

Dragsted et al. [20] followed 1,308 patients in Denmark and reported an overall 5-year survival rate of 58%, although once again certain subgroups had much poorer survival (e.g., cancer, medical and older patients). In Sweden, Zaren and Bergstrom [21] looked at 980 adult patients admitted to the ICU, and at the end of one year 73.6% survived compared to 96% for the normal population. The authors concluded that follow up was only required for one year.

In Scotland, it took four years for the survival of 1,168 critically ill patients to match that of a normal population by which time 55% of patients survived [22]. Results from East Anglia confirm that the survival of critically ill patients does not match a normal population for at least two and a half years (Fig. 4) [17].

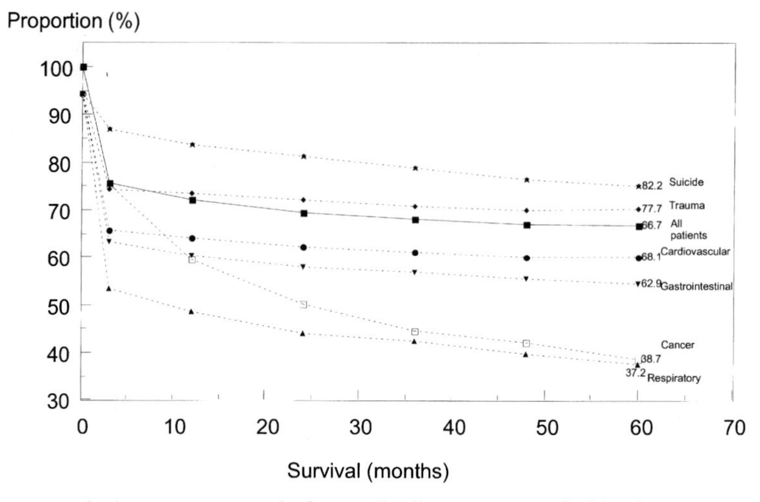

Fig. 3. The long-term survival of critically ill patients stratified by diagnosis (modified from Niskanen et al. [19]).

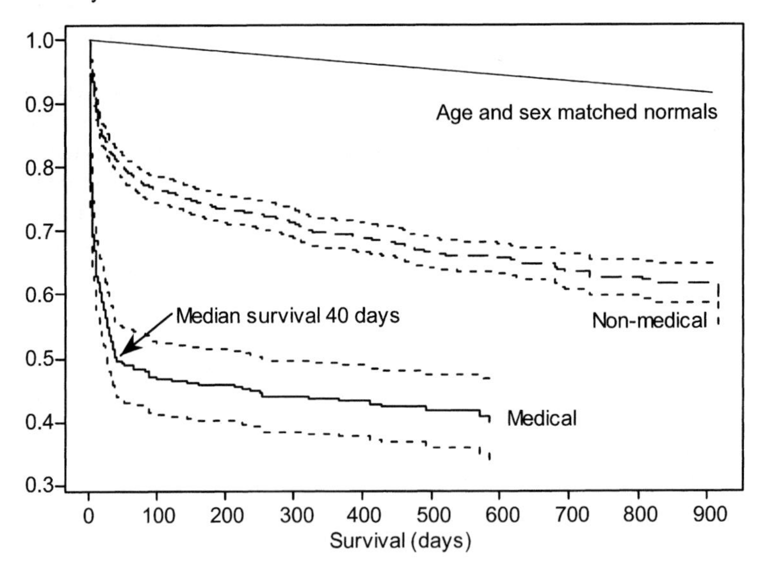

Fig. 4. The survival of critically ill patients divided into those referred from medical and non-medical specialties (95% confidence intervals shown). Note the median survival of medical patients is only 40 days. Neither survival curve matches that of an age and sex matched normal population

In summary, these studies indicate that in most patient groups it is possible to determine when the survival curve of ICU patients matches that of the general population (accepting that this may not in fact be a valid comparison). Overall, depending upon the population studied, the follow-up time required for satisfactory results may be anywhere between one and four years for entire cohorts of critically ill patients but may be more variable if certain subgroups are examined.

Non-Mortality Outcome Measures

Non-mortality outcome measures are vitally important to the surviving patients as they encompass all the aspects of life that concern the patient. While the patient is critically ill on the ICU, the most frequently asked question is whether or not the patient is going to survive. However, having left the ICU, the patients and their relatives become more interested in how the patient is going to survive. The long-term consequences of critical illness now become prominent and these are reflected in the non-mortality outcome measures.

Problems with Non-Mortality Outcome Measures

Critical care is a relatively modern specialty and so the consequences, both physical and mental, of life threatening critical illness are also new. Attempts to measure these are hampered by a number of difficulties. First, such assessment needs the selection of special tools or measurement devices. Generally such measurement tools have been designed for use in other areas of medicine or different populations of patients. The performance of such tools may not be as good in a new population, such as critical illness survivors, when compared with the patient group for whom the tool was designed. Second, the results obtained will depend upon case-mix, patient selection and the confounding influences of socio-economic changes that affect the whole population. For example, Figure 5 represents the theoretical recovery of pre-morbid quality of life in the survivors of critical illness.

The line representing recovery following cardiac surgery exceeds pre-morbid levels because surgery had a therapeutic effect and the patient's quality of life is improved. The other two lines represent two patients recovering following emergency aortic aneurysm repair. One patient made a good recovery in terms of quality of life but the other, as in the clinical example above, suffered a stroke two months after ICU discharge. This resulted in a dense hemiparesis, and despite some recovery, significantly impaired long-term quality of life. Quality of life after the stroke will be poor but unless precise details about the timing of the stroke are elicited, this poor recovery of quality of life will be ascribed to the aneurysm repair and associated critical illness. Third, the rate of recovery of the individual components such as quality of life and functional outcome following critical illness is unknown. It is unlikely that the rates of physical recovery and quality of life are identical and follow the same time course. There will be a balance between allowing as full a recovery of quality of life as possible and avoiding other socio-economic influences which impinge upon quality of life but may only be indi-

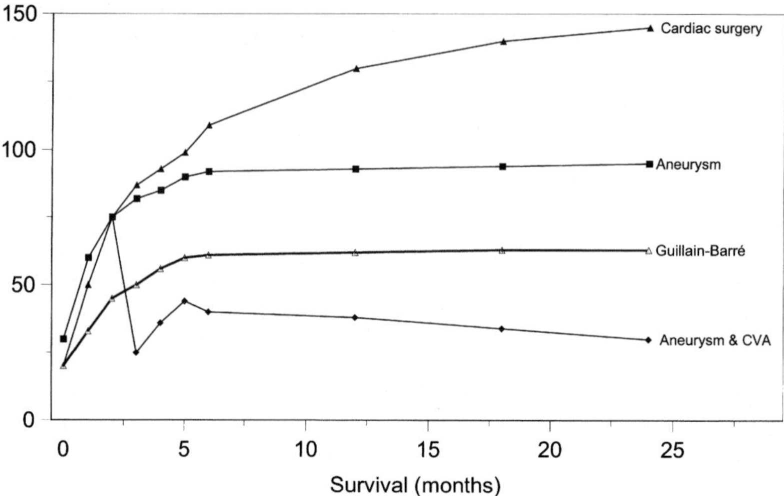

Fig. 5. Theoretical recovery of premorbid quality of life after cardiac surgery and emergency aneurysm repair. CVA: cerebrovascular accident

rectly associated with critical illness. Major life events such as marriage, divorce, unemployment may make the interpretation of changes in quality of life in relation to intensive care much more difficult (and hence dangerous). Not enough is known about the recovery of quality of life to make recommendations concerning appropriate measurement points. Many of the non-mortality outcome measures have been designed for or applied to patients with chronic diseases such as hypertension and arthritis. Theoretically, clinical changes in such conditions should be gradual rather than the faster recovery usually expected after critical illness. The responsiveness of tools designed for more chronic and stable conditions may not be adequate for critical care. Finally, any changes need to be compared to a suitable baseline as there is little evidence to suggest that ICU patients have the same distribution of pre-morbid physical and psycho-social attributes as the general population. Medical and nursing staff should not offer their own assessment of a patient's quality of life as these have been shown to be erroneous [23]. Only very close relatives or partners who care for the patients are really qualified to act as proxy respondents, and even then surrogate answers are more reliable in the physical rather than the psycho-social domains [24–26].

Non-Mortality Outcome Measures

A number of non-mortality outcome measures have been used following intensive care and these may be broadly categorized into six classes:

1) *Physical impairment and disability.* Physical impairment and disability will be common after severe trauma but its measurement may not be appropriate for

other causes of critical illness. Because ventilation is a key therapeutic modality on the ICU, measures of physical impairment have concentrated on the respiratory system and have included spirometry, diffusing capacity and bronchoscopy. Alas, these outcome measures have rather limited application in outcome analysis except for those patients admitted with acute lung injury and other causes of severe respiratory impairment.

2) *Functional status.* Functional status measures may be broadly classified as disease specific or general measures. The New York Heart Association classification [27] has been used in critically ill patients but this tool was originally designed for patients suffering from congestive cardiac failure. The classification grades physical activities. Generic measures of functional status include the activities of daily living (bathing, dressing, toileting, moving, continence, and feeding) [28] and these have been modified into the instrumental activities of daily living (using the telephone, shopping, using transport, cooking, housekeeping, taking medicine, and handling finances) [29]. Unfortunately most outcome measures examining functional status were developed for use in other fields. For example, Katz's activities of daily living were originally developed from results obtained from elderly patients with fractured neck of femur. The application of the activities of daily living as a primary outcome measure to critical care survivors may therefore be flawed.
3) *Mental function.* As with functional status, mental function outcome measures may be divided into generic measures including the Profile of Mood State (POMS) [30]. This scale was developed to assess mood in psychiatric outpatients. The scale assesses mood by ranking 65 adjectives on a five-point scale. The Hospital Anxiety and Depression Scale (HADS) was developed in non-psychiatric patients to measure mood disorders and depression [31]; it contains 14 items asking about depression and anxiety. Disease specific mental function tests include the Impact of Events Scale [32] and this assesses psychological distress following trauma. Mental function assessment has not been closely nor frequently measured after critical illness.
4) *Neuro-psychological function.* This measures cognitive function and examples include Trailmaking Tests A and B [33], Wisconsin Card Sorting Test [34], and Benton's test for visual retention [35]. The tests are generally complex and used as part of a battery of investigations assessing neuro-psychological function; because the tests are complex, they usually require face to face interviews. They measure attention, perception, cognitive flexibility, information processing, and visual memory. These tests have been used for patients with head injury, but are probably rather limited for the general ICU patient because of their complex application.
5) *Measures of recovery.* The extent of recovery may be measured in a multi-item scale such as the Glasgow Outcome Scale which has four grades of recovery (good, moderate disability, severe disability, and vegetative state) [36]. The scale was originally intended to assess recovery six months after head injury. Simple single items scales such as returning to work or independent living have been used but their simplicity limits their usefulness as there are many grades of employment and varying levels of support available to maintain independence.

6) *Quality of life.* Measures of quality of life have been widely used outside critical care. Such measures may be disease specific or general. In the critical care setting, quality of life has been most frequently measured using tools such as the Sickness Impact Profile [7], Nottingham Health Profile [6] and the Short Form 36 [5]. Gill and Feinstein [37] randomly selected 75 articles reporting quality of life and found that 136 out of 159 of the instruments used had been used only once. When assessing critical care, investigators frequently fail to report the psychometric properties (validity and reliability) of the instrument they use and rarely report the steps they have taken to ensure adequacy of the sample size. Investigators should be encouraged to select the tools that are specifically designed for the area of outcome in which they are interested (physical impairment, functional status, mental or neuro-psychological function, recovery or quality of life).

Non-Mortality Outcomes

Although the outcome measures listed above have been used in critical care survivors, apart from quality of life and functional status measures, such non-mortality outcomes may not actually measure what troubles the patients. While follow-up clinics have only recently been established and are few in number, their results do provide an insight into the problems experienced by patients. During critical illness it is possible to lose 2% of the body's muscle mass per day. Not only does this lead to severe weakness and fatigue but also poor muscle co-ordination and difficulty swallowing and coughing. Anxiety and depression are common and this may strain relationships with partners and limit social interaction. More severe psychological upset may present as nightmares and delusions. These may be consequences of the initial trauma or the results of the psychological disturbances that developed in the ICU. The patient's lack of memory, compounded by a lack of understanding or explanation may aggravate these disturbances. Such non–mortality consequences of critical illness will certainly impinge on quality of life. Therefore it may be more fruitful initially to look at specific outcomes perceived as problems by the patient rather than attempt to interpret the results of global non-mortality outcome measures.

Conclusion

Unfortunately there are still many problems and inadequacies with our understanding and appreciation of outcomes following critical care. Until follow-up of patients is standardized in terms of duration, it will be difficult to fully explore the influences that affect survival. Many non-mortality outcome measures have been used but their application to critical care survivors may not have been appropriate. Follow-up clinics have identified the types of long-term problems experienced by patients and it may be more appropriate to rigorously quantify these problems prior to investigating global changes in quality of life or functional status.

References

1. Vincent JL, Bihari DJ, Suter PM, et al (1995) The prevalence of nosocomial infection in intensive care units in Europe. Results of the European Prevalence of Infection in Intensive Care (EPIC) Study. EPIC International Advisory Committee. JAMA 274: 639–644
2. Giraud T, Dhainaut JF, Vaxelaire JF, et al (1993) Iatrogenic complications in adult intensive care units: a prospective two-center study. Crit Care Med 21: 40–51
3. Beckmann U, Baldwin I, Hart GK, Runciman WB (1996) The Australian Incident Monitoring Study in Intensive Care: AIMS-ICU. An analysis of the first year of reporting. Anaesth Intensive Care 24: 320–329
4. Schelling G, Stoll C, Haller M, et al (1998) Health-related quality of life and posttraumatic stress disorder in survivors of the acute respiratory distress syndrome. Crit Care Med 26: 651–659
5. Davidson TA, Caldwell ES, Curtis JR, Hudson LD, Steinberg KP (1999) Reduced quality of life in survivors of acute respiratory distress syndrome with critically ill control patients. JAMA 281: 354–360
6. Ware MK, Snow KK, Kosinski M, Gandek B (1993) SF-36 Health survey: manual and interpretation guide. The Health Institute, New England Medical Center, Boston
7. Hunt SM, McEwen J, McKenna SP (1985) Measuring health status: a new tool for clinicians and epidemiologists. J R Coll Gen Pract 35: 185–188
8. Bergner M, Bobbitt RA, Carter WB, Gilson BS (1981) The Sickness Impact Profile: development and final revision of a health status measure. Med Care 19: 787–805.
9. Li TS, Tubiana R, Katlama C et al (1998) Long lasting recovery in CD4 T cell function and viral load reduction after highly active antiretroviral therapy in advanced HIV-1 disease. Lancet 351: 1682–1686
10. Forrest DM, Russell JA, Montaner JSG (1999) Focus on *Pneumocystis carinii* pneumonia in the intensive care unit. Curr Opin Crit Care 5: 368–375
11. Sprung CL, Geber D, Eidelman LA et al. (1999) Evaluation of triage decisions for intensive care admission. Crit Care Med 27: 1073–1079
12. Metcalfe MA, Sloggett A, McPherson K (1997) Mortality among appropriately referred patients refused admission to intensive-care units. Lancet 350: 7–11
13. Atkinson S, Bihari D, Smithies M, Daly K, Mason R, McColl I (1994) Identification of futility in intensive care. Lancet 344:1203–1206
14. Esserman L, Belkora J, Lenert L (1995) Potentially ineffective care. A new outcome to assess the limits of Critical Care. JAMA 274: 1544–1551
15. Cox DR, Oakes D (1994) Analysis of survival data. Chapman and Hall, London
16. Goldhill DR, Sumner A (1998) Outcome of intensive care patients in a group of British intensive care units. Crit Care Med 26: 1337–1345
17. Lam S, Ridley SA (1999) Critically ill medical patients, their demographics and outcome. Anaesthesia 54: 845–852
18. Wallis CB, Davies HTO, Shearer AJ (1997) Why do patients die on general wards after discharge from intensive care units? Anaesthesia 52: 9–14.
19. Niskanen M, Kari A, Halonen P (1996) Five-year survival after intensive care – comparison of 12,180 patients with the general population. Finnish ICU Study Group. Crit Care Med 24: 1962–1967
20. Dragsted L, Qvist J, Madsen M (1990) Outcome from intensive care IV. A five year study of 1308 patients: long term outcome. Eur J Anaesthesiol 7: 51–61
21. Zaren B, Bergstrom R (1988) Survival of intensive care patients I: prognostic factors from the patients' medical history. Acta Anaesthesiol Scand 32: 93–100
22. Ridley SA, Plenderleith L (1994) Survival after intensive care. Comparison with a matched normal population as an indicator of effectiveness. Anaesthesia 49: 933–935
23. Uhlmann RF, Pearlman RA, Cain KC (1988) Physicians' and spouses' predictions of elderly patients' resuscitation preferences. J Gerontol 43: M115–121
24. McCusker J, Stoddard AM (1984) Use of a surrogate for the Sickness Impact Profile. Med Care 22: 789–795

25. Rothman ML, Hedrick SC, Bulcroft KA, Hickman DH, Rubenstein LZ (1991) The validity of proxy-generated scores as measures of patient health status. Med Care 26: 115–124
26. Rogers J, Ridley S, Chrispin P, Scotton H, Lloyd D (1997) Reliability of the next of kin's estimate of critically ill patients' quality of life. Anaesthesia 52: 1137–1143
27. Criteria Committee of the New York Heart Association (1964). Nomenclature and criteria for diagnosis of disease of the heart and blood vessels. Little Brown & Co, Boston
28. Katz S, Ford AB, Moskowitz RW, Jackson BA, Jaffe MW (1963) Studies of illness in the aged. The index of ADL: A standardized measure of biological and psychosocial function. JAMA 185: 914–919
29. Inouye SK, Peduzzi PN, Robison JT, Hughes JS, Horwitz RI, Concato J (1998) Importance of functional measures in predicting mortality among older hospitalized patients. JAMA 279: 1187–1193
30. McNair DM, Lorr M, Droppleman LF (1992) EdITS Manual for the Profile of Mood States. Educational and Industrial Testing Service, San Diego
31. Zigmond AS, Snaith RP (1983) The Hospital Anxiety and Depression Scale. Acta Psychiat Scand 67: 361–370
32. Horowitz M, Wilner N, Alvarez W (1979) Impact of Events Scale: A measure of subjective distress. Psychosom Med 41: 209–218
33. Reitan RM (1958) Trail-making manual for administration, scoring and interpretation. Indiana University Medical Center, Indianapolis
34. Heaton RK (1981) Wisconsin Card Sorting Test manual. Psychological Assessment Resources, Odessa
35. Benton AL (1984) Revised Visual Retention Test: Clinical and Experimental Application. Psychological Corporation, New York
36. Jennett B, Snoek J, Bond MR, Brooks N (1981) Disability after severe head injury: observations on the use of the Glasgow Outcome Scale. J Neurol Neurosurg Psychiatry 44: 285–293
37. Gill TM, Feinstein AR (1994) A critical appraisal of the quality of quality-of-life measurements. JAMA 272: 619–626

Techniques for Acquiring Information

Comparing ICU Populations: Background and Current Methods

J.E. Zimmerman, E.A. Draper, and D.P. Wagner

Key Messages

- Intensive care unit (ICU) scoring systems provide case mix adjusted benchmarks which can be used to compare mortality rates among hospitals
- Differences between observed and predicted hospital mortality are often due to factors other than the quality of ICU therapy
- Patient characteristics that have a significant influence on hospital mortality are not fully accounted for in current ICU scoring systems
- The prognostic impact of identical patient risk factors varies within the healthcare systems of different regions and countries
- Future ICU prognostic systems will be more complex and more accurate; they will require automated data collection and periodic adjustment for changes in therapy over time

Several years ago an international course was developed to assist in the planning and optimal use of intensive care. The course was organized in response to rising costs and increasing demands for ICU services in the host country, and was attended by ICU physicians and government officials representing national and regional health funding agencies. The participants described and compared patient demographics, clinical characteristics, and ICU resource use for 7,609 to 16,662 ICU admissions; and then compared observed and predicted mortality rates for the three countries. ICU admissions from the host country were significantly more often nonoperative, had more comorbid conditions, particularly metastatic cancer, and a higher severity of illness. The host country's ICUs provided less technologic monitoring and similar amounts of therapy on the first ICU day, but ICU stay was twice as long as in the two other countries. Observed hospital mortality was similar to predicted in two countries but significantly higher (21.2%) than predicted (19.6%) in the host country.

Many ICU physicians from the host country questioned the possibility of comparing patients and practices from three different countries; and the accuracy of the equation used to predict mortality. They emphasized that differences in ICU length of stay and in observed vs. predicted mortality might be accounted for by differences in duration of prior therapy, interhospital transfer practices, diagnoses, comorbidities, ICU discharge practices, and the infrequent use of do not resuscitate (DNR) orders. Many expressed concern that the government officials in attendance would not recognize these limitations.

Introduction

To evaluate critical care services, outcome data must be collected and then compared to a performance benchmark or standard. The outcomes that are examined include mortality, complication rates, hospital and ICU length of stay, staffing level, or the use of treatment resources. A simple comparison of these outcomes, however, is frequently unsatisfactory because the characteristics of patients treated in different ICUs are not the same. In addition, the ICUs that are compared will often differ because of variations in hospital referral patterns, teaching status, and location. To meaningfully evaluate ICU performance, therefore, data comparisons must be adjusted for variations in both patient and hospital characteristics.

When comparing ICU outcomes, three approaches have been used to adjust for patient and institutional characteristics. First, the outcomes of a single ICU can be examined over time. If there is no significant change in patient characteristics, differences in performance can be meaningfully compared. Examples of change over time comparisons include assessments of mortality and resource use before and after changes in ICU organizational structure [1, 2]. Second, an ICU's outcome data can be compared with that of units with similar characteristics. Useful comparisons are possible when the hospitals, ICUs, and patients are similar. For example, comparing length of stay and the process of care after cardiac surgery has been possible because the hospitals, ICUs, and operative procedures are reasonably similar [3,4]. Third, an ICU scoring system can be used to compare observed outcomes to a case-mix adjusted standard. ICU scoring systems use statistical techniques to predict outcomes that are prospectively adjusted to reflect differences in hospital and patient characteristics such as diagnosis, severity of illness, and other known outcome determinants. The patient data on which these case–mix adjusted outcome predictions are based provide a standard or benchmark which is then compared to the observed measure of ICU performance. In addition to comparing ICU outcomes to an average standard, benchmarking can also identify ICUs with the best outcomes and provide insights about the clinical practices associated with their superior performance.

Background

The 1970s: You Can't Predict Mortality

Variations in severity of illness are a major reason why comparison of outcome data across ICUs requires adjustment for patient differences. In the early 1970s, methods for adjusting clinical outcomes for patient differences were limited to a few specific disorders. For trauma patients severity was defined by the type and extent of injury using the Injury Severity Scoring System [5]; for burn injuries by the extent of third degree burn area using the Burn Index [6]; and for head injury patients by the impact of the injury on neurological function using the Glasgow Coma Score (GCS) [7]. Each of these severity measurements correlated with hospital mortality rates, but each was limited in explanatory power and patient applicability.

In the late 1970s the use of physiological measures was a new approach to defining severity. Using physiological measurements was helpful because abnormalities are common to many acute diseases and the extent of derangement represented an objective and reproducible way to measure severity. Two major approaches were used to choose the physiological measures and decide on the importance or weight for each one. The first approach was to collect physiological information during treatment. The physiological patterns of survivors and non-survivors were contrasted and the measures weighted based on how often specific physiological values were associated with survival versus death. These methods were used by Siegal et al. [8] in septic shock, by Shoemaker et al. [9] for postoperative patients, and by Teres et al. [10] in developing the Mortality Prediction Model (MPM I). The second approach was to select and weight the physiological measures before treatment. Selection and weighting was based on prior studies and expert opinion. This was the method used in developing the Acute Physiology, and Chronic Health Evaluation (APACHE I) system [11].

In addition to measuring severity of illness, APACHE I was also used to predict group mortality [12]. To do this a multivariate regression equation was developed using information on age, gender, chronic health status, a 34 item acute physiology score, and the organ system dysfunction responsible for ICU admission. Regression coefficients were obtained using data for 613 ICU patients at the George Washington University Hospital and used to predict the number of deaths among 795 ICU patients at five university hospitals [12]. There was close agreement between observed and predicted death rates at the five hospitals. These results were later confirmed by similar analyses for 1,260 emergency ICU admissions at five United States and seven French tertiary care hospitals [13], and at 14 hospitals in the United States, France, Spain and Finland [14].

The 1980s: We Must Simplify

Knowledge gained in the 1970s produced reliable methods for severity measurement and risk stratification. These scoring systems, however, required multi-institutional validation; and APACHE I was too complex for use in clinical trials or for evaluating performance in individual ICUs. APACHE II was introduced in 1985 and incorporated major changes to the original APACHE system [15]. The number of physiological variables was reduced from 34 to 12 and higher scores were assigned to renal and neurological variables; scoring for emergency operative status was added, and chronic health evaluation was changed to reflect the impact of aging, and chronic cardiac, pulmonary, renal, or liver disease. The APACHE II score ranged from 0 to 71 with an increasing score reflecting an increased severity of disease and a higher risk of hospital death. In addition, an equation to predict risk of death was developed and coefficients published to reflect the prognostic impact of the APACHE II score, emergency surgery, and 49 disease categories.

The Simplified Acute Physiology Score (SAPS) was introduced in 1984 and measured severity using weights for physiologic variables similar to those used in

APACHE II. SAPS, however, emphasized simplifying severity scoring rather than predicting hospital mortality [16]. The 14 variable MPM 24 hour model and an 11 variable MPM 48 hour model also emphasized simplicity, but focused on predicting risk of death rather than severity scoring [17]. MPM also used a different analytic approach. Instead of using an expert panel to select and weight predictor variables, MPM used objective statistical reduction techniques to identify a smaller subset of the strongest outcome predictors.

During the later part of the 1980s and early 1990s APACHE II, MPM, and SAPS were used to describe ICU populations, to predict mortality for ICU patient groups, and to compare severity in clinical trials. There were growing concerns, however, about errors in prediction caused by differences in patient selection [18,19] and lead time bias [20]. There were also concerns about the size and representativeness of the databases used to develop the three systems, and about poor calibration within patient subgroups [21, 22] and across geographical locations [23].

Table 1. Variables used by the APACHE III, MPM II admission, MPM II 24, 48, 72 hour, and SAPS II systems for predicting hospital mortality

Prior Health Status	
APACHE III	7 comorbidities plus age
MPM II admission	3 comorbidities plus age
MPM II 24, 48, 72 hr.	2 comorbidities plus age
SAPS II	3 comorbidities plus age
Physiological Measures	
APACHE III	6 vital signs, 11 laboratory tests
MPM II admission	3 vital signs
MPM II 24, 48, 72 hr.	2 vital signs, 3 laboratory tests
SAPS II	5 vital signs, 7 laboratory tests
Timing and Selection for ICU	
APACHE III	7 locations; length of stay before ICU
MPM II admission	CPR, ventilator at or before ICU
MPM 24, 48, 72 hr.	not used
SAPS II	not used
ICU Admission Diagnosis	
APACHE III	78 diagnoses or disease categories
MPM II admission	5 acute diagnoses
MPM II 24, 48, 72 hr.	2 acute diagnoses
SAPS II	not used
Other Information	
APACHE III	4 hospital characteristics medical, elective, or emergency surgery
MPM II admission	medical or unscheduled surgery
MPM II 24, 48, 72 hr.	medical or unscheduled surgery constants for 24, 48, and 72 hours
SAPS II	medical, scheduled, or unscheduled surgery

APACHE III, Acute Physiology and Chronic Health Evaluation; MPM II, Mortality Probability Models; SAPS II, Simplified Acute Physiology Score; CPR, cardiopulmonary resuscitation.

The 1990s: The Limits of ICU Comparisons

Between 1991 and 1993 the three major scoring systems were refined and updated using the knowledge and experience gained during the 1980s. As a result of these refinements each system became more complex. The increase in complexity is shown in Table 1 which displays the type and number of predictor variables used in APACHE III, MPM II, and SAPS II [24–26]. The reference databases on which predictions are based reflect more contemporary (1988–1992) treatment results, include more patients (12,997–19,124), and more ICUs (42–140). Although each system predicts hospital mortality rate, the capabilities of APACHE III were expanded to include outcomes such as ICU and hospital length of stay, TISS score, risk for active therapy, use of pulmonary artery catheters, laboratory studies, and duration of mechanical ventilation. Each system was internally validated using a development and validation set, and within each database the systems demonstrated excellent discrimination (ability to identify patients who live or die), and calibration (correlation between predicted and observed mortality).

During the late 1990s studies using APACHE III [27–32], SAPS II [32, 33–37], and MPM II [36,38] frequently revealed an observed mortality that was different from expected. Each system predicted a mortality rate that was adjusted for differences in the variables included in each system. The predicted mortality provided a benchmark that was based on the effectiveness of therapy at the time and places where the systems were developed. These predictions, however, were not adjusted for unmeasured variables, for the passage of time, or for differences in the process, amount, or timing of treatment. Most of these studies detected differences between observed and predicted mortality which were explained using one or more of the following approaches:

1) Inadequate predictive equations. If the observed and predicted mortality were not uniform across all ranges of risk the system was poorly calibrated and it was concluded that the system is inaccurate.
2) Predicted mortality was treated as a 'gold standard'. When observed mortality exceeded predicted it was concluded that care must be suboptimal.
3) Observed outcome was treated as a 'gold standard'. When multiple prognostic systems were tested, the 'best' system had a predicted mortality that was closest to observed. Unfortunately APACHE II, a benchmark based on 1979 to 1981 treatment standards, was often selected.
4) Factors that might account for differences between observed and predicted mortality were analyzed and, if possible, identified.

Fortunately, most studies used the later approach and as a result have provided information that should lead to improvements in comparing ICU patients and in prognostic accuracy. Based on available information, the ability to accurately predict hospital mortality is based on the following factors: First, data must be available and reliably collected. Second, data collection must be accurate and reproducible. Third, there must be adequate adjustment for variables known to influence mortality, such as patient selection, lead time bias, diagnosis, physiologic reserve, physiologic abnormalities, and environmental factors such as geographic location, hospital characteristics and practices. Fourth, the reference database must be broadly representative and the predictive equation accurate with regard to discrimination, calibration, and ability to account for mortality differences among subgroups. Fifth, the patient sample must be large enough to avoid randomness and have the power to detect clinically significant differences between observed and predicted mortality. Sixth, average treatment results must be similar to those for patients within the reference database. It is unlikely, however, that treatment results will be identical because quality of therapy differs among hospitals, before and after ICU admission, and over time. Nonetheless, when a prognostic system satisfies the first five criteria it can be used to compare effectiveness with the benchmark established by the reference database.

Which Variables Should Be Compared?

Based on the knowledge and experience gained from the studies using APACHE III [27–32], SAPS II [32, 33–37] and MPM II [36, 38], it is possible to identify prognostic variables that may require modification or should be investigated in future studies (Tables 2–4). Some of these variables have been shown to influence hospital mortality, but are not included in each of the current models. Others have not yet been tested in multi-institutional studies, but on the basis of recent studies appear to be strong candidates for future testing. Some variables reflect patient characteristics, others are environmental, but none should directly reflect the type, process, or amount of treatment. This is because comparison of observed and predicted mortality is intended to reflect the outcome from treating a single episode of critical illness.

Patient Characteristics That Influence Outcome

Chronic Health Status

APACHE III, SAPS II, and MPM II each account for the adverse impact of increasing age on hospital mortality. Compared to physiologic abnormalities and other prognostic factors the weighting and relative explanatory power of age is relatively small, a finding that has been demonstrated in multiple studies of survival from critical illness. Each prognostic system also considers comorbid conditions (Table 1). Metastatic cancer is common to each system, and cirrhosis and hematologic malignancy (leukemia/multiple myeloma) are included in both MPM II and APACHE III. During model development, 34 comorbid conditions were tested for inclusion in APACHE III and 12 for inclusion in SAPS II. Conditions such as diabetes, severe impairment of activities of daily living; and chronic cardiovascular pulmonary and renal diseases were tested for their independent impact on hospital mortality, but did not meet statistical requirements for inclusion. Although each of these variables are known to influence hospital mortality, it is likely that their significance was diminished by the impact of physiological variables or diagnostic information that either directly or indirectly reflect these

Table 2. Studies using APACHE III mortality predictions and proposed reasons for differences between observed and predicted hospital mortality.

Study Location	Year	Patients	ICUs	SMR	ROC	H–L X^2 Statistic	Proposed reasons for calibration differences
United States (Cleveland) [27]	1991–1995	116,340	38	0.90	0.90	C^2=2407	Early discharge to skilled nursing facilities, patient selection (more beds, more low severity admissions), unmeasured variables, earlier treatment withdrawal
United States [28]	1993–1996	37,668	285	1.01	0.89	C^2=48.7	Inaccurate disease labeling, faulty assessment of GCS, changes in treatment outcomes over time
United Kingdom [29]	1993–1995	12,793	17	1.25	0.89	C^2 = 333	Differences in case mix, patient selection (fewer beds more high severity admissions), lead time bias (due to delayed ICU admission), earlier ICU discharge, manual vs. automated data collection
United Kingdom [30]	1993–1996	1,144	1	1.35	0.85	H^2=130	Differences in patient selection, comorbidity, admission criteria, disease labeling, less pre–hospital care & trauma experience, lead time bias
Brazil [31]	1990–1991	1,734	10	1.67	0.82	C^2=400	Lack of ICU equipment, beds, nurse preparation, poor ward care, selection bias, lead time bias
Germany [32]	1991–1994	2,661	1	1.13	0.85	C^2=48.4	More medical and emergency surgery patients, GCS not accurate for 43% of patients, selection bias(frequent interhospital transfer) lead time bias, longer hospital stay

SMR=standardized mortality ratio; ROC=reciever operating curve area; GCS=Glasgow coma score; H–L X^2 statistic= Hosmer Lemeshow statistic; critical value for X^2 is 16.9 for p=.05, with 9 degrees of freedom. For a fixed difference between observed and predicted X^2 will increase with sample size.

comorbidities. It should be noted that the comorbidities included in each prognostic system have an impact on immunologic status and their prognostic importance probably reflects the association of infection with ICU and hospital mortality. Based on past findings it seems unlikely that future scoring systems will be substantially improved by adding items reflecting chronic health status.

Physiological Measures

In contrast to age and comorbidities, physiological measures account for the largest proportion of explanatory power of APACHE III and SAPS II for hospital mortality. In aggregate, APACHE III, SAPS II, and MPM II use a total of 21 physiological measurements, but only heart rate, blood pressure, and a modified GCS are common to each system. The MPM II models are less reliant on physiological measures and in aggregate use only three vital signs and three laboratory tests. APACHE III uses 17 physiological measures compared to 12 measures for SAPS II. Variables that are unique to each system include hematocrit, albumin, glucose, and creatinine in APACHE III; and potassium and prothrombin time in SAPS II. It is unlikely, however, that simply adding measures that are unique to another system will improve accuracy. This is because, except for hematocrit and prothrombin time, the remaining unique variables were tested and did not meet statistical criteria for inclusion during model development. Future studies, therefore, should test hematocrit and prothrombin time as potential predictor variables. In addition, measures such as platelet count [39] and pupillary reactions [40] have been shown to have an independent impact on mortality and also deserve future testing.

Improving the weighting and accuracy of measuring the GCS would greatly enhance prognostic accuracy for each system. Recent evidence suggests that the GCS requires additional weighting for head trauma patients [28]. In addition, several studies have demonstrated scoring difficulties in measuring GCS for as many as 43% of patients [28, 31, 32]. The GCS measurement problem appears to be caused by the wide variation across ICUs in the use of deep sedation and paralysis, treatments that can make accurate scoring impossible. Because no severity weighting is applied when GCS cannot be assessed, the effect is to underpredict hospital mortality for patients whose GCS might otherwise reflect a substantial neurological deficit. Such problems are particularly common among trauma, neurological, and respiratory patients [28, 32]. Because there is no better measure of neurological function, data collectors should use the following approach to minimize errors in recording GCS:

1) The GCS should be obtained for as many patients as possible. Frequent inability to record GCS due to sedation is often a sign of poor data reliability.
2) Carefully adhere to definitions provided in the original description of the GCS. Avoid scoring until hypotension or hypoxemia have been stabilized, and use an ocular score of 1 for patients with severe periorbital swelling.
3) If the patient is sedated or paralyzed but an accurate GCS was previously recorded use that score. This approach was specified for SAPS II and should now be used for each system [26].

Table 3. Studies using SAPS II mortality predictions and proposed reasons for differences between observed and predicted hospital mortality.

Study Location	Year	Patients	ICUs	SMR	ROC	H-L X^2 Statistic	Proposed reasons for calibration differences
Italy [33]	1994	1,393	99	1.14	0.80	C^2=71	Insufficient diagnostic data, imprecise variable definitions, lead time bias, international and regional differences in case-mix/therapy
Portugal [34]	1994–1995	982	19	1.02	0.82	C^2=32.7 H^2=49.7	Insufficient diagnostic data, imprecise variable definitions, international and regional differences,
Austria [35]	1997	1,733	9	0.85	0.81	C^2=91.8 H^2=89.1	Unmeasured case mix differences, unreliable GCS assessment
12 European Countries [36]	1994–1995	10,027	89	1.15	0.82	C^2=218.2	Insufficient diagnostic data, unmeasured clinical and nonclinical variables, changes in effectiveness of therapy over time
Tunisia [37]	1994–1995	1,325	3	1.27	0.84	H^2=73.8	Differences in patient selection (fewer ICU beds), resource limitations, international differences, unmeasured case mix differences
Germany [32]	1991–1994	2,661	1	1.16	0.85	C^2=20.5	Unmeasured case mix differences, unreliable GCS assessment, lead time bias, longer hospital length of stay.

SMR=standardized mortality ratio; GCS = Glasgow coma score; ROC = reciever operating curve area; H–L X^2 statistic = Hosmer Lemeshow statistic; critical value for X^2 is 16.9 for $p=.05$, with 9 degrees of freedom. For a fixed difference between observed and predicted X^2 will increase with sample size.

4) If there is a suspicion that neurological status has changed and sedation or paralysis can be safely reduced, repeat GCS assessment after therapy is reduced.
5) If direct measurement is impossible, record a GCS of 15. Although risk will be underestimated, it will cause a systematic error that might be corrected by recalibration.

Diagnosis

Tables 2–4 demonstrate that insufficient diagnostic data or inaccurate disease labeling were frequently proposed as reasons for differences between observed and predicted mortality [28, 30, 33–37]. This reflects a widely held belief that a patient's ICU admission diagnosis provides important prognostic information. For example, a recent study of 37,668 ICU admissions reported an observed hospital mortality rate of 3.3% for asthma compared to 37.5% for noncardiac pulmonary edema, and 18.2% for gastrointestinal bleeding due to varices compared to 8.4% for bleeding due to diverticulitis or angiodysplasia [28]. For each of the above diagnoses, specific disease labeling provided more accurate prognostic information than could be achieved by aggregating patients into medical, respiratory, or gastrointestinal subgroups. The same study also demonstrated improved prognostic accuracy when mortality rates for combined diagnoses such as unstable angina and acute myocardial infarction or bacterial and viral pneumonia were predicted separately, and when residual organ system categories were disaggregated into specific diagnostic categories [28]. Unfortunately, developing coefficients for specific diseases requires a very large reference database. In addition, imprecise diagnostic labeling and difficulty choosing a single diagnosis are also a source of error in predicting mortality risk. These issues will be discussed further in the section on data reliability.

Selection for ICU Care

When a prognostic system is used to predict mortality in a new population it is important that the reference database from which the estimated patient risks are derived contains only patients chosen by similar selection criteria. The APACHE III, SAPS II, and MPM II databases were all created using consecutive ICU admissions to a diverse group of hospitals in the US, Canada, and Europe. Unfortunately, the decision to admit a patient to ICU is not uniform among hospitals, and admission source, particularly the transfer of a patient from another hospital to an ICU, is associated with a higher mortality rate [41, 42].

Several studies have suggested that variations in selection criteria for ICU admission may have caused differences between observed and predicted mortality (Tables 2–4). One study suggested a selection bias due to frequent admission of low severity patients because of the ready availability of beds [27], but

Table 4. Studies using MPM II mortality predictions and proposed reasons for differences between observed and predicted hospital mortality.

Study Location	Year	Patients	ICUs	SMR	ROC	H–L X^2 Statistic	Proposed reasons for calibration differences
Tunisia [38]							
MPM II_0	1994–1995	1,325	3	0.91	0.85	C^2=36.7 H^2=19.9	Unmeasured case mix differences, treatment differences including lack of full-time intensivist lack of nursing education skill and motivation
MPM II_{24}	1994–1995	1,325	3	1.14	0.88	C^2=38.0 H^2=29.6	
12 European Countries [36]							
MPM II_0	1994–1995	10,027	89	0.85	0.78	C^2=437.1 H^2=368.2	Inadequate diagnostic data, failure to adjust for prior location and other unmeasured clinical and nonclinical variables, changes in quality of treatment over time

SMR=standardized mortality ratio; ROC=reciever operating curve area; H–L X^2 statistic= Hosmer Lemeshow statistic; critical value for X^2 is 16.9 for p=.05, with 9 degrees of freedom. For a fixed difference between observed and predicted X^2 will increase with sample size.

others suggested that selection bias was caused by too few beds and consequent delays in ICU admission [29–31, 37]. Selection bias has also been attributed to differences in the frequency of interhospital transfer [31, 36, 37] and in the reasons for transfer [32]. In an independent US database, APACHE III adjusted well for the prognostic implications of the selection differences reflected by patient location before ICU admission [28]. Studies from Europe and developing countries, however, suggest that the selection variable of APACHE III does not adequately adjust for international differences in selection for intensive care.

Lead Time Bias

When data for all ICU admissions are not obtained at approximately the same time in the course of an acute illness or within a similar time period after major surgery, prognostic estimates will be inaccurate because physiological measures reflect different phases of critical illness [18, 19]. Adjustment for differences in patient location before ICU admission (selection) allows for some of these differences, but cannot account for delays in interhospital transfer, or for extensive amounts of intensive care therapy on hospital wards before the patient physically arrives in ICU [20, 43]. Based on this knowledge, adjustments for prior location and for the length of hospital stay before ICU admission were included as prognostic variables in APACHE III [41]. These adjustments work well in the US [28], but international differences in lead time have been proposed as a potential explanation for differences between observed and APACHE III predicted mortality in Europe and Brazil [29–32]. Failure to account for selection and lead time bias were also proposed as reasons for miscalibration in studies using SAPS II and MPM II [33, 36, 38]. Based on this knowledge, prognostic systems should account for location before ICU admission and the length of hospital stay before ICU admission. It seems likely that adjustment for these variables will be required at the national level. At present, however, no method has been proposed to adjust for differences between observed and predicted mortality that might be related to the quality or process of care before ICU admission [30, 44] or after ICU discharge [45]. Accounting for such treatment differences, however, should not be necessary since the outcome of interest is mortality from a single episode of critical illness.

Environmental Factors that Influence Outcome

Hospital Practices

Hospital practices that are not directly related to the quality of ICU and hospital care also influence hospital mortality. One example is the discharge of ICU patients directly to skilled nursing or long term acute care facilities. These ICU patients are typically stable, but at discharge still require mechanical ventilation or dialysis and skilled nursing care. The number of long term acute care facilities in the US has increased substantially during the last 10 years, but their availability and the transfer practices of individual hospitals vary widely. Direct transfer of these patients from ICU to long term acute care facilities can markedly reduce observed hospital mortality [27]. This is because these 'chronically critically ill patients' are at high risk for death after transfer [46]. Frequent transfer of such patients, therefore, can result in substantial overprediction of hospital mortality.

Variations in the frequency of limiting or withdrawing therapy must also be considered when comparing observed and predicted hospital mortality. These practices vary among hospitals [47], and have also increased over time [47, 48]. Interhospital differences in treatment withdrawal practices can have a marked, but variable influence on observed mortality. Among otherwise identical patients, observed mortality will be higher at hospitals where lifesupport withdrawal is frequent compared to hospitals where withdrawal is infrequent. In two recent analyses, differences in the frequency of treatment withdrawal, and in withdrawal among high versus low risk patients were thought to have a marked and varied impact on observed versus predicted mortality [28, 49]. Studies in the US using APACHE III have also shown a small but significant difference in hospital mortality that is associated with hospital size and teaching status [28, 41]. The exact reasons for these differences are uncertain, but should be examined in future studies.

Hospital Length of Stay

An ICU patient's risk of dying in the hospital is influenced by how long that patient remains in the hospital. APACHE III mortality predictions are adjusted for this influence using coefficients derived from a regression analysis of hospital length of stay among survivors [41]. This analysis incorporated all patient specific predictor variables, forecast a predicted hospital length of stay, and then calculated the mean difference between observed and predicted hospital length of stay for each ICU. Compared to hospitals where mean length of stay for survivors was within 1.6 days of predicted stay, shorter stays (1.6 days < predicted) decreased the multivariate odds ratio of death to 0.7; and longer stays (1.6 days > predicted) increased the odds ratio of death to 1.2.

Because this adjustment is unique to US hospitals it has not been possible to adjust for the impact of hospital length of stay on mortality in international studies using APACHE III. The potential importance of this adjustment is emphasized in Figure 1 which displays as much as a four fold difference in mean hospital length of stay after acute myocardial infarction in six countries. That similar variations exist within large ICU databases is suggested by reports of a 11.6 to 12.0 day mean hospital length of stay in the US [27, 28], 17.1 days in Brazil [31], 25.6 days in Germany [32], and 14.8 to 22.8 days in 10 European countries [26]. This information suggests that future studies of mortality among ICU patients should report hospital length of stay, and also investigate the impact of differences in hospital length of stay on mortality.

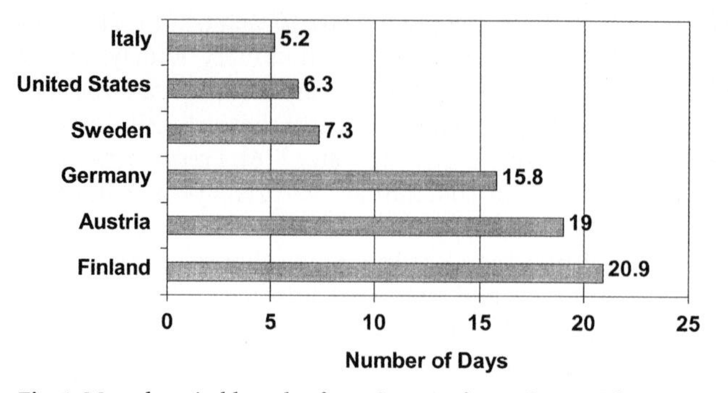

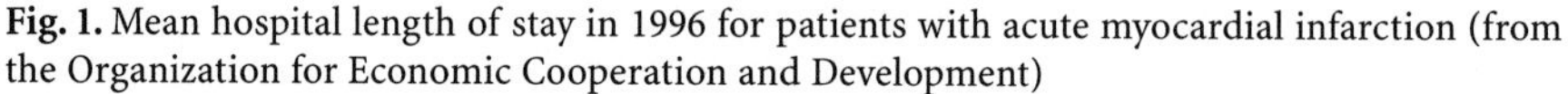

Fig. 1. Mean hospital length of stay in 1996 for patients with acute myocardial infarction (from the Organization for Economic Cooperation and Development)

Geographical Location

Many of the studies shown in Tables 2–4 either explicitly or implicitly suggest that APACHE III, SAPS II, and MPM II do not adequately adjust for national differences in intensive care. In addition, studies in the US [28,41] and Italy [33] have demonstrated differences in hospital mortality across geographic regions despite adjustment for patient differences. It is uncertain whether these mortality differences reflect national and regional variations in critical care practices, socioeconomic differences, variations in disease labeling, patient selection and lead time bias, frequency of treatment withdrawal, or duration of hospital stay. For example, in the US differences between observed and predicted hospital mortality evaporated after adjustment for hospital length of stay for survivors. It seems doubtful that each of the above differences could be accounted for by simply customizing current systems using national databases [36, 50, 51]. Instead, national and regional differences in each prognostic variable should be reported; examined for a significant independent impact on hospital mortality, and if significant added to the predictive model.

Changes Over Time

Reductions in mortality from critical illness are usually related to the introduction of new drugs (e.g., thrombolytic agents), new technologies (e.g., non-invasive positive pressure ventilation [NIPPV]) or new techniques (e.g., low tidal volume ventilation in acute respiratory distress syndrome [ARDS]). We all believe in medical progress, but attributing a lower observed versus predicted mortality to changes in treatment effectiveness over time is overly simplistic. Reductions in mortality due to improvements in treatment effectiveness are usually disease specific, e.g., thrombolytic therapy for acute myocardial infarction. For some diseases, however, it may be difficult to attribute improved mortality to therapy alone. For example, should the improved outcome for parasitic pneumonia [28] be attributed to better ICU therapy for *Pneumocystis carinii* pneumonia, to improved therapy for human immunodeficiency virus (HIV) infection, or to recent changes in the definition of acquired immunodeficiency syndrome (AIDS)? Although medical progress usually improves survival, some changes over time tend to increase observed mortality, e.g., the recent increase in frequency of withdrawal of life support. In the United States we now adjust for the prognostic impact of changes in practices and therapy every one to two years by examining observed and APACHE III predicted mortality for each ICU admission diagnosis and adjusting coefficients as needed.

Data Accuracy and Reliability

If a prognostic scoring system cannot be applied reproducibly in a different population it will not perform accurately, irrespective of how well the system examines the variables that influence outcome [52]. The accuracy of outcome prediction is therefore in part determined by inter (between) observer reliability, i.e., the difference in quantifying data when different individuals score the same patient. A high degree of interobserver reliability was reported by the developers of APACHE III [24], SAPS II [26], and MPM II [25]. Interobserver reliability was excellent for discrete measures such as age and other demographic information; and for physiological measures that require little or no judgement on the part of data collectors. In contrast, interobserver reliability was lower for variables that require choosing the most deranged physiological measurement (e.g., temperature), or calculation (e.g.. PaO_2/FiO_2); and even lower for agreement on GCS parameters. Independent studies that have used APACHE III, SAPS II, and MPM II [27, 34, 36] have also reported good interobserver reliability during data collection, but have confirmed that interobserver reliability deteriorates for measures such as GCS [32, 53], ICU admission diagnosis, and physiological variables that require calculation [53, 54].

We believe that the reliability of data collection can and has been improved [27, 28, 55]. Because current prognostic systems have become more complex it is no longer possible to replicate methods directly from journals [56]. It is our experience that a comprehensive instruction manual is needed to precisely describe methods and definitions. This instruction manual is supplemented by on-site data collector training, an instructional video, training exercises, direct data collection supervision, and ongoing telephone assistance. After data for 100 to 200 patients is collected, formal interobserver reliability testing is performed for a 10% random sample. In addition, emphasis is placed on careful design of data collection forms, the use of software based error checking for manually collected data, and automated data collection. A recent study of prognostic scoring using an automated ICU information system versus manual data collection showed that automation improved the detection of physiological abnormalities [57]. This resulted in increased severity scores, which in turn increased predicted mortality. Automation improves the reliability of collecting laboratory data; and of recording comorbidity and ICU admission diagnosis through the use of computerized pick lists. Computer software also calculates mean arterial pressure and PaO_2/FiO_2 and oxygen delivery values and assists in identifying the most abnormal physiological values.

Conclusion

During the past three decades there has been significant progress in predicting group mortality for ICU patient groups. Although simplification of prognostic scoring is a desirable goal, current information suggests that improvements in prognostic accuracy will require the addition of more prognostic variables. As in the past, independent studies have suggested a substantial number of variables that require further testing. We believe that each prognostic model should adjust for variables that significantly influence outcomes, and that simple re-calibration is insufficient to adjust for the absence of proven outcome predictors. Unfortunately, as the number of predictor variables increase, data reliability and ease of use decreases. We believe that technology, not simplification, is the answer to this challenge. Accurate predictive models, however, can only provide a benchmark not a true 'gold standard'.

The Rest of the Story

The course participants believed that a common data set made it possible to compare patients' resource use and outcomes in the three countries. Because the cultures, ICU policies, and health care systems varied markedly across the different countries, the participants believed that country-specific efforts were essential to provide national standards, which could then be compared internationally. Shortly after the course, leaders of the host country's national and regional governments met with the course's ICU physician organizers and representatives of the national intensive care society. Subsequent to this meeting the government and intensive care society supported collection of a nationally representative ICU data set and the development of a customized mortality predictive equation. In 1999, the host country's ICU society made data collection instruments and automated calculation of predicted mortality available over the Internet. ICUs now compare their observed and predicted mortality rates and use this information to assess individual ICU performance.

References

1. Carson SS, Stocking C, Podsadecki T, et al (1996) Effects of organizational change in the medical intensive care unit of a teaching hospital: a comparison of "open" and "closed" formats. JAMA 276:322–328
2. Manthous CA, Amoateng YA, Al-Kharrat T, et al (1997) Effects of a medical intensivist on patient care in a community teaching hospital. Mayo Clin Proc 72:391–399
3. Engleman RM (1996) Mechanisms to reduce hospital stays. Ann Thorac Surg 61: S26–S29
4. Cheng DCH, Karske J, Peniston C, et al (1996) Early tracheal extubation after coronary artery bypass graft surgery reduces costs and improves resource use. Anesthesiology 85:1300–1310
5. Baker SP, O'Neil B, Haddun W, Long WB (1974) The injury severity score: a method for describing patients with multiple injuries and evaluating emergency care. J Trauma 14:187–196
6. Feller I, Tholen D, Cornell RG (1980) Improvements in burn care, 1965 to 1979. JAMA 244:2074–2078

7. Teasdale G, Jennett B (1974) Assessment of coma and impaired consciousness: a practical scale. Lancet ii: 81–84
8. Siegel JH, Goldwyn RM, Friedman HP (1971) Patterns and processes in the evaluation of human septic shock. Surgery 70:232–240
9. Shoemaker WP, Chang P, Czer L (1979) Cardiovascular monitoring in post-operative patients. Crit Care Med 7: 237–241
10. Teres D, Brown RB, Lemeshow S. (1982) Predicting mortality of intensive care unit patients: the importance of coma. Crit Care Med 10: 86–94
11. Knaus WA, Zimmerman JE, Wagner DP, Draper EA, Lawrence DE (1981) APACHE – acute physiology and chronic health evaluation: a physiologically based classification system. Crit Care Med 9: 591–597
12. Knaus WA, Draper EA, Wagner DP, et al (1982) Evaluating outcome from intensive care: a preliminary multihospital comparison. Crit Care Med 10: 491–496
13. Knaus WA, LeGall JR, Wagner DP, et al (1982) A comparison of intensive care in the U.S.A. and France. Lancet ii: 642–646
14. Wagner DP, Draper EA, Abizanda-Campos R, et al (1984) Initial international use of APACHE an acute severity of disease measure. Med Decis Making 4: 297–313
15. Knaus WA, Draper EA, Wagner DP, Zimmerman JE (1985) APACHE II – a severity of disease classification system. Crit Care Med 13: 818–829
16. Le Gall JR, Loirat P, Alperovitch A, et al (1984) A simplified acute physiology score for ICU patients. Crit Care Med 12: 975–977
17. Lemeshow S, Teres D, Pastides H, Avrunin JS, Gage RW (1985) A method for predicting survival and mortality of ICU patients using objectively derived weights. Crit Care Med 13: 519–525
18. Escarce JJ, Kelly MA (1990) Admission source to the medical intensive care unit predicts hospital death independent of APACHE II score. JAMA 264:2389–2394
19. Borlase BC, Baxter JK, Kenney PR, Forse RA, Benotti PN, Blackburn GL (1991) Elective intrahospital admissions versus acute interhospital transfers to a surgical intensive care unit: cost and outcome prediction. J Trauma. 31: 915–919
20. Dragsted L, Jorgenson J, Jensen NH, et al (1989) Interhospital comparisons of patient outcome from intensive care: importance of lead time bias. Crit Care Med 17: 418–422
21. Rowan KM, Kerr JH, Major E, McPherson K, Vessey MD (1993) Intensive Care Society's study in Britain and Ireland – II: Outcome comparisons of intensive care units after adjustment for case mix by the American APACHE II method. Br Med J 307:977–981
22. Jacobs S, Chang RWS, Lee B, Lee B (1988) Audit of intensive care: a 30 month experience using the APACHE II severity of disease classification system. Intensive Care Med 14:567–574
23. Sirio Ca, Tajimi K, Tase C, et al (1992) An initial comparison of intensive care in Japan and the United States. Crit Care Med 20: 1207–1215
24. Knaus WA, Wagner DP, Draper EA, et al (1991) The APACHE III prognostic system. Risk prediction of hospital mortality for critically ill hospitalized adults. Chest 100:1619–1636.
25. Lemeshow S, Teres D, Klar J, Avrunin JS, Gehlbach SH, Rappoport J (1993) Mortality probability models (MPM II) based on an international cohort of intensive care unit patients. JAMA 270: 2478–2486
26. Le Gall JR, Lemeshow S, Saulnier F (1993) A new simplified acute physiology score (SAPS II) based on a European/North American multicenter study. JAMA 270:2957–2963
27. Sirio CA, Shepardson LB, Rotondi AJ, et al (1999) Community-wide assessment of intensive care outcomes using a physiologically based prognostic measure. Chest 115:793–801
28. Zimmerman JE, Wagner DP, Draper EA, Wright L, Alzola C, Knaus WA (1998) Evaluation of acute physiology and chronic health evaluation III predictions of hospital mortality in an independent database. Crit Care Med 26:1317–1326
29. Pappachan JV, Millar B, Bennett D, Smith GB (1999) Comparison of outcome from intensive care admission after adjustment for case mix by the APACHE III prognostic system. Chest 115:802–810

30. Beck DH, Taylor BL, Millar B, Smith GB (1997) Prediction of outcome from intensive care: a prospective cohort study comparing acute physiology and chronic health evaluation II and III prognostic systems in a United Kingdom intensive care unit. Crit Care Med 25:9–15
31. Bastos PG, Sun X, Wagner DP, Knaus WA, Zimmerman JE, The Brazil APACHE III Study Group (1996) Application of the APACHE III prognostic system in Brazilian intensive care units: a prospective multicenter study. Intensive Care Med 22:564–570
32. Markgraf R, Deutschinoff G, Pientka L, Scholten T (2000) Comparison of acute physiology and chronic health evaluation (APACHE II and III) and simplified acute physiology score (SAPS II): a prospective cohort study evaluating these methods to predict outcome in a German interdisciplinary intensive care unit. Crit Care Med 28: 26–33
33. Apolone G, Bertolini G, D'Amico R, et al (1996) The performance of SAPS II in a cohort of patients admitted to 99 Italian ICUs: results from GiViTI. Intensive Care Med 22:1368–1378
34. Moreno R, Morais P (1997) Outcome prediction in intensive care: results of a prospective, multicenter, Portuguese study. Intensive Care Med 23:177–186
35. Metnitz PGH, Valentin A, Vesely H, et al (1999) Prognostic performance and customization of the SAPS II: results of a multicenter Austrian study. Intensive Care Med 25:192–197
36. Moreno R, Miranda DR, Fidler V, Schilfgaarde RV (1998) Evaluation of two outcome prediction models on an independent database. Crit Care Med 26:50–61
37. Nouira S, Roupie E, El Atrouss S, et al (1998) Intensive care use in a developing country: a comparison between a Tunisian and a French unit. Intensive Care Med 24:1144–1151
38. Nouira S, Belghith M, Elatrous S, et al (1998) Predictive value of severity scoring systems: comparison of four models in Tunisian adult intensive care units. Crit Care Med 26:852–859
39. Vanderschuern S, Weerdt A, Malbrain M, et al (2000) Thrombocytopenia and prognosis in intensive care. Crit Care Med 28:1871–1876
40. Hamel MB, Goldman L, Teno J, et al (1995) Identification of comatose patients at high risk for death or severe disability. JAMA 273:1842–1848
41. Knaus WA, Wagner DP, Zimmerman JE, Draper EA. (1993) Variations in mortality and length of stay in intensive care units. Ann Intern Med 118:753–761
42. Borlase BC, Baxter JK, Benotti PN, et al (1991) Surgical intensive care unit resource use in a specialty referral hospital: I. Predictors of early death and cost implications. Surgery 109:687–693
43. Porath A, Eldar N, Harman-Bohem I, Gurman G (1994) Evaluation of the APACHE II scoring system in an Israeli intensive care unit. Isr J Med Sci 30:514–520
44. Boyd O, Grounds RM (1993) Physiological scoring systems and audit. Lancet 341: 1573–1574
45. Goldhill DR Sumner A (1998) Outcome of intensive care patients in a group of British intensive care units. Crit Care Med 26:1337–1345
46. Seneff MG, Wagner DP, Thompson D, Honeycutt C, Silver M (2000) The impact of long term actue care facilities on the outcome and cost of care for patients undergoing prolonged mechanical ventilation. Crit Care Med 28: 342–350
47. Jayes RL, Zimmerman JE, Wagner DP, Knaus WA (1996) Variations in the use of do-not resuscitate orders in ICUs. Chest 110:1332–1339
48. Pendergrast TJ, Luce JM (1997) Increasing incidence of witholding and withdrawal of life support for the critically ill. Am J Respir Crit Care 155:15–20
49. Egol A, Willmitch B (1998) Witholding and withdrawing care affects severity adjusted outcome data. Crit Care Med 26:A25 (Abst)
50. Zhu BP, Lemeshow S, Hosmer DW, Klar J, Avrunin J, Teres D (1996) Factors affecting the performance of the models in the mortality probability model II system and strategies of customization: a simulation study. Crit Care Med 24:57–63
51. Teres D, Lemeshow S (1999) When to customize a severity model. Intensive Care Med 25:140–142
52. Justice AC, Covinsky KE, Berlin JA (1999) Assessing the generalizability of prognostic information. Ann Intern Med 130:515–524
53. Chen LM, Martin CM, Morrison TL, Sibbald WJ (1999) Interobserver variability in data collection of the APACHE II score in teaching and community hospitals. Crit Care Med 27:1999–2004

54. Holt AW, Bury LK, Bersten AD, Skowronski GA, Vedig AE (1992) Prospective evaluation of residents and nurses as severity score data collectors. Crit Care Med 20:16898–1691
55. Rosenthal GE, Harper DL (1994) Cleveland health quality choice: a model for collaborative community based outcomes assessment. J Comm J Qual Improv 20:425–442
56. Langham J, Goldfrad C, Rowan K (1998) Can case mix adjustment methods be replicated directly from the publication. Intensive Care Med 24 (Suppl 1): S23 (Abst)
57. Bosman RJ, Oudemans van Straaten HM, Zandstra DF (1998) The use of intensive care information system alters outcome prediction. Intensive Care Med 24:953–958

A Hospital-Wide System for Managing the Seriously Ill: A Model of Applied Health Systems Research

K. Hillman, A. Flabouris, and M. Parr

"For it happens in this, as the physicians say it happens in hectic fever, that in the beginning of the malady it is easy to cure but difficult to detect, but in the course of time, not having been either detected or treated in the beginning, it becomes easy to detect but difficult to cure." (Niccolo Machiavelli, The Prince)

Learning Points

- In-hospital cardiac arrests are often proceeded by a slow and potentially reversible deterioration in the patient's condition
- The Medical Emergency Team (MET) is a hospital-wide concept aimed at early identification and management of the seriously ill patient using simple clinical criteria
- Ward-based outcome indicators should include measures of potential preventability such as deaths, cardiorespiratory arrest, and intensive care unit (ICU) admissions without prior referral to the MET
- Introduction of the MET concept requires a change in culture of the whole hospital
- The practice of intensive care medicine is about process rather than location

In 1982 at a large tertiary hospital, a 20 year old injured motor cyclist was admitted to a general ward after being resuscitated in the emergency department. He had a fractured pelvis and left femur. While traction was being applied later that evening he had a cardiac arrest and did not respond to cardiopulmonary resuscitation (CPR). The case was discussed the following day and postulated reasons for the sudden death included fat embolism, and the sudden rupture of an undiagnosed aortic dissection. In fact, the clinical charts clearly demonstrated he had slowly deteriorated in the general ward and simply bled to death. The pulse rate had risen, the blood pressure decreased, the respiratory rate increased and finally the level of consciousness had slowly decreased. Autopsy confirmed this.

Introduction

We have had many similar patients admitted from the general wards who had slowly deteriorated without adequate management. Interestingly the attending nursing staff usually charted the deterioration perfectly and often the nursing staff shared their concerns with junior medical staff. However, the system did not seem to respond rapidly enough to the seriously ill on general wards, nor was there sufficient expertise, skills or supervision when medical assistance eventually arrived. This is a saga extending over almost 20 years, of how the principles of health systems research were used to address this issue. It is a saga of the specialty of intensive care moving out of its four walls and realizing that outcome is determined as much by the level of care delivered before and after the ICU as it is by the interventions within the ICU.

Early Management of Ischemia

Shock is described as inadequate cellular perfusion. We usually measure the extent of shock in terms of hypotension and signs of overt ischemia to individual organs such as oliguria, decreased level of consciousness and poor peripheral perfusion. However, these are late signs and ischemia can also occur in the splanchnic beds [1], liver [2], and even the cerebral circulation [3], despite apparently normal vital signs. Early ischemia, even if it is seemingly minor, can lead to measurable cellular dysfunction [4]. More overt ischemia can, of course, predispose to organ dysfunction such as acute respiratory distress syndrome (ARDS) [5], as well as multiple organ failure (MOF) [6], resulting in severe complications and death.

A common model of ischemia occurs as a result of trauma. Ischemia can occur soon after the traumatic event and unless detected and managed rapidly, can result in MOF and death [7]. This has focused our attention on the importance of rapid resuscitation in the management of trauma. The organization of a system to optimize trauma management involves components such as initial stabilization, transport to a major trauma center, activation of a team with personnel trained in resuscitation, as well as rapid investigation and definitive treatment [8]. The organization of trauma management in order to rapidly correct ischemia and hypoxia has resulted in a significant reduction in preventable deaths [9].

Despite our knowledge about the dangers of even minor degrees of ischemia [6], and the beneficial impact of organized and early intervention in patients with severe trauma, there have been few other systematic attempts to organize early intervention for all at-risk patients. While not involved in specific systems, specialized sections of a hospital such as ICUs, high dependency units (HDUs), operating rooms (OR), and emergency departments, provide a 24 hour environment where at-risk patients are rapidly attended to. A combination of comprehensive monitoring and supervision by staff with expertise in the management of the seriously ill should guarantee early recognition and rapid correction of ischemia.

However, other environments such as the general wards of hospitals may not provide that level of care [10]. Up to 80% of patients who suffer an in-hospital cardiac arrest have readily detected changes in vital signs within the eight hours preceding the arrest [11]. Other studies have suggested that up to 41% of admissions to ICUs were potentially avoidable [12] and that patients admitted from the general wards had a higher mortality than those from the OR, emergency department or recovery room [13].

A matched group of septic patients initially managed on the general wards had a higher mortality than those initially managed in the ICU [14]. The lack of a systematic approach to at-risk patients may explain the large numbers of potentially preventable deaths in hospital [15, 16]. Peter Safar, one of the pioneers of modern resuscitation, said as long ago as 1974: "the most sophisticated intensive care often becomes unnecessarily expensive terminal care when the pre-ICU system fails"[17].

System Failure in Acute Hospitals

Why are acute hospitals, particularly the general wards, so dangerous for patients? For a start, medical practitioners are not necessarily trained, as undergraduates, in even the basic aspects of how to manage the seriously ill [18, 19]. Nor is training in resuscitation consistent in the postgraduate period [20]. The exceptions may be in areas such as anesthesiology, intensive care medicine or emergency medicine, where formal training in all aspects of advanced resuscitation should occur. It follows, therefore, that most hospital-based specialists may also not be competent in the practice of acute medicine [21], as they do not receive formal training at an undergraduate or postgraduate level and do not have the opportunity to practice and maintain the skills they were not formally taught in the first place. This lack of training in, and awareness of, acute medicine is one of the factors resulting in poor systematic 24 hour cover for acute hospitals [22], despite the fact that in–hospital emergencies occur in an unpredictable fashion at any time of the day or night [23, 24].

The situation is exacerbated by specialists 'owning' patients. At best, 'ownership' guarantees one person has responsibility for co-ordination and managing every aspect of the patient's care. However, 'ownership' may also be driven by economic motives or perhaps it is simply as a result of territorialism. This means that systems that cross professional and functional boundaries are difficult to establish, often fuelled by fear of losing 'control' by the owning specialist.

The fact that there is little in the way of an organized system to provide 24 hour early detection and management of life-threatening emergencies, may contribute to the large number of potentially preventable cardiorespiratory arrests [11] admissions to the ICU [12,13] and deaths [15,16] that occur in hospitals.

A model is described here for hospital-wide provision of emergency care 24 hours a day based on the Medical Emergency Team (MET) concept [24–26]. The system comprises early identification of at-risk patients, an emergency response based on those criteria, resuscitation by a multidisciplinary team with at least one member with formal training in all aspects of advanced resuscitation; evaluation of the effectiveness of the system, and a mechanism where all members of the hospital are educated and aware of the system and are provided with feedback as to its effectiveness in order to adjust and improve it as necessary. The system is based on a MET, which replaces the hospital cardiac arrest team. The model has become known as the MET, even though the 'team' is only one aspect of the overall system. The simultaneous implementation and evaluation of this concept highlights the difficulties of health systems research but also the satisfaction that can be gained from reorganizing existing health resources in a more efficient fashion.

The MET Criteria

The MET criteria identify a patient who is at-risk of serious deterioration and requires emergency management. Initially, over 30 criteria were used to identify at-risk patients. These have gradually been refined to 8 simple criteria (Table 1), based on abnormalities of commonly measured vital signs such as pulse rate, respiratory rate, blood pressure, and level of consciousness.

The MET criteria assume all at-risk patients deteriorate in a similar way (Fig. 1). Patients ultimately die of physiological abnormalities, rather than specific diagnoses or anatomical pathology. Ischemia and/or hypoxia are final common pathways, eventually leading to cardiorespiratory arrest and death. Along the way, patients respond by changes in vital signs: such as increasing or decreasing pulse and respiratory rates, either as a primary or secondary event; decreasing blood pressure; or losing consciousness. No matter whether the cause of the deterioration is disease related (e.g., pneumonia) or syndrome related (e.g., shock), deterioration is along largely predictable pathways. The aim of the MET criteria is to detect this predictable deterioration and identify at-risk patients before severe complications occur. Initially, biochemical abnormalities were also included in the criteria, but they made an otherwise simple system more complex and had a low rate of identifying at-risk patients. The adverse effects of abnormal biochemistry such as hyper- and hypokalemia are usually manifested by changes in vital signs and the credibility of the MET system was being compromised by being over-called for abnormal pathology results without adverse clinical manifestations.

Table 1. MET calling criteria

Threatened airway
Respiratory rate <5 or > 36
Cardiorespiratory arrest
Pulse rate <40 or >140
Systolic blood pressure <90
Repeated or prolonged seizures
Fall in Glasgow coma score (GCS) > 2 points
Worried

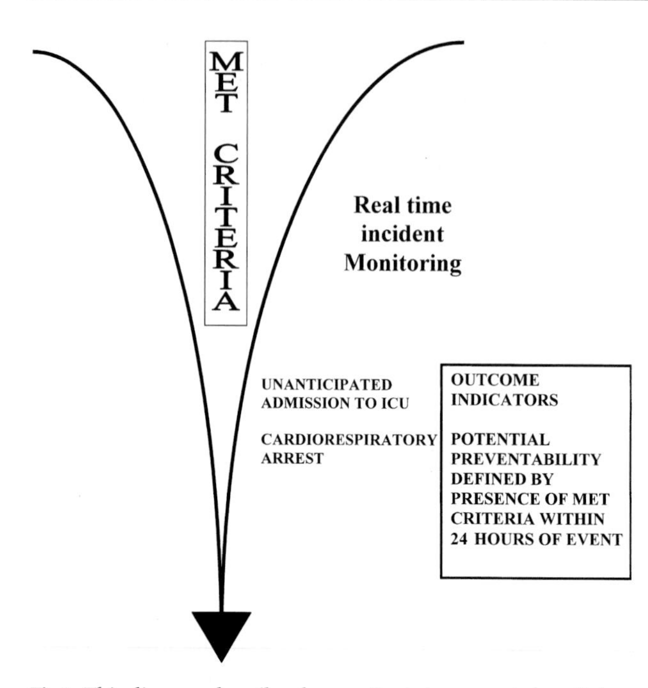

Fig. 1. This diagram describes how patients in an acute hospital usually pass through the MET criteria as their condition deteriorates and they go on to have a cardiorespiratory arrest, die or be unexpectedly admitted to the ICU. The MET criteria (Table 1) provide the basis for response as well as being part of evaluation. If the MET criteria precede an unexpected death, ICU admission or cardiorespiratory arrest, it was potentially preventable and should be analyzed further

Convulsion is the only diagnostic criteria remaining as part of the MET criteria. Not only are convulsions distressing for attending staff but can predispose to immediately life-threatening sequels, such as airway compromise, hypoxia, pulmonary aspiration and permanent neurological damage [27]. Convulsions are also a marker for significant physiological disturbances.

In order to encourage staff to maintain a low threshold for calling the MET, a 'worried' category was also included. Ward hospital staff normally have no system for summoning immediate assistance when they have a 'feeling' that their patient is deteriorating, unless, of course, the patient actually dies, when they then can call the cardiac arrest team. Often attempts are made to contact junior medical staff of the responsible medical team. The junior staff may be delayed or lack appropriate skills and knowledge to manage an acute medical emergency in the ward. This situation is not unlike the circumstance that existed for the management of acute trauma prior to the introduction of trauma teams and systems. In fact, it is often part of a hospital's culture that you must not call the cardiac arrest team until you are sure the patient is unequivocally dead! Junior nurses are made to feel inadequate if they call too early and members of the cardiac arrest team can even reinforce their own sense of importance by abusing more junior medical and nursing staff for calling for near-death situations, rather than for genuine cardiorespiratory arrests. The calling criteria need to be set at a low enough threshold to identify an appropriate population of at-risk patients, without causing major disruption to hospital function; but not at such a high level that serious complications as a result of delay in management, would result. Obviously it is better to err on the side of over-calling. The 'worried' category empowers staff to call earlier rather than later. Our own analysis shows that 19% of patients for whom a 'worried' call is made, are admitted to ICU as a result of that call.

It is important that members of the MET are instructed never to denigrate or abuse staff for calling the MET and in fact are encouraged to actively support staff who utilize the worried criteria, for being astute enough to detect serious illness at an early stage. This reinforces a culture within the hospital of concern for seriously ill and at-risk patients. At the same time, delayed calling is discouraged and cardiorespiratory arrest is seen as a potential failure of the system. In this way, the MET criteria can themselves drive a cultural change in a hospital, from one of separate islands of care and 'ownership' to a widespread awareness and systematic response for all at-risk patients.

The MET Response

Just as the best trauma systems are designed to minimize ischemia and hypoxia, so should other systems, designed to deal with medical emergencies. In fact, one could argue it is at least as important to restore, for example, the circulating volume of a shocked patient with diabetic ketoacidosis, as it is to resuscitate a young, otherwise fit, patient with trauma. This is especially so for patients with chronic health problems who already have compromised organ function, such as cardiovascular disease and renal dysfunction. The next challenge in establishing a safe health system for at-risk patients was to guarantee an appropriate response. Once triage criteria for defining an at-risk patient have been agreed upon, then there must be a rapid and skilled response in order to limit organ damage.

Most trauma systems now have a trauma team with members who have skills in maintaining the airway, breathing, and circulation [28]. Trauma teams now resuscitate according to up-to-date guidelines such as The Advanced Trauma Life Support (ATLS®) system [29]. Participants in the trauma team are usually trained in all aspects of advanced resuscitation according to these ATLS® guidelines. While the importance of early intervention in a limited number of medical emergencies such as acute myocardial infarction is recognized [30], there is little in the way of guaranteeing personnel fully trained in advanced resuscitation at all times in every acute hospital. Even if training was adequate, there is little regard paid to the systematic provision of trained medical staff over a 24 hour period in acute hospitals. Apart from the concept of the specialist 'hospitalist' in North America [31], the system for caring for the acutely ill in our hospital wards is largely based on in-house trainee medical staff or on-call specialists who may or may not be appropriately trained, or regularly manage critically ill patients. Whatever the level of response to a hospital emergency, it is crucial that at least one member of the team is formally trained and regularly practices in advanced resuscitation skills.

A crucial part of the MET system is to provide these trained personnel at all times. The MET system was developed at Liverpool Hospital in Sydney, Australia. Liverpool Hospital is an integral part of the South Western Sydney Area Health Service (SWSAHS) which has one 547 bed tertiary referral hospital (Liverpool Hospital), 2 rural hospitals (71 beds and 116 beds) and 3 metropolitan hospitals (183, 191 and 442 beds). Twenty-four hour medical cover varies from full-time trainees in intensive care medicine in the tertiary referral hospital, to off-site general practitioner cover in one of the small rural hospitals. There are junior medical staff rotating through the metropolitan hospitals for periods from 3–12 months. In order to provide 24 hour advanced resuscitation cover that meets the needs of all hospitals, the following principles were agreed on:

1) Ten to fifteen trained staff from each hospital were necessary to provide at least one member of staff with advanced resuscitation skills covering each hospital for all shifts, allowing for leave and holidays.
2) Because the training involves a 6 month self-directed learning package, only full-time staff and not staff on short term (less than 1 year) rotation could be considered for training.
3) As there were insufficient medical staff permanently working in hospitals at all times of day and night, nursing staff were considered for training. Nursing staff from the emergency department and ICU with postgraduate qualifications were preferred but not essential.
4) Each hospital nominated their own staff, within these guidelines for training and arranged their own rosters to cover their hospital at all times.

Training in Advanced Resuscitation

Medical practitioners do not have a monopoly on the skills and knowledge necessary for advanced resuscitation. In fact, Kenneth Calman, the chief medical officer in the UK argued that a doctor's most unique and valuable role is in diagnosis [32]. Paramedics, nursing staff and even lay people can be trained in many aspects of advanced resuscitation [33–35]. Unfortunately most so-called resuscitation training focuses on cardiopulmonary resuscitation (CPR) [36]. Each hospital has its own variation of training in CPR with varying amounts of resources being allocated for training. However, the outcome from in-hospital cardiac arrest has changed little over the last 30 years and it has been estimated that it costs approximately $400,000 (US) per life saved to operate in-hospital CPR programs [37].

Other initiatives in advanced resuscitation training include a Fundamental Critical Care Support (FCCS) program, developed to provide basic principles of critical care and to offer guidance for decision making in the early management of the critically ill patient [38]. The course is aimed to assist the non-intensivist in the initial 24 hours of management of the critically ill patient if specialist expertise is not readily available and is limited in that it concentrates more on intensive care medicine, such as the ongoing need for mechanical ventilation and monitoring, rather than initial resuscitation.

It is imperative that each acute hospital address the need to have at least one person available at all times who can practice all aspects of advanced resuscitation. This will become more important as bed numbers decrease, hospital length of stay declines, and alternatives to hospital admission are explored, resulting in acute hospitals having to manage an increasing population of critically ill [39].

To complement the early warning MET criteria and in line with the principles previously outlined to meet the needs of each hospital in the provision of a 24 hour service for hospital emergencies, the Advanced Resuscitation Course (ARC) was established to train staff. The features of the ARC include:

1) A 6 month self-directed course done largely within the candidates own time.
2) The theoretical content of the course is covered in a specially prepared manual [40].
3) The specialized skills associated with advanced resuscitation are taught largely within the trainee's own hospital and include intubation, central line insertion and initial ventilatory skills, with each candidate having to perform a minimum number under supervision. The anesthesiology department conducts much of the teaching in the OR setting. Increasingly, mannequins are also being used for instruction. A total of 76 skills required for the practice of advanced resuscitation, have been identified.
4) A multiple choice questionnaire is given before and after the 6 month course, testing acute medicine knowledge. This was developed and validated by emergency medicine and intensive care specialists.
5) A 3 day evaluation course is held at the end of each 6 month period which includes skill testing, tutorials and simulated emergencies. If the candidate passes, they are given their ARC certificate and permitted to practice advanced resuscitation in the own hospital.
6) Ongoing education, support and re-certification then becomes part of the program.
7) The program is organized across the health area by one intensive care nurse and a clerical assistant. Medical staff from the tertiary hospital ICU support teaching and supervision of the course. So far 96 candidates have enrolled in the course from five hospitals. Of those, 60 have qualified. Forty-four of the successful candidates are nurses and 16 are medical officers.

Auditing the System

Once a system has been established – in this case to manage seriously ill and at-risk patients throughout an acute hospital – then outcome indicators should ideally be developed to monitor that system. Not only do measurements have to be made, but the data needs to be widely distributed to those who can appropriately adjust and improve the system. This process is the basis for what is called, amongst other things, continuous quality management (CQM) [41].

Many separate departments within a hospital attempt to measure and monitor their performance. The standardized mortality ratio (SMR) is often used to estimate the quality of care in an ICU. Predicted hospital mortality is compared with actual hospital mortality after the admission data is adjusted for factors such as case mix, age, and chronic health status [42]. Even using SMRs with data collected from ICUs, true mortality may be concealed as a result of lead time bias [43,

44]. Lead time bias is related to delays or inappropriate treatment prior to admission to the ICU and the effect this would have on eventual mortality. In other words, mortality is related to factors other than the care given within the four walls of the ICU. The severity of illness on admission to the ICU may be related more to inappropriate management prior to ICU admission and, therefore, be testing the whole hospital system rather than simply the ICU component.

Other hospital departments and specialties may have other ways of determining the outcome of the seriously ill patients that they manage. However, there is little in the way of measurements which estimate the standard of care of the seriously ill across the whole hospital system involving various departments, functions and professions. The measurement of the standard management of trauma care from the prehospital setting to eventual outcome in the community is one of the few exceptions.

One of the few ways we have of measuring the quality of care given to the seriously ill across the whole hospital is by focusing on mortality [45]. Attempts have been made to adjust hospital death rates in order to make them a more accurate tool for measuring hospital care [46]. Random audit of patient notes have also been used to analyze hospital mortality [15,16]. These studies show that up to 27% of in-hospital deaths have been estimated to be preventable. However, the usual methodology for analyzing hospital mortality is time consuming, expensive and often involves clinicians subjective opinion about preventability. For these reasons, mortality is not often systematically used as a practical tool for measuring the quality of an acute hospital.

Using the MET System to Measure Hospital Quality

The MET system lends itself to measuring the effectiveness of the system itself as well as identifying potentially preventable events. The hospital-wide outcome indicators chosen for the MET system are deaths, unanticipated admission to the ICU and cardiorespiratory arrest rates (Fig. 1). Patients may, of course, develop serious illness and not suffer any of these complications. However, outcome indicators have to be achievable using available resources. The indicators need to make intuitive sense to clinicians as well as to other levels of the health system. Using deaths, unanticipated admission to ICU, and cardiorespiratory arrest rates, assumes that if patients are discharged without these serious complications, then the system, while not perfect, at least ensured their discharge alive from hospital, without complications serious enough to require admission to the ICU.

Use of Outcome Indicators to Indicate Potential Preventability

The presence of MET criteria within the 24 hours prior to the three outcome indicators which were not acted upon by initiating a MET response, may be used as a measure of potential preventability. A review of the patients' notes and charts would indicate whether MET criteria had been noted and whether or not appropriate action had been taken when the MET criteria were first recorded. Utilizing this 24 hour period greatly reduces the workload needed to determine hospital outcome indicators as only the final entries in the patient's case notes, covering the 24 hour period prior to the three events, have to be reviewed in any detail. Again it is a matter of balancing available resources with objectives. Interviews with attending staff may reveal whether the patient could have fulfilled MET criteria without them being recorded. However, this is not only time-consuming but may defeat the purpose of the audit by making staff feel defensive and encouraging inaccurate answers.

Hospital Outcome Indicators and End-of-Life Decisions

The MET system is not designed to be used to resuscitate patients who are terminally ill and for whom resuscitation measures are deemed as futile. The term 'do not resuscitate' (DNR) refers specifically to patients who are terminally ill and may require CPR [47]. CPR in these circumstances obviously would represent inappropriate use of resources, as well as providing unfair hope to the patient and relatives; and in most cases would be futile anyway. It may be equally futile to provide early resuscitation, in the form of a MET response and the associated resuscitation measures, to terminally ill patients. The MET system can help drive a systematic cultural change in acute hospitals by encouraging clinicians to make an explicit diagnosis of dying in terminally ill patients, and thus discussing the withholding of futile resuscitation attempts, including that of CPR, may not be in the patient's interest.

'Not for MET' (NF-MET) is a slightly different concept compared to 'not for resuscitation' (NFR). NF-MET may imply that death is imminent and MET associated resuscitation measures are not indicated, whereas NFR may imply that active management is still continuing but if it fails to the extent that cardiorespiratory arrest occurs, then CPR will not be attempted. Not all terminally ill patients need to be NF-MET. It is important for each hospital to think carefully about these issues and discuss the implications of all that these terms imply and then develop their own procedures for their application. There is a perceived need that we should be more explicit, both amongst ourselves as clinicians, as well as with patients and their friends and relatives about prognosis and end of life wishes expressed by the patient. We are often reluctant to make a diagnosis of dying in the acute hospital setting.

The MET outcome indicators can be a catalyst for this process. Patients who have no NF-MET or NFR order and who have died or had a cardiorespiratory arrest can be labeled as 'unexpected'. This label is used to flag patients for auditing purposes as well as to assist in driving debate and discussion about the appropriateness of a MET call for that particular patient.

In our experience of the MET system, the MET team often acts as the surrogate end of life decision making body. When, for example, the patient is obviously suffering a quite predictable end of life event, for which a MET is called, the MET has to negotiate with the admitting team about whether active management is appropriate in these circumstances. Often it is not. The MET system in this situation is making explicit a decision making process which ideally should have occurred and been discussed at an earlier time with the patient and relatives.

Summary of MET Outcome Indicators (Table 2)

The three outcome indicators represent one dimension of an acute hospital's quality. The indicators are relatively easy to collect and are 'flagged', indicating possible cases where management across the hospital system may have been less than optimal and opportunities for improvement possible.

The indicators can be modified according to each hospitals' needs. By not including patients from the emergency department, OR or recovery room in 'Unanticipated admission to the ICU', we are assuming that management in these environments is optimal. In other words, we are assuming that patients managed in environments which are monitored, and who are cared for by staff trained in advanced resuscitation should not be flagged for further audit as the system could not be improved without enormous cost anyway. The MET concept, in theory, would provide little benefit in these environments. Other outcome indicators should be used to monitor quality of care in these areas. Other sites such as high dependency units (HDUs) or coronary care units (CCUs) may also be excluded from unanticipated admissions to ICU. In doing so, we are saying that the MET system would add little benefit to these areas and including them in the audit process would achieve little. Similarly age limits can be used to define these indicators. For example, the MET system may not be appropriate for neonates. The MET system has not formally been developed or tested in a pediatric setting and other outcome indicators may be more appropriate.

Completing the Quality Circle

Much data are already demanded of clinicians and the health system. These data are often not made readily available to clinicians in an easy to understand and timely fashion, disappearing into 'data graveyards'. In order to maintain the accuracy of data and commitment of clinicians to collecting them, data must be analyzed and fed back in an easily understood fashion. The clinicians delivering health care are the main determinants of system improvement. In order to improve the system, clinicians need to have data on how their system currently performs.

The cost of collecting the outcome indicators needs to be minimal and their impact on clinical practice, maximal. The outcome indicators used as part of the MET system are deaths, cardiorespiratory arrests and unanticipated admission to the ICU. Each potentially measures the potential effectiveness of the MET system as well as estimating dimensions of hospital quality, particularly its ability to manage the seriously ill in a systematic way.

Table 2. Summary of MET outcome indicators

Unexpected deaths	=	Total deaths	–	deaths with a DNR order
Unexpected cardiorespiratory arrests	=	Total number of cardiorespiratory arrests	–	cardiorespiratory arrests with a DNR order
Unanticipated admissions to ICU	=	All in-hospital admissions to ICU	–	patients admitted from the OR or emergency department

The outcome indicators are 'flags'. These indicate patients for whom the system may have operated more effectively. They do not specifically indicate which part of the system failed. That is left to individual clinicians, wards or departments to determine by examining the circumstances of the patient's event in more detail.

As part of the MET system, data on each patient are fed back to all clinicians that they have been responsible for managing patients who have suffered a death, cardiorespiratory arrest or unanticipated admission to the ICU. Data are also provided on whether this patient had MET criteria within 24 hours of those events and whether these criteria were appropriately acted on or not. The clinician then has a measurement tool for assessing, on a system-wide basis, the management of their own patients. They also presumably have control over a large part of that system and can implement appropriate strategies to improve the system.

The data are then de-identified and aggregated as deaths without an NFR order, unanticipated ICU admissions and cardiac arrests. This information can then be tailored for distribution to all levels of the hospital system (e.g., ward, medical team, medical service, division, etc.), so that different dimensions of quality can be estimated. The crude numbers, as well as 'unexpected' and 'potentially preventable' numbers, can then be examined either individually or as trends. Similarly, aggregated data on a larger scale can be examined across a whole hospital, health region or even country. Hospitals can be matched for factors such as age, case mix and emergency department admissions and used for benchmarking purposes.

Accountability and Acute Hospitals

Accountability is increasingly becoming important in health care delivery. Until recently we only had good information on the cost of health care, with little information on the quality of care. Now the funders and users of health care are demanding more information on the quality of health care. This has made many clinicians defensive. First, there is sometimes a reluctance to be more accountable. But, second, and a very practical point, there are very few clinical indicators which unequivocally and accurately measure clinical practice. Data can easily be misinterpreted. Some American cities publish comparative surgical mortality in order to give consumers and health funders information about the relative standards of individual surgeons. This simplistic approach does not take into account adjusted risk factors and as a result is rejected by clinicians. Nor does it take into account the many components of a system which the admitting surgeon may not have direct control over. Nevertheless accountability and transparency can be positive agents for change and clinicians need to take the initiative in developing indicators which accurately reflect the outcome of clinical practice.

Disseminating the System

We normally disseminate products in health by means such as publications, conferences and 'word of mouth'. In order to facilitate this process a professionally produced 15 minute video on the MET system has been produced and an accompanying manual published [48]. Implementing a new system is more difficult than prescribing a new drug or performing a new procedure, and tools such as the video and manual are aimed generically at all hospital staff – doctors, nurses and administrators – with step-by-step guidelines on how to implement the MET system. More details on this information are available from the MET Research & Training Unit, The Simpson Centre for Health Service Innovation, The Liverpool Health Service, Locked Bag 7103, Liverpool BC, NSW, 1871.

Conclusion

The MET concept provides a framework for managing seriously ill and at-risk patients across an acute hospital. It is an extension of intensive care and emergency medicine, but operating outside their usual four walls. It provides a means of identifying those at-risk of serious deterioration. The system provides rapid resuscitation with skilled personnel at all times and it provides a means of measuring the quality of care of the seriously ill as well as giving clinicians ownership of that data so they can adjust and improve the system as necessary. The MET concept represents a move from the traditional doctor/patient relationship with its focus on individual wards, departments and professions to a systematic, integrated, co-ordinated and patient focused approach to the seriously ill. Using relatively few extra resources, the MET concept may improve the outcome of the seriously ill. The MET concept represents a move away from the expensive magic bullets which have had little impact on ICU to an early intervention and preventative approach.

The MET system is an example of clinician driven health re-engineering and health systems research. The MET system was established by a multidisciplinary team of clinicians supported by local hospital managers as well as by local and federal governments. Simultaneously the system is being evaluated by a multidisciplinary team of clinicians, statisticians, epidemiologists and informatics experts. Health systems research must by definition be multidisciplinary as well as closely engaging evaluation and implementation.

The MET concept also highlights the arbitrary boundaries between an intensive care environment and elsewhere in an acute hospital. The level of illness which requires an ICU bed has not, as yet, been defined. Nor indeed has what exactly is an ICU bed and how that definition varies between and within countries. When is it safe to manage a patient outside the intensive care environment?; and what is the place of intensive care step down beds?

The concept of triage is readily applied to patients as they enter a hospital through an emergency department. A level of risk is assigned and the patient then managed appropriately in terms of intervention and timing. A similar system needs to be operating with acute hospitals. We need to assign levels of risk to the critically ill and triage them to appropriate environments within the hospital and provide them with certain minimum standards of care within those environments. It seems there is an urgent need to consider these issues from the critically ill patient's perspective in order to guarantee appropriate 24 hour care for all the critically ill and potentially critically ill in our acute hospitals.

References

1. Price HL, Deutsch S, Marshall BE (1966) Hemodynamic and metabolic effects of hemorrhage in man with particular reference to the splanchnic circulation. Circ Res18:469–474
2. Gottlieb ME, Sarfeh IJ, Stratton H, Goldman ML, Newell JC, Shad DM (1983) Hepatic perfusion and splanchnic oxygen consumption in patients postinjury. J Trauma 23:836–843
3. Schmoker J, Zhuang J, Shackford SR (1991) Hemorrhagic hypotension after brain injury causes an early and sustained decrease in oxygen delivery despite normalization of systemic oxygen delivery. J Trauma 31:1038
4. Rhee P, Langdale L, Mock C, Gentilello LM (1997) Near-infrared spectroscopy: Continuous measurement of cytochrome oxidation during hemorrhagic shock. Crit Care Med 25:166–170
5. Demling RH (1993) Adult respiratory distress syndrome: Current concepts. New Horiz 1:388–401
6. Biffl WL, Moore EE (1996) Splanchnic ischaemia/reperfusion and multiple organ failure. Br J Anaesth 77:59–70
7. Faist E, Baue AE, Dittmer H, Heberer G (1983) Multiple organ failure in polytrauma patients. J Trauma 23:775–787
8. Pagliarello G, Dempster A, Wesson D (1992) The integrated trauma program: A model for cooperative trauma triage. J Trauma 33:198–204
9. Shackford SR, Hollingworth-Fridlund P, Cooper GF, et al (1986) The effect of regionalization upon the quality of trauma care as assessed by concurrent audit before and after institution of a trauma system. J Trauma 26:812–820
10. Garrad C, Young D (1998) Suboptimal care of patients before admission to intensive care. Is caused by a failure to appreciate or apply the ABCs of life support. Br Med J 316:1841–1842
11. Schein RMH, Hazday N, Pena M, Ruben BH, Spring CL (1990) Clinical antecedents to in-hospital cardiopulmonary arrest. Chest 98:1388–1392
12. McQuillan P, Pilkington S, Allan A, et al (1998) Confidential inquiry into quality of care before admission to intensive care. Br Med J 316:1853–1858
13. Goldhill DR, Sumner A (1998) Outcome of intensive care patients in a group of British intensive care units. Crit Care Med 26:1337–1345
14. Lundberg JS, Perl TM, Wiblen T, et al (1998) Septic shock: An analysis of outcomes for patients with onset on hospital wards versus intensive care units. Crit Care Med 26:1020–1024
15. Brennan TA, Leape LL, Laird N, et al (1991) Incidence of adverse events and negligence in hospitalised patients: Results of the Harvard Medical Practice Study I. N Engl J Med 324:370–376
16. Wilson RMcL, Runciman WB, Gibbert RW, Harrison BT, Newby L, Hamilton JD (1995) The quality in Australian Health Care Study. Med J Aust 163:458–471
17. Safar P (1974) Critical Care Medicine – Quo Vadis? Crit Care Med 2:1–5
18. Harrison GA, Hillman KM, Fulde GWO, Jacques TC (1999) The need for undergraduate education in critical care – Results of a Questionnaire to Year 6 Medical Undergraduates, University of New South Wales and recommendations on a curriculum in Critical Care. Anaesth Intensive Care 27:53–58
19. Buchman TG, Dellinger RP, Raphaely RC, Todres ID (1992) Undergraduate education in critical care medicine. Crit Care Med 20:1595–1603
20. Redmond AD (1987) Training in resuscitation. Arch Emerg Med 4:205–206
21. Thwaites BC, Shankar S, Niblett D, Saunders J (1992) Can consultants resuscitate? J R Coll Physicians Lond 26:265–267
22. Spear SF (1986) Life-threatening emergencies: Patterns of demand and response of a regional emergency medical services system. Am J Prev Med 2:163–168
23. Hillman KM, Beehan SJ (1998) Acute hospital medical staffing during the night shift. Aust Health Rev 21:163–173
24. Lee A, Bishop G, Hillman KM, Daffurn K (1995) The medical emergency Team. Anaesth Intensive Care 23:183–186

25. Hourihan F, Bishop G, Hillman KM, Daffurn K, Lee A (1995) The medical emergency team: A new strategy to identify and intervene in high risk patients. Clin Intensive Care 6:269–272
26. Hillman KM, Bishop G, Lee A, et al (1996) Identifying the general ward patient at high risk of cardiac arrest. Clin Intensive Care 7:242–243
27. Nashef L, Brown S (1996) Epilepsy and sudden death. Lancet 348:1325–1325
28. Deane SA, Gaudry PL, Pearson I, Misra S, McNeil RJ, Read C (1990) The hospital trauma team: A model for trauma management. J Trauma 30:806–812
29. Committee of Trauma American College of Surgeons (1993) Advanced trauma life support. American College of Surgeons, Chicago
30. Mitchell JM, Wheeler WS (1991) The golden hours of myocardial infarction: Non-thrombolytic interventions. Ann Emerg Med 20:540–548
31. Wachter RM, Goldmann DR (1999) The hospitalist movement in the United States. Ann Intern Med 130:338–387
32. Calman K (1995) The profession of medicine. Br Med J 309:1140–1143
33. Smale JR, Kutty K, Ohlert J, Cotter T (1995) Endotracheal intubation by paramedics during in-hospital CPR. Chest 107:1655–1661
34. McKee Dr, Wynne G, Evans TR (1994) Student nurses can defibrillate within 90 seconds. Resuscitation 27:35–37
35. Moore JE, Eisenberg MS, Cummins RO, Hallstrom AP, Litwin P, Carter W (1987) Lay persons use of automated external defibrillators. Ann Emerg Med 16:101–104
36. Birnbaum ML, Robinson NE, Kuska BM, Stone HL, Fryback DG, Rose JH (1994) Effect of advanced cardiac life-support training in rural community hospitals. Crit Care Med 22: 741–749
37. Lee KH, Angus DC, Abramson NS (1996) Cardiopulmonary resuscitation: What cost to cheat death? Crit Care Med 24:2046–2052
38. Dellinger RP (1996) Fundamental critical care support: another merit badge or more? Crit Care Med 24:556–557
39. Hillman KM (1999) The changing role of acute-care hospitals. Med J Aust 170:325–328
40. Anonymous ()Advanced Resuscitation Course Manual. The MET Research & Training Unit, South Western Sydney Area Health Service, Sydney.
41. Berwick DM (1989) Continuous improvement as an ideal in health care. N Engl J Med 320:53–56
42. Knaus WA, Draper EA, Wagner DP, Zimmerman JE (1985) APACHE II: A severity of disease classification system. Crit Care Med 13:818–829
43. Tunnell RD, Smith GB (1997) The quality of pre-ICU care influences outcome of patients admitted from the ward. Clin Intensive Care 8:104
44. Dragsted L, Jorgensen J, Jensen NH, et al (1989) Interhospital comparisons of patient outcome from intensive care: Importance of lead-time bias. Crit Care Med 17:418–422
45. Dubois RW, Rogers WH, Mosley JH, Draper D (1987) Hospital inpatient mortality. Is it a predictor of quality? N Engl J Med 1674–1680
46. Keeler EB, Rubenstein LV, Kahn KL, et al (1992) Hospital characteristics and quality of care. JAMA 268:1709–1714
47. Anonymous (1998) Ethics Manual. Fourth edition. American College of Physicians. Ann Intern Med 128:576–594
48. Implementation of the MET System into your Hospital (2000) The MET Research & Training Unit, South Western Sydney Area Health Service, Sydney

Funding and Support

D. R. Miranda

Learning Points

- It cannot be expected that the first steps in health services research will be initiated internally (peripherally), i.e., by the hospital or the intensive care unit (ICU). They need to be externally (centrally) stimulated and financed
- External funding should only consider projects addressing questions which require the use of professional skills and research methodologies specific to different disciplines
- Each research proposal, as well as the various phases of its development through analysis and reporting, should be able to show a true multidisciplinary input. Otherwise, external funding should be rejected/withdrawn
- The ICU is one of the major beneficiaries of health services research in the unit. The ICU should therefore contribute financially to the cost involved in learning and improving. External financing should never cover 100% of the cost of health services research

The EURICUS-II study explored the effect of a managerial based intervention on clinical outcome. The intervention aimed at increasing collaborative practice between physicians and nurses. This prospective, randomized and controlled study (RCT) started in 72 ICUs from 12 European countries. During the first month of research, the number of enrolled ICUs fell drastically, both in the intervention and in the control groups. There were two main reasons given for this reduction: 1) the intervention would reduce the time available for necessary patient care, in light of staff shortages, etc; 2) we are already very good at collaborative practice. Actually, these arguments, used by some to explain withdrawal, were almost unanimously voiced by all participating ICUs when the study was initially presented to them.

Forty-two ICUs completed the 10-month period of research. The results of the study (unpublished data) have shown that the intervention: 1) was associated with a significant decrease in the incidence of adverse events, organ failure and mortality; 2) was perceived as improving collaborative practice.

Introduction

The characteristics of health care research have changed significantly over the last decade. The most relevant change, perhaps, concerns the deliberate search for a link between the ability to discover with the ability to produce. As Cresson puts it "we are moving from research based on performance for its sake, to research which focuses on the social and economic problems which face society today" [1]. Health care, seen from the point of view of society, therefore involves the contribution of more disciplines than medicine alone. And this is where health services research, the focus of this book, becomes important.

As is clearly illustrated in the example above, physicians and nurses are trained to concentrate 100% of their best knowledge and efforts to direct patient care. In principal there is nothing wrong with this approach. Yet, it has been shown on several occasions that non-medical aspects of the organization and management of care play a significant role in the outcome of medical care. It is therefore important, without loosing the patient as the center of their attention, that health care professionals perform, and support, collaborative health services research together with non-medical disciplines. As it was, seen from the perspective of the health care professional with the patient central, health services research revolves around patient care (Fig. 1).

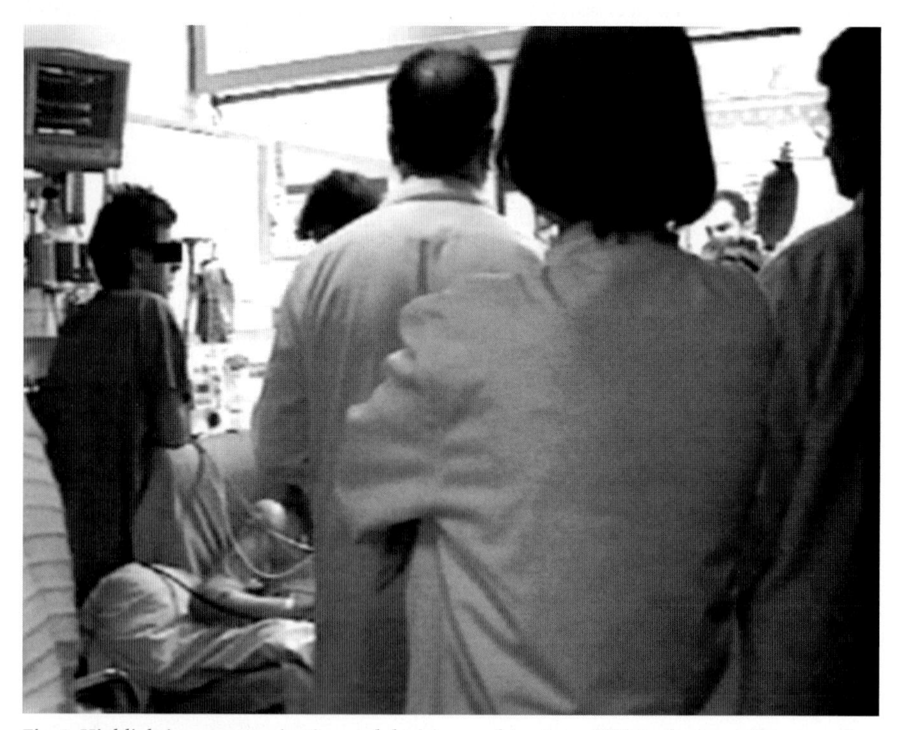

Fig. 1. Highlighting communication and decision-making in an ICU. In the morning, more than two visitors at a time are allowed

Because an immediate understanding of its needs cannot be expected, external financing is necessary for the gradual introduction of health services research to the professional environment of health care. Generally speaking, experience will show that without having tried it out first, none of the medical and non-medical disciplines to be involved in health services research are readily used to the interdisciplinary discussion, study, and solving of problems. External support is therefore necessary, at least at the start of the first health services research programs. These two issues will be presented in this chapter.

Since 1986, the Foundation for Research on Intensive Care in Europe (FRICE) has been conducting multicenter and multinational studies in European ICUs, from a health services research perspective. The need for health services research was particularly felt when it became clear that the planning of, and the decisions involving health care could not (should not) be exclusively dependent on the health care professionals (physicians, nurses, etc). Other disciplines, such as economics, epidemiology, decision-theory, organization and management, psychology, sociology and statistics, should also be at the forefront of studying planning and decision making concerning health care.

The research field that FRICE has cultivated in particular is that of the Organization and Management of Health Care. An important portfolio of research in this field was developed, of which the EURICUS-projects (European ICU Studies) are the most relevant and known worldwide. Given its complexity, the EURICUS project was divided into complementary studies. Three studies have already been designed and performed or are in progress. The studies have been accepted as Concerted Actions in the Biomed Research Programs of the European Commission. More information about this research program can be accessed on the web site: http://www.frice.nl.

The intensive care unit (ICU) is an excellent laboratory for health services research for several reasons. First, as a result of the multidisciplinary nature of many of the issues involved (e.g., medical, economic, ethical). Second, because the collection of data can be maximized in a short period of time, given the high frequency of actions and interactions occurring. In addition, the patient populations, and the applied processes of care, form a rather clear identifiable package, from admission until discharge. Finally, because of the conflicting relevance attributed to the ICU by society (e.g., high expectations, high cost, unclear results).

The rest of this chapter will be based on the experience we have acquired from the EURICUS studies.

Funding

In Europe, the role of the European Union (EU) is predominant in developing and harmonizing research that best serves the Communities of the Union. Besides helping to select and guide the research to be conducted, the EU attributes itself the role of extracting added value from the coordination of national initiatives. This view is clearly expressed in the strategies adopted by the European Commission (EC) for funding research amongst the Member States.

It is fair to say that communication and exchange of experience and knowledge amongst the various research groups in Europe, was perhaps one of the major targets of the first research programs (the BIOMED programs) designed by the EC [2]. These objectives were very successfully attained; today, an important share of the scientific 'space' in Europe is independent of National boundaries. In the Fifth Framework Program (FP5), launched by the EC in 1998, this strategy is further developed, stimulating the contribution of specialists from different scientific fields, together with industrial researchers, users, and political and economic decision-makers, by the definition of research themes and key actions [3].

A budget of 15 billion Euros (1 Euro = 0.9 US Dollar, May 2000) was created to finance the FP5. Therefore, the EC is by far the single largest provider, and the most powerful policy-maker for research in Europe [3].

The 15 billion Euros are to be distributed among:

Thematic Programs

1. Quality of life and management of living resources (16%; 6 key actions)
2. Promoting a user-friendly information society (24%; 4 key actions)
3. Competitive and sustainable growth (18%; 4 key actions)
4. Energy, environment and sustainable development (14%; 6 key actions)
5. Energy, environment and sustainable development – EURATOM (7%; 2 key actions)

A substantial percentage (between 5% and 23%) of the budget allocated to each program is reserved for: "...generic research and activities to support infrastructures. The generic activities aim to build up the knowledge base in selected areas of strategic importance. The support of infrastructures, intended to ensure the optimal use of European and national scientific and technical installations, and to permit their rational and economically efficient development through transnational cooperation" [3].

Horizontal Programs

1. Confirming the international role of Community research (3%)
2. Promoting innovation and the participation of small and medium enterprises (2%)
3. Improving human research potential and the social-economic knowledge base (9%; 1 key action)
4. Joint Research Center (7%; EC and EURATOM actions)

The key actions address 23 issues identified as high-priority social and economic problems. Targeting objectives, these actions assure a multidisciplinary approach, involving researchers, industry, users, etc. In fact, the rationale behind the choice of the key actions is very much that of health services research. In addition, the key actions have two important additional objectives: a) the integration of research, and the development of demonstration and training activities; b) a better coordination of research between the Member States.

The Quality of Life and Management of Living Resources Program

The strategic elements of the program are 6 key actions and 7 generic activities.

The key actions are: food, nutrition and health; control of infectious diseases; the 'cell factory'; environment and health; sustainable agriculture, fisheries and forestry, and integrated development of rural areas including mountain areas; the aging population and disabilities.

The generic research activities are: chronic and degenerative diseases, cancer, diabetes, cardiovascular diseases and rare diseases; research into genomes and diseases of genetic origin; neuroscience; public-health and health services research; research related to persons with disabilities; biomedical ethics and bioethics in the context of respect for fundamental human values; social-economic aspects of life sciences and technologies.

This program, the only one dedicated exclusively to health care, has a budget of about 2.5 billion Euros, of which about 15%–20% (around 550 million Euros) are allocated to generic research activities. If this amount of resources was divided equally among the consigned generic activities, about 100 million Euros would be available for subsidizing research in public health and in health services research during the period of time covered by the program.

The vision and the design of FP5, concerning health care, is much improved in comparison to the former research programs. In addition to the larger allocation of resources to the program, the most significant difference relates to the integration of the traditional concepts of health care (illness, cure and care) in a broader context of 'life and health' (see key activities of Theme 1 above). If the EC is able to stimulate the development of collaborative research across these targeted areas, the new vision will have succeeded.

Implementation Modalities

Besides 'fellowships', 'accompanying measures', 'clusters' and 'bursaries' (for more details see [4]), the program is to be implemented in projects of two types:

- *Concerted actions:* These are intended to coordinate 'research and technological development (R&D)' tasks, between teams of researchers. Concerted actions aim to stimulate the exchange of experience, and to expand the research efforts of the different teams, so that a critical mass of knowledge is reached and reported. Concerted actions can be considered when pooling of data would facilitate common interpretation of facts and contribute to the development of harmonized standards, procedures, methodologies, processes or common research instruments. In fact, concerted actions are projects for the coordination of research (already) performed at national level. The subsidy concerns only the coordination costs; in other words, the costs involved with the research activities at national level are not covered by the subsidy. Estimations carried out by the EC, concluded that the cost of the coordination covered by the concerted actions is about 5% of the total cost of the research involved.

Table 1 presents the summary of the coordination costs of, for example, EURICUS-II. In this prospective RCT, an organizational and managerial intervention (for increasing the collaborative practice between nurses and physicians in the ICU) was implemented in 40 units of 10 European countries. The coordination subsidy of the EC was 510,000 Euros. These funds were divided among: workshops and exchange of staff for preparing, implementing and assessing the progress of the research made; central coordination activities related to project logistics; pooling, handling, analysis and reporting of the data collected.

According to the 5% estimated for coordination cost, the total calculated cost of EURICUS-II was about 10 million Euros. These costs corresponded to the coordination of the project at a national level; to the implementation of the study at a unit level; to the research activities of the various teams involved that could not be included in the coordination tasks.

Concerted actions can also be subsidized for the development of 'thematic networks' [4].

- *Shared-cost actions:* In many aspects similar to concerted actions, shared-cost actions are intended to support the development of products (instruments, prototypes, etc.,) that need to be tested (demonstration projects) before being spread (and eventually commercialized). The important difference in relation to concerted actions, is that shared–cost actions receive a higher contribution of EC resources (around 50% of eligible costs). Understandably, this new (more subsidized) modality of implementation received the attention of researchers in the last round of project submissions (attracting around 90% of all submissions entered!). In fact, many proposals submitted as shared-cost actions would have been more appropriately submitted as concerted actions. This misuse of earmarked community resources (which will probably be corrected in the next round of project-submissions) comes from the traditional understanding that research in health care has necessarily to be supported by exter-

Table 1. Breakdown of costs of EURICUS-I study (the subsidized % of costs incurred by the participants in the study are in parentheses)

	Euros
Labor e.g., coordination, data management, analysis & reporting	326,404.01 (12%)
Exchange & Mobility e.g., meetings, exchange of staff, site visits	129,070.13 (90%)
Support Services e.g., hardware/software, printed matter, mailings, newsletters	94,858.82 (62%)
Overheads	60,421.05 (42%)
Total	610,754.01 (39%)

nal parties. The salutary change that the EC wants to introduce in this traditional attitude of the Health Care Systems of the Member States, however, is that each health care system, and sub-system, should reserve, and allocate, funds for the performance of research activities concerning the improvement of their own effectiveness and efficiency. Concerted actions and shared-cost actions intend to introduce and give structure to this type of research.

Besides their specific content (scientific quality, innovation, adequacy, etc.), these projects have to comply with two important principles: 1) Provide added value to the European Community; 2) Not be possible without the contribution of different Member States.

Updated information on the EC Research Program is available at: www.cordis.lu/fp5

Other Funding

The funding of research at a national level is very different among the European countries. The differences concern both the expressed vision (if any) of the research programs and the amount of resources allocated to them. To our knowledge, there are actually no 'true' health services research programs centrally subsidized in any of the European countries. Medical technology assessment (MTA) programs have been centrally stimulated in several countries. However, the vision, and the mission of MTA programs (e.g., cost-effectiveness and/or cost efficiency studies of targeted technologies, or courses of treatment), are by definition different of those of health services research (the multidisciplinary understanding of processes involved in health care).

The non-existence of health services research programs at a national level is associated with the weakness of central guidance often found in modern society. More prone to making decisions with anticipated success (e.g., standardizing the cost of drugs), the central authorities 'leave to the periphery' the approach to more delicate issues, such as collaborative practice between different disciplines. The point we want to make here, is that it cannot be expected that significant developments in health services research will originate at the so-called periphery (e.g., at the hospital); professionals will not easily change their behavior unless stimulated (and rewarded!) in the appropriate direction. In addition, and because of its proper nature, the development of health services research requires the contribution of different (academic) disciplines. This is not easily conducted by organizations at the 'periphery'. In fact, it would be fair to say that health services research funding does not exist in the hospitals of the countries of the EU.

Support

The study of health care issues, from a health services research perspective, requires an extraordinary effort of coordination. This coordination has three main objectives:

1. that the study takes place as designed, within the stated deadlines. The study, and its design, must be formulated and agreed by all participants. This should not become a major issue of concern, if the preparatory tasks before implementation are done appropriately. The same is not true regarding project deadlines. The involved teams have different research agendas, and different work flexibility, usually in relation to their own availability of resources. Strategies should be utilized to effectively enhance commitment, such as frequent reports, memos, phone calls, and the structured preparation of (co-authored) regular newsletters. The chosen strategies 'cannot fail', as they should comply with two principles: 'any failed deadline is a major problem'; and, 'nobody should wait for anybody'. The research groups should therefore agree, at the beginning of the study, that it will be preferable to reshape (re-evaluate) the study, or to eliminate a contribution, in the case of non-compliance to the agreements made.
2. that the individual research teams of the involved disciplines can contribute in entire scientific freedom and independence. This is the most crucial, and most difficult, aspect of the health services research approach. Society has not yet succeeded in acquainting the various disciplines with each other (besides being blocks of knowledge, disciplines are also social blocks). Inadequate professional contact between disciplines makes it rather difficult for them to understand each other (concerning for example social role, methodologies, professional language, etc.). It takes several years before professionals of different disciplines are able to can work effectively with each other. The classical situation (very much present in several projects subsidized by the EC) is that one discipline takes the lead in the interactive research process, therefore, decreasing the degree of input by the other disciplines (with obvious bias, from a health services resaerch perspective).

   The strategy followed by FRICE to fulfill this objective is summarized below. It should however be said, that the way in which inter-professional contacts are exchanged (particularly during meetings of the research groups) is essential to the success of the task. This inter-professional exchange should not (in our opinion cannot successfully) be conducted by a member of any of the participating disciplines. The chairman of these meetings should therefore be an independent scientist, with professional experience in the task of guiding people towards common objectives.
3. that the final integration of all contributions is the appropriate answer to the formulated question(s) of the study.

The System Approach

"A system is a collection of interrelated entities such that both the collection and the interrelationships together reduce local entropy (degree of disorder)" [6]. Systems can be closed, in which the input of the system is its own output (e.g., some physiologic processes), or open, in which case the input of a (sub)system is the output of another (sub)system; e.g., the patient condition produced in the operating room (output) is the input condition for the ICU. Therefore, although the treatment of a clinical condition may correspond to the professional interference in a closed system, the overall care of the patient is submitted to the functioning of various open (sub)systems.

The importance of the system approach in health care, is that the focus on one individual element of the system has to take into consideration the other elements in the system to which that element is interrelated. The size and complexity of the system can be large (e.g., the National Health Care System), but it can also be limited (e.g., mechanical ventilation in the ICU). Another important aspect of the system approach, is that interdependent elements in the system may belong to the domain of different disciplines (e.g., medicine, economics).

The overall assumption of the system approach is that the total system (and its outcome) is different from the simple sum of the entities (and their outcomes) comprising the system [7]. The magnitude of the mismatch (the total is not the sum of the parts), depends on the interrelations between the entities. In other words, the interrelations determine the role, and the relative weight, of each element of the system. Some of these interrelations are quantitative (e.g., related to physiologic parameters, staffing, financial resources, etc). Others are qualitative (e.g., related to organizational commitment, culture, professional education, etc).

The system approach allows the inclusion of both quantitative and qualitative interrelations in the same model [6,8]. Figure 2 depicts the research model of the EURICUS-projects, following the general system theory [9]. As can be seen in the figure, the input and output are used as reference in the study of the throughput.

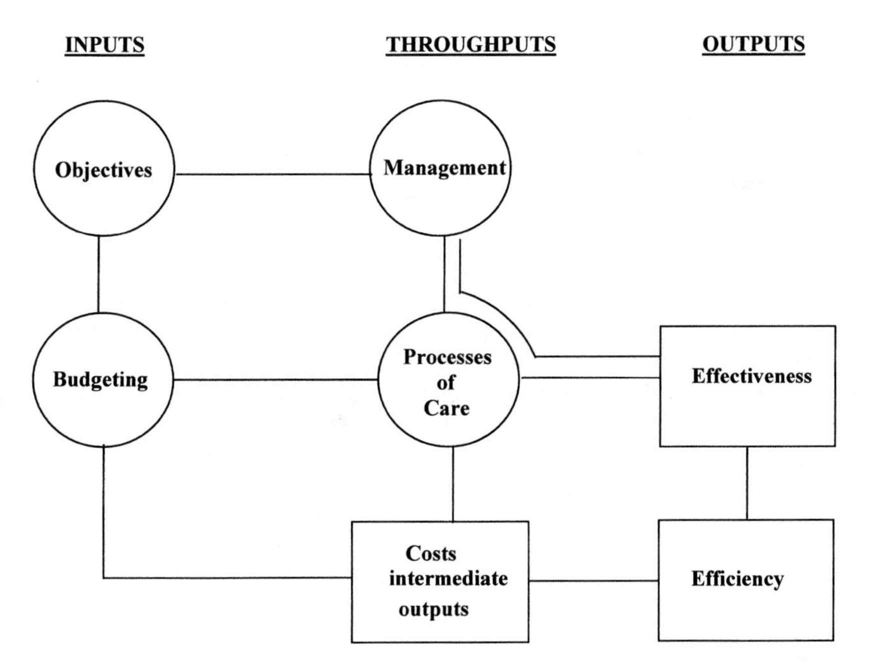

Fig. 2. Basic research model of the EURICUS program, studying the organization and management of the ICU from a health services research perspective [5]

The analysis of (sub)systems should be always approached from two perspectives [7]:

1) a focus on the elements of the system: studying the pieces composing each element under analysis, and understanding their interrelationships. This analysis is obviously necessary for it increases the detail of our knowledge about the system. It is however not sufficient, as it blurs the overview, and the understanding of the total system;
2) focus on the interrelationships of the elements within the system.

The Support Tasks in Health Services Research

The search for the optimal mix of individual team contribution with a strong central coordination, should be a constant concern in any health services research project. Participating teams will have to work together, as well as individually, at selected moments in the development of the project:

1. Study preparation must obviously involve a multidisciplinary, team approach and must include:
   - definition of the problem and of the research areas (disciplines) involved
   - formulation of the hypothesis and of the research model
   - design and setting of the study
   - methodology to follow, with focus on the instruments to be used.

Considering only the support tasks, the preparation of the study has to focus on the role that each individual-team will play in the various research phases of the study. The contribution of each research discipline will preferably be handled as a substudy of the project. The EURICUS-I study (or the effect of organization and management on the effectiveness and efficiency of ICUs), for example, included five substudies: patients and facilities, organization, personnel, culture, and finances [5]. The final research model will therefore address how the hypothesis formulated by each discipline will contribute to the testing of the overall hypothesis of the study.

The full preparation of a health services research project, before it can be implemented in the field, entails complex coordination tasks (bringing the various disciplines to reach a consensus), and is time consuming (about one year for each EURICUS project). Frequent discussion of issues among the disciplines must occur with at least two carefully planned plenary meetings: one for discussing the project and the work to be done; another for assessing the final work plan before its implementation. Each of these meetings has to be divided into three distinct parts: inventory (e.g., issues to be addressed, definitions, etc.); discussion (e.g., methodology, research tasks for each team, etc.); and final arrangements (deadlines, who does what, etc.). In the EURICUS studies, these meetings take about two and a half days, of which the two first parts take one day each. It is our strong conviction that this investment is very much necessary for the successful development of health services research projects. In each of these parts, general consensus has to be reached. The chairman of the meeting plays a key-role in these discussions. Whenever consensus is impossible, a group of experts is formed to report at a later date.

In order to strengthen the scientific interaction between the research teams, at the same time as supporting the coordination tasks, FRICE has established a Methodology Group (MG) to serve in the EURICUS projects. The MG, including respected methodologists and statisticians, operates independently as a subgroup of the Steering Committee of the studies.

2. The first analysis of the data collected has to be performed by each individual team, independently, and blindly, regarding the data of the other teams. This includes three steps:
   - general analysis of own data
   - preparing and testing own variables
   - selection of the variables that best explain the variance of the sub-study data

This step is followed by another multidisciplinary exercise:

3. The integration of the data collected concerning the different sub-studies. This integration includes:
   - selection of the variables testing the general hypothesis. The number of variables that can be included in the testing is obviously dependent on the size of the sample under analysis. In EURICUS-I, for example, although data concerning a large number of variables were collected, only 10 variables (the best two of each sub-study) were included in the formal analysis of the hypothesis of the study. This was because the data, to be analyzed at ICU level, only concerned 89 units.
   - cross exploration of data: understanding associations; generating new hypotheses.
4. Reporting, is the obvious final multidisciplinary exercise.

All the above steps need to be centrally coordinated. Central coordination, besides communication tasks (with the field and between sub-studies) also the creation of a well-staffed unit for building up the database, and for pooling, handling, management and analysis of the data.

Conclusion

Health services research (a true multidisciplinary approach to systems and methods of working) has become the method of choice for the planning, evaluation and improvement of health care systems.

At least during the initial phase, the implementation of health services research needs to be guided by a robust mechanism of coordination, so that the impact of the contribution of one discipline is not overshadowed by another.

References

1. Cresson E (1998) A turning point for community research. RTD Info 21, p3. European Commission, Brussels
2. The Fourth Framework Programme (1993) The European Commission, Brussels

3. The Fifth Framework Programme (1998) The European Commission, Brussels
4. Work Programme (1999) The quality of life and management of living resources. The Fifth Framework Programme. The European Commission, Brussels
5. Reis Miranda A, Ryan DW, Schaufeli WB, Fidler V (1997) Organization and Management of Intensive Care. A Prospective Study in 12 European Countries. Springer Verlag, Heidelberg
6. Hitchins DK (1992) Putting systems to work. John Wiley & Sons, Chichester, New York
7. Veld J (1992) Analyse van organisatieproblemen. Een toepassing van denken in systemen en processen. Stenfert Kroese Uitgevers, Antwerp
8. Checkland P, Scholes J (1990) Soft systems methodology in action. John Wiley & Sons, Chichester, New York
9. Boulding KE (1956) General systems theory: the skeleton of science. Management Science, pp 197–208

Hypothesis Generation: Asking the Right Question, Getting the Correct Answer

D. C. Angus and P. Pronovost

Learning Points

- To be valuable, a research question must be important, must lead to new knowledge, must be relatively simple to understand, and must be practical to implement
- In critical care, research is largely driven by the healthcare industry, whose definition of 'important' may not coincide with that of the patient or society
- The threats to finding a correct answer to a research question are random and systematic errors. Both can be minimized by correct study design
- Large-scale randomized controlled trials (RCTs) evaluating the efficacy of new therapies in critical care may be more successful if:
  - Sample size is increased
  - Entry criteria are based on well-demarcated disease processes rather than loosely-defined syndrome definitions
  - Potentially confounding co-interventions are better standardized through greater use of protocols
- Important adjuncts to the traditional efficacy RCT include effectiveness studies, observational studies, cost-effectiveness studies, and studies that evaluate longer-term patient-centered outcomes

Today, the critical care literature is challenging the status quo with considerable vigor. Arguably, every practicing intensivist was trained to manage hypoxic, shocked patients with central hemodynamic monitoring and full ventilatory support. Yet, recent evidence suggests that central hemodynamic monitoring with the pulmonary artery catheter may be harmful and our traditional approach to mechanical ventilation likely also kills. These findings are only examples from the rapidly expanding medical literature that is of variable quality and frequently contradictory. Assessing and intergrating new evidence in an environment that demands careful cost control coupled with the provision of up-to-date, optimal care is the new ground zero for the modern clinician. Requisite skills for these tasks go beyond clinical acumen and include a basic understanding of clinical epidemiology, health economics, and health services administration and research.

Introduction

With its state-of-the-art, often futuristic technologies, intensive care has long been touted as an example of '21st century' medicine. Yet, as we now enter that century, intensive care arguably finds itself with a reputation somewhat tarnished. For example, the pulmonary artery catheter, a mainstay in the management of the critically ill, has been recently associated with harm to intensive care unit (ICU) patients [1]. Similarly, emerging data regarding mechanical ventilation practice suggests that for years we may have been harming our patients with excessive tidal volumes and ventilatory pressures [2,3]. And although we have made considerable in-roads in our understanding of the pathophysiology of sepsis and multiple systems organ failure, our field is littered with potential therapies that failed to improve outcomes in clinical trials.

Not only have there been problems with our search for safe and effective therapies and interventions, but also there have been issues regarding how we staff our ICUs. There is an ever growing body of literature demonstrating wide variation in practice styles, with many studies showing that these variations are associated with clinically meaningful differences in outcomes [4]. Despite these uncertainties, we continue to spend more and more money on intensive care, much of which is consumed in the care of an increasingly elderly population, often with controversy over the value of this care. Furthermore, we have been accused of often providing inadequate care at the end-of-life [5] and there has been a call for less technology and more compassion in our practice.

These concerns force us to consider more carefully the value ICU care has for patients, payers, and society. This requires first that we conduct evaluation of new and existing therapies with the highest scientific rigor. These evaluations should include consideration of how our therapies impact on outcomes valued by patients and society. We must also determine the financial consequences of both our interventions and the overall delivery of critical care services, and we must measure how well scientific breakthroughs actually translate into improved practice and patient outcomes.

In this chapter, we will briefly discuss the importance of asking the right question; review the sources of errors in clinical research and how these impact patient selection, sample size determination, and study protocols; discuss the various outcome measures used in clinical research; and discuss issues in the selection of study design including experimental (randomized) and observational studies as well as cost-effectiveness analyses and decision models.

Asking the Right Question

The How ...?

In the quest for value, the critical care researcher must begin by asking the right question. Four characteristics of the right question are that it must be important, it must lead to new knowledge, it must be relatively simple to understand, and it must be practical to implement [6]. The common management quote "the answer is in the question" directly applies to clinical research. Indeed, the specific research question determines what answers we will obtain as well as the requirements for the study design and conduct. For example, studies evaluating efficacy of a therapy are best conducted using a randomized design, studies evaluating incidence rates are best conducted with a cohort study, and studies evaluating a rare outcome are best using a case control study.

The Who ...?

Although the researcher is free to choose the research question, the questions that are actually asked (or tested) are driven by the agendas of numerous stakeholders. One set of stakeholders is national government funding agencies, such as the Medical Research Councils in the United Kingdom, Canada and Australia and the National Institutes of Health (NIH) in the United States. Priorities for these government agencies may have important ramifications for critical care research. For example, the NIH is organized into several sections, none of which focus specifically on critical care. Consequently, there is no coordinated federal program to help develop a focused research agenda or further critical care research.

Another key stakeholder that has influenced the critical care research agenda is the pharmaceutical industry. The vast majority of large multicenter trials of sepsis and acute respiratory distress syndrome (ARDS) have been funded by pharmaceutical companies who are interested in learning whether their proprietary products influence short-term mortality in critical illness. These studies are explicitly targeted at gaining regulatory approval for the product under study. Although such studies are common in all fields of medicine, the concern for critical care is that they are the predominant type of large clinical trial, resulting in a research agenda that is driven principally by the financial concerns of the pharmaceutical industry.

The critical care clinical researchers may also be the principal stakeholders influencing a research question though these questions generally are translated into smaller trials. A notable exception is the Canadian Critical Care Trials Group, which has conducted several large randomized controlled trials (RCTs) assessing important clinical questions such as the optimal transfusion threshold [7]. The stakeholders who have the least impact on the current research agenda are patients and families. However, as healthcare consumers gain more voice and influence at national levels, we can expect greater pressure on the primary funding stakeholders to request studies that consider more explicitly patient and family preferences.

Getting a Correct Answer: Reducing Error

After formulating a question, the researcher conducts the study and the results can be 'true', due to random error, or due to systematic error. The risk for both random and systematic error can be greatly reduced through appropriate study design.

Random Error

Random error can be defined as unexplained fluctuations [8]. A hypothesis test is subject to two types of random error: type I (false positive), and type II (false negative). A type I error occurs when there is no treatment effect and the investigator wrongly concludes that there is one. A type II error occurs when there is a treatment effect and the investigator wrongly concludes that there is none. Power is the probability of finding a treatment effect if one exists and is equal to 1 – probability of a type II error. The risk of a type one error is easy to control in the study design and is determined by the critical value, or the point above which a test will be deemed statistically significant. If the value of a test statistic is above the critical value, we would conclude that there is a treatment effect (reject the null hypothesis).

The concept of a critical region is graphically represented in Figure 1, which shows the distribution of a treatment effect (Δ) under the null hypothesis (H_0) and the alternative hypothesis (H_a). The short vertical line represents the critical value. A p value quantifies the risk of a type I error and is interpreted as the probability of observing this result or one more extreme if the null hypothesis were true. Thus, the p-value helps the investigator evaluate the evidence for or against the null hypothesis (not the alternative hypothesis) and not the magnitude of the treatment effect [8]. The risk of a type I error can increase when multiple tests are performed, either when investigators analyze data during the course of the trial (such as when determining if the study should be terminated) or when many outcomes or treatment groups are analyzed. By having preplanned stopping rules, we can reduce the risk of type I error.

The risk of a type II error is dependent on three factors: the critical value, the size of the treatment effect (difference between the control group (H_0) and the treatment group (H_a) in Figure 1), and the width of the distribution of the out-

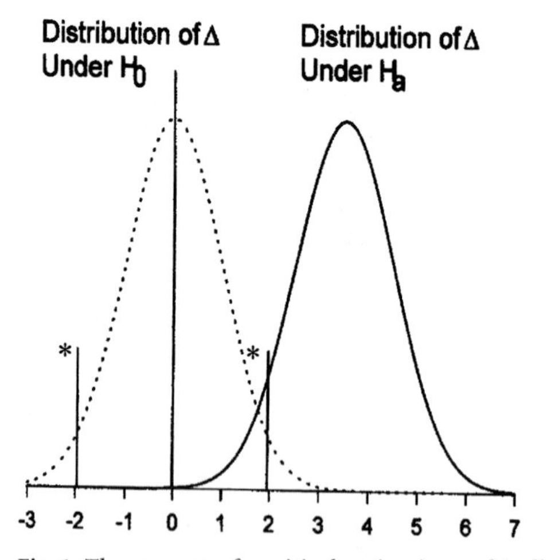

Fig. 1. The concept of a critical region is graphically represented showing the distribution of a treatment effect (Δ) under the null hypothesis (H_0) and the alternative hypothesis (H_a). The short vertical line represents the critical value. (Adapted from [8] with permission)

come in the treatment group often called the alternative hypothesis (H_a) [8]. As discussed above, the investigator chooses the critical region and also determines the size of the treatment effect that is clinically relevant and plausible to achieve. When calculating the sample size for a study, we can estimate that the therapy will have a large treatment effect and reduce the required sample size. However, the study would be underpowered to detect smaller treatment effects that may be clinically relevant, often resulting in a negative study that is underpowered and difficult to interpret. In critically ill patients, the required sample size may be difficult to estimate due to misclassification or the erroneous classification of an individual or value into a category other than the one assigned (See later section on 'Selecting the right patients and the problem of poor case definition').

Systematic Error: Bias and Confounding

The other component of error is systematic error. Unlike random error, systematic error has a direction and magnitude. Though these may be difficult to quantitate, systematic error is usually easy to detect and can often be controlled with rigorous study design [8]. Bias is a process at any stage of research tending to produce results that depart systematically from the truth. There are many sources of bias in clinical research and Sackett has provided us with a classification system for biases [9]. To simplify this concept, we can classify bias into selection bias, information bias, and statistical bias. The first two are generally correctable with attention to study design, while statistical bias is generally correctable with use of alternative statistical tests.

Selection bias occurs when patients in the treatment group are different from patients in the control group. Randomization is the best means to reduce selection bias because randomization will balance both known and unknown confounders equally between the treatment and control groups. A confounder is a variable, such as age, that is associated with treatment and outcome, and thus may distort the relationship between treatment and outcome. When a study is observational (Fig. 2), we must carefully evaluate for selection bias generally through the use of risk adjustment.

We usually think of patient characteristics as confounding variables. However, characteristics of the hospital or ICU may also be confounders. For example, high-risk surgery patients who do not have daily rounds by an ICU physician have a 3-fold increased risk of in-hospital mortality [10]. Imbalances between the treatment and control groups in patients that have daily rounds by an ICU physician can easily mask most treatment effects and such differences must be accounted for in the study design. This can be accomplished by restricting the choice of the ICUs to study, matching, or stratifying by ICU characteristics, and using constrained randomization [8, 11]. Another type of bias is information bias, which refers to imperfect information on disease (outcome), exposure, or confounders. One common type of information bias is assessment bias where the investigator assesses the outcome differently for the treatment and control groups. Masking (blinding) can significantly reduce assessment bias [8].

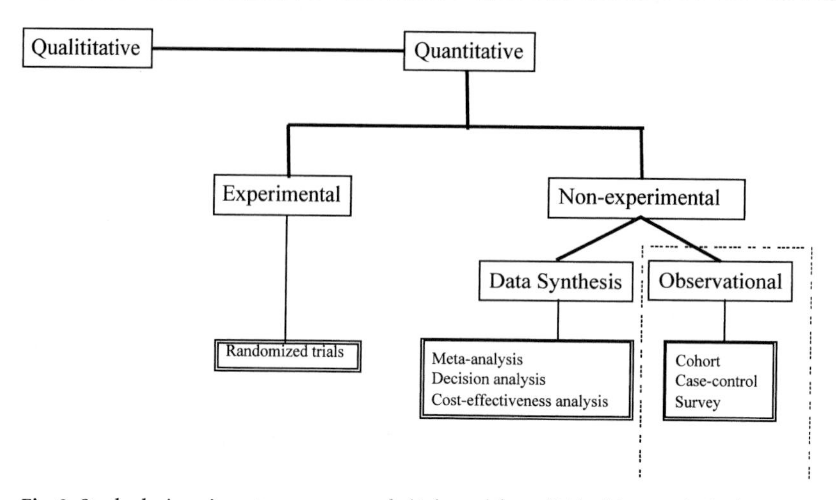

Fig. 2. Study designs in outcomes research (Adapted from [11] with permission)

Although the term 'double blinded' is used liberally as a seal for quality in a clinical trial, double blinding requires that neither the patients nor the investigators are aware of treatment assignment. This requires that the therapies look, feel and taste the same and that the therapy does not cause changes in some other parameter (such as gastric pH increasing with H_2 blockers) that may inform the investigators of the treatment assignment [12]. The need to blind the investigator is increased when outcomes are subjective. Blinding may be especially difficult in research on acutely ill patients because the treatment is often an invasive procedure (surgery or pulmonary artery catheter) that is difficult to blind.

Getting a Correct Answer: Selecting the Right Patients and the Problem of Poor Case-Definition

Currently, to identify patients for sepsis and ARDS studies, researchers consider a constellation of clinical and laboratory data [13-15]. Through mechanisms such as consensus conferences, investigators have standardized the criteria to diagnose these diseases and may have enhanced the reliability with which we then identify these patients. Nevertheless, there remain significant problems with the accuracy and validity of our definitions leading to misclassification and an increased risk for type II error [16, 17].

To illustrate, we can compare sepsis to acute myocardial infarction, a condition for which there have been several successful interventional trials. Acute myocardial infarction is relatively easy to confirm early in the disease process, and the extent of the infarction is easy both to measure (by serum markers, electrocardiogram [EKG], and cardiac imaging studies), and to correlate with outcome. Sepsis, on the other hand, is a vague term and lacks explicit diagnostic tests to confirm the diagnosis. As a result, it is easy to misclassify septic patients as nonseptic and nonseptic patients as septic. Furthermore, the subsequent course and outcome of the septic patient is not necessarily correlated with the management of, and recovery from, the event, making it difficult to differentiate between those who 'died of', as opposed to 'died with', sepsis.

To improve the selection process and better screen and stratify patients, researchers have suggested using a risk score to select patients in a medium range of risk (e.g., 30-80% risk of hospital mortality) who are most likely to benefit [18-20]. Others have argued that we need to identify patients earlier in the disease process, during the prodromal period, known as the systemic inflammatory response syndrome (SIRS), if we are to maximize the chance of eliciting a significant effect.

Intuitively, early intervention seems likely to provide the most promising results [21]. Unfortunately, several problems remain with this concept. First, SIRS as an early marker of sepsis is both insensitive and nonspecific [22]. Second, just like sepsis, SIRS is based on a rather broad set of criteria of clinical and laboratory data not closely linked to an underlying physiologic event [22]. Third, perhaps as a consequence of the broadness of its definition, studies of the prevalence and outcome of SIRS have reported different estimates of mortality and the rates of sepsis, severe sepsis, and septic shock [23-27]. Fourth, there is increasing evidence that SIRS is only one of several clinical presentations in patients at risk of developing sepsis [28]. As a result of these problems, studies that enroll patients with SIRS will misclassify patients with sepsis (sensitivity problem) and without sepsis (specificity problem), leading to a further increase in sample size and, consequently, cost and logistic problems for the study.

Thus, an option to better delineate which patients to study will be to develop rapid tests that allow a more accurate determination of the specific underlying pathophysiologic process. An alternative is to develop risk stratification models that separate modifiable and nonmodifiable risks (Fig. 3). Such risk models might include, for example, the response of physiologic parameters to standard therapy.

Getting a Correct Answer: Determining Sample Size

When determining the sample size for a study, we generate an estimate of a therapy's effect that ought to be both large enough to be clinically relevant and small enough to be plausibly achievable.

What is a Clinically Relevant Effect Size?

Clinical relevance is subjective, varies with different stakeholders, and is difficult to consider in isolation from other influencing factors. Such factors include: prior beliefs and assumptions regarding the anticipated cost and side-effects of the therapy; the nature of the underlying clinical problem; the availability of healthcare resources; the difficulty inherent in conducting a study to detect small changes; the available funding for the study [29]. Consequently, clinical relevance varies widely between studies.

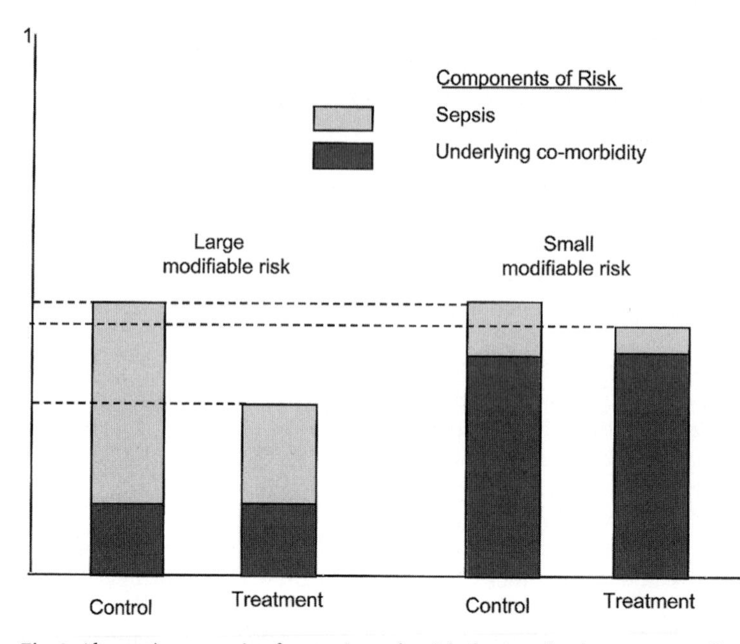

Fig. 3. Alternative scenarios for sepsis study with therapy that has a strong effect on sepsis process (Adapted from [29] with permission)

A striking example of a 'fluctuating' effect size can be seen examining the GUSTO (Global Utilization of Streptokinase and tPA for Occluded Coronary Arteries) studies. The recent GUSTO III study of alternative tissue plasminogen activators (tPA) in the treatment of acute myocardial infarction was powered to detect a relative change in mortality of at least 20% [30]. This study failed to find a difference between therapies and the investigators concluded the two therapies were equivalent. The choice of a 20% difference in mortality was deemed clinically relevant in the accompanying editorial [31]. Yet, the GUSTO investigators powered an earlier study (GUSTO I) [32], comparing the first generation tPA to streptokinase, to detect a relative change of 12.5% (absolute change of 1% from 8% to 7%). Though this study was successful and led to the subsequent widespread adoption of tPA in clinical practice over the cheaper and marginally less effective streptokinase, it would have been deemed ineffective had the investigators used their subsequent GUSTO III estimate of clinical relevance.

What is Plausibly Achievable?

To estimate the effect size the therapy might plausibly achieve, investigators must adopt a Bayesian consideration of prior evidence [33]. When designing a cardiology trial, investigators can look to size and design characteristics of the multiple successful prior studies, often of similar therapeutic agents. However, with the exception of the recent successful studies of low-volume ventilation strategies, intensivists have no such references to call upon and must infer a plausible effect. Prior phase III trials in the critically ill are virtually all negative and human data on the therapy in question are usually only available for phase I studies of healthy volunteers or for phase II studies designed principally to evaluate the safety, toxicity, and dosing of the therapy – not to measure effect. Frequently, phase I and II studies are unavailable and investigators must rely on animal studies that are most often conducted on animals without chronic illness. The treatment effect achieved in these studies may be significantly reduced when studying animals (and people) with chronic diseases [21, 34].

The implications for sample size in clinical studies are profound. The typical phase III RCT in sepsis and ARDS has been conducted on less than 1,500 patients and often only several hundred patients are studied. Typically, these studies are designed with the assumption that septic patients have a hospital mortality of around 40% and that the therapy under consideration will reduce the mortality by 25%, an absolute change of 10% (mortality decreased from 40% to 30%). When constructed to have 80% power, this would require 750 patients, and, at 90% power, 1,200 patients. The GUSTO I study [32] on the other hand, required 40,000 patients to detect a 12.5% relative difference (1% absolute difference) at 90% power. If we apply the same relative change to a sepsis trial (i.e., to drop mortality from 40% to 35%), we need 3,000 patients at 80% power and 3,700 at 90% power. A sepsis study designed to detect a similar absolute change (i.e., a 1% drop from 40% to 39%) would require 76,000 patients at 80% power and 100,000 patients at 90%.

There is no *a priori* reason to believe that therapies for sepsis are significantly more efficacious than therapies for acute myocardial infarction. Rather, the critical care researcher usually estimates large treatment effects because smaller effects (and the accompanying increase in sample size) may be practically or financially impossible. The decision whether to conduct an RCT, weighing its likely cost against the benefit derived from the information it would yield, can be modeled using simulation techniques. Such decision-making models might better quantitate which trials we can and cannot afford to do.

Getting a Correct Answer: Using Protocols to Control the Process of Care

There is wide variability in how clinicians manage patients with critical illness such as sepsis or ARDS. For example, it is unclear whether the patient with ARDS should be managed 'wet' or 'dry' or be positioned prone or supine. Similarly, the decision whether to use pressors or fluids in the management of septic hypotension is made differently by different clinicians. This variation in the management of a critically ill patient, leads to 'noise' that may quickly obliterate any 'signal' of effect from the therapy under study, increasing the risk for type II error.

While the use of protocols may reduce noise in a study, protocols may introduce systematic error. In weaning trials, for example, the particular weaning protocol used may force a minimum length of stay that differs for the treatment and control groups [35]. Nevertheless, the appropriate use of protocols to reduce the signal-to-noise ratio ought to help reduce systematic error and type II error.

The use of such protocols, however, moves the care of the patient further away from daily practice, reducing the generalizability of the studies' findings. Most RCTs are efficacy studies in that they evaluate how something works in an artificial world where many variables are controlled, often with the use of protocols. While this control is necessary to maintain the internal validity of the study, it may limit our ability to apply the results of the clinical trial to a population of patients outside the trial. On the other hand, effectiveness studies evaluate how a treatment works 'in the real world', have less internal validity (i.e., ability to make an inference without systematic error), and have increased generalizability or external validity.

This difference between efficacy studies and effectiveness studies and the potential problem of assuming the generalizability of an RCT is illustrated by carotid endarterectomy surgery. The Asymptomatic Carotid Atherosclerosis Study (ACAS) [36], an efficacy study, found that the 30-day mortality for asymptomatic patients having carotid endarterectomy was 1/1000. Coincident with the publication of this trial, there was a significant increase in the rate of this operation [37]. However, an effectiveness study revealed that the mortality for asymptomatic patients having a carotid endarterectomy was 1/100, ten times greater than in the clinical trial [38]. This difference in mortality is likely due to the strict entry criteria for the RCT, as patients with comorbid diseases, patients over 79 years old, and hospitals and surgeons with poor outcomes were excluded.

This example demonstrates the need for observational studies to ensure that results achieved in RCTs are being achieved in daily clinical practice. This difficulty replicating trial results may be particularly problematic in populations of critically ill patients when the success of the intervention may depend on provider and hospital factors such as the organization of the ICU [10].

Getting a Correct Answer: Choosing the Right Outcome

When designing a study, the researcher must select a primary outcome variable. This variable is usually determined by the research question and is used to estimate power and sample size. We will briefly review outcome measures commonly used in clinical research in the ICU (Table 1).

Mortality

Short-term, all-cause mortality has traditionally been used as the endpoint in clinical trials of critical illness because critical illness is thought to be acute. The two traditional short-term measures have been in-hospital mortality and a fixed time-point mortality (e.g., day 28 or day 30) [39–44]. The short-term mortality rate may arbitrarily fail to capture the duration of the episode of critical illness. For example, a patient with severe sepsis and ARDS may still be critically ill and require life support at day 28 yet be called a survivor even though he may die within one or two weeks following the endpoint. When using a fixed time period, the estimation of other end points (especially resource utilization) is also problematic [45]. Furthermore, because it is difficult to distinguish between patients

Table 1. Outcome measures used in critical care research

Outcome measure	Time Frame	Advantage	Disadvantage
Short-term mortality	In-hospital, 28 day	Likely linked to processes of care/easy to obtain	May be less informative than long-term mortality
Long-term mortality	6 month, 1 year	More relevant because it captures entire risk period	Difficult to obtain. Patients lost to follow up
Morbidity: physiologic	Generally in-hospital	Has biologic plausibility	Often a weak relationship between physiologic measure and outcome
Morbidity: economic	Generally in-hospital such as length of stay	Easy to obtain	Distorts cost-effectiveness ratio. Should generally be avoided as measures of morbidity
Morbidity: quality of life	Could be short or long term	Important to patients	Methodologic issues in measuring quality of life in critically ill patients remain
Cost efficacy	Short or long term	Less risk for error due to internal validity	Difficult to generalize
Cost effectiveness	Short or long term	More closely represents 'real world'	Greater risk for error
Patient-centered outcomes	Long-term	Important to patients and includes functional status, quality of life, satisfaction with care	Generally unexplored in critical care research, methodologic issues (such as instrument development) remain

who die with, versus from, critical illness, it may be difficult to distinguish between all-cause mortality and cause-specific mortality.

A critical care patient cohort should be followed until the episode of critical illness has resolved. However, the duration of critical illness is generally unknown and follow-up for several months beyond enrollment can be expensive and time-consuming. A pragmatic solution is to better delineate the relationship between short-term and long-term mortality in epidemiologic studies, which may lead us to a better understanding of the implications of differences in short-term mortality.

Morbidity

Much of the value of critical care may be derived from the mitigation of morbidity. Unfortunately, critical care may save a life only to produce a survivor with low quality of life and high reliance on continued, expensive healthcare. For this reason, measures of outcome other than mortality are important. There are several approaches to evaluate morbidity. First, we can use a 'physiological' approach; morbidity can be recorded by assessing change in organ function [46, 47]. Second, morbidity can be considered in terms of economics (e.g., hospital costs, lost wages, cost of home help, or new requirement for chronic dialysis) [48, 49]. Third, the impact of illness on quality of life can serve as a measure of morbidity [48-55]. Of these three, the first is gaining favor in critical care, the second continues to be used confusedly, and the third is gaining favor outside of critical care.

Measuring Costs as Well as Clinical Outcomes

The reasons to perform a cost-analysis are to help determine whether a new therapy is worth using with respect to existing therapies, and whether existing resources should be allocated to pay for a new therapy [56]. Thus, a cost analysis could estimate the likely costs and effects in the community and express those estimates in units comparable to other cost analyses [57]. Incorporating into an RCT the elements necessary to generate cost-effectiveness estimates is somewhat complicated.

Cost-effectiveness or cost-efficacy? Until we have conducted RCTs that show a positive result, we are likely to focus on efficacy trials. In other words, we will do our best to obtain a study result that is 'true' (free from random and systematic error). If a cost analysis is part of the trial, and the estimate of effect is generated from the trial, then the cost analysis will be a cost-efficacy ratio, rather than a cost-effectiveness ratio. The differences in such ratios are not trivial [58]. If the investigator is interested in cost-effectiveness, the study design can be adapted to measure effectiveness [56–58].

Alternatively, the costs and effects generated from the study can be entered into an economic decision model and exposed to a sensitivity analysis driven by observational data about current practice patterns and assumptions of likely use of the therapy if approved. Such models could determine the impact of loosening patient eligibility criteria (treating additional patients not likely to benefit), treating patients with alternative therapies, and prescribing the therapy inappropriately. Recent guidelines from the US Public Health System Panel on Cost-effectiveness in Health and Medicine (PCEHM) should lead to improved standardization and comparability of such models in healthcare [59].

Difficulty with combined end-points: The unit of effect, or utility, recommended by the PCEHM is quality-adjusted survival [57]. This allows comparison of different cost analyses to each other. We rarely measure quality of life directly. Rather, we estimate quality of life using simulation modeling. Unless there is a belief that the two treatment arms will affect quality of life differently (an assumption largely untested), the error associated with such estimates will largely be a function of the effect of the therapy on survival. On the other hand, if we do not set mortality as the primary end-point, we run the risk of creating uncertainty not over the magnitude of effect but of whether there is an effect at all.

To illustrate, the recent NINOS study of inhaled NO in the treatment of hypoxic distress of the newborn was powered for the combined end-point of extracoporeal membrane oxygenation (ECMO) or death [60]. The study was terminated when an overwhelming difference in this combined end-point was measured. However, there was no significant difference in mortality. When constructing a cost-effectiveness model, it is unclear how to treat ECMO [61]. Theoretically, ECMO is a resource, and is thus associated with a cost. Therefore, it should be placed in the numerator. Death, on the other hand, is placed in the denominator. In short, the combined end-point is split. Once split, we re-introduce the uncertainty (i.e., no statistical significance) of whether inhaled NO achieved an effect. A cost model can still be constructed and exposed to a sensitivity analysis where the model is tested across the confidence boundaries of the costs and effects [61].

An even more complicated situation may occur with the use of organ-failure-free days. For example, using ventilator-free days (VFDs) in an ARDS trial, we may create a scenario where we have a significant decrease in VFDs with no significant change in mortality. What would this mean in terms of costs and effects? VFDs are poor proxies for cost since they do not account for potential differences in the length of stay of non-survivors (all non-survivors receive a value of zero even though a therapy may well delay the onset of death by temporarily ameliorating the illness). Therefore, VFDs should not be placed in the numerator. They may also be poor proxies for survival since those alive but ventilated at the end of follow-up are counted as equal to non-survivors, regardless of whether they are subsequently weaned and discharged home alive. Thus, we have a single significant end-point, the meaning of which is unclear with regard to both costs and effects. Such data may leave clinicians and policy-makers uncertain over the implications of the trial, and with a need for further trials.

Patient-Centered Outcomes: Patient centered outcomes such as quality of life, functional status, and satisfaction with care are increasingly being used in clinical research including critical care [62]. Nevertheless, several methodological issues remain. First, we must continue to develop valid instruments that can discriminate between 'diseased and nondiseased' patients and that are responsive to changes in a critically ill patient population. Second, we need to conduct epidemiologic studies to define the 'natural history' of critical illness on quality of life and functional status. These will likely come about by routinely measuring patient-centered outcomes on critically ill patients. Third, we will need to decide how to incorporate predictions of quality of life and functional status into patient care. This third issue is similar to the concerns with incorporating mortality prediction models to individual patient care. Though the probabilities in individual patients are uncertain, such information may help patients and families make informed clinical decisions.

Getting a Correct Answer: Choosing the Right Study Design

A randomized design provides the strongest evidence to make an inference about the efficacy of a therapy. This is largely because randomization balances both known and unknown confounders equally between treatment and control groups, eliminating the risk of selection bias. Indeed, when randomization is coupled with blinding (masking) to reduce the risk of assessment bias, the risk for systematic error is significantly reduced. Because of this, we believe randomization should be incorporated into a study design whenever possible. Nevertheless, there are ethical, practical, and logistical reasons why randomization is sometimes not possible, and in these cases, alternative study designs must be sought.

Observational Outcomes Studies as Alternatives to RCTs

A framework for the approach to study design is provided in Figure 2. The principal alternative to the RCT involves observation rather than experiment, and we have become much more sophisticated in the design and execution of observational outcomes studies. In critiquing such studies, rather than making the knee-jerk response 'just a retrospective study', we should consider carefully whether the study result is subject to random and systematic error. This critique must evaluate the source of data, the risk of type I and type II errors, the method of risk adjustment, the risk for additional confounding variables, and the risk for misclassification.

There are several techniques that attempt to account for known confounding variables, including matching, stratification, and regression modeling. All have advantages and disadvantages, and it is incumbent on the investigators to defend the rationale for their choice and present evidence supporting how well their technique performed [63]. Nonetheless, with observational studies the reader must ask the question, "Is there anything unaccounted for in this study that I believe could explain the magnitude and direction of effect otherwise attributable to the intervention?"[11].

It may appear that the alternative to randomization is quite burdensome. However, observational outcomes studies are very powerful tools for addressing many questions that RCTs cannot address, including measuring the effect of harmful substances (e.g., smoking and other carcinogens), organizational structures (e.g., payer status, open versus closed ICUs), or geography (e.g., rural versus urban access to healthcare). In addition, some questions cannot be studied with an RCT for ethical reasons. Furthermore, we should even be prepared to deal with situations such as the carotid endarterectomy story, where a well-conducted RCT and a well-conducted observational outcome study yield opposite results, and conclude that both studies are correct. Experimental and observational studies are needed to help inform clinical and policy decision making.

Conclusion

To ask the right question, and get a correct answer, is a challenge that requires a multi-part solution. First, to strengthen the likelihood of asking 'good' questions, we must specify a research agenda that is carefully debated, and not simply reactive to the particular needs of one stakeholder. Second, the funding for these questions must be adequate to at least address priorities and must be allocated on the merit of these priorities. Third, we must select the appropriate study design for the question asked, appreciating that the RCT may often not be the ideal approach. Fourth, when conducting RCTs, we should consider carefully the ramifications of decisions we make regarding patient selection, nature of intervention, and standardization of the process of care. Fifth, where appropriate, we should consider complimenting evidence from RCTs with alternative studies, such as well-designed observational outcomes studies or decision models. Sixth, regardless of study design, we should consider inclusion of patient and society valued outcomes such as long-term survival, quality of life, and direct and indirect costs of care. With this expanded, and more proactive, approach to the clinical research agenda in critical care, we can look forward to acquiring information that is more relevant, more accurate, and more focused on improving the value of critical care services for patients, providers, payers, and policy makers.

References

1. Connors AFJ, Speroff T, Dawson N V, et al (1996) The effectiveness of right heart catheterization in the initial care of critically ill patients. JAMA 276:889–897
2. Amato MB, Barbas C S, Medeiros D M, et al (1998) Effect of a protective-ventilation strategy on mortality in the acute respiratory distress syndrome. N Engl J Med 338:347–354
3. The NIH/NHLBI ARDS Network (1999) Low tidal ventilation is routinely used in patients with early acute lung injury. Am J Respir Crit Care Med 159:A694–A694 (Abst)
4. Pronovost P, Angus D C (1999) Determining the value of critical care. Clin Pulm Med 6:302–308
5. SUPPORT Principal Investigators (1995) A controlled trial to improve care for seriously ill hospitalized patients: the study to understand prognoses and preferences for outcomes and risks of treatments. JAMA 274:1591–1598
6. Kahn CR (1994) Picking a research problem. The critical decision. N Engl J Med 330:1530–1533
7. Hebert PC, Wells G, Blajchman M A, et al (1999) A multicenter, randomized, controlled clinical trial of transfusion requirements in critical care. Transfusion Requirements in Critical Care Investigators, Canadian Critical Care Trials Group. N Engl J Med 340:409–417
8. Piantadosi S (1997) Clinical trials: A methodological perspective. John Wiley and Sons, New York

9. Sackett DL (1979) Bias in analytic research. J Chronic Dis 32:51–63
10. Pronovost PJ, Jencks M, Dorman T et al (1999) Organizational characteristics of intensive care units related to outcomes of abdominal aortic surgery. JAMA 281:1310–1312
11. Rubenfeld GD, Angus DC, Pinsky MR, et al (1999) Outcomes research in critical care: Results of the American Thoracic Society Critical Care Assembly Workshop on outcomes research. Am J Respir Crit Care Med 160:358–367
12. Cook DJ, Fuller HD, Guyatt GH, et al (1994) Risk factors for gastrointestinal bleeding in critically ill patients. N Engl J Med 330:377–381
13. Bone RC, Balk R A, Cerra F B, et al (1992) Definitions for sepsis and organ failure and guidelines for the use of innovative therapies in sepsis. Chest 101:1644–1655
14. Angus DC, Kramer DJ (1993) Bacteremia and sepsis: Clinical perspectives. In: Pinsky MR, Dhainaut JF (eds) Pathophysiologic Foundations of Critical Care Medicine. Williams and Wilkins, Baltimore, pp 96–111
15. Bernard GR, Artigas A, Brigham KL, et al (1994) The American-European Consensus Conference on ARDS. Definitions, mechanisms, relevant outcomes, and clinical trial coordination. Am J Respir Crit Care Med 149:818–824
16. Knaus WA, Sun X, Nystrom O, Wagner DP (1992) Evaluation of definitions for sepsis. Chest 101:1656–1662
17. Rubenfeld GD, Doyle RL, Matthay MA (1995) Evaluation of definitions of ARDS. Am J Respir Crit Care Med 151:1270–1271
18. Knaus WA, Harrell FE J, Fisher CJ, et al (1993) The clinical evaluation of new drugs for sepsis. A prospective study design based on survival analysis. JAMA 270:1233–1241
19. Marshall JC, Cook DJ, Christou NV, Bernard GR, Sprung CL, Sibbald WJ (1995) Multiple organ dysfunction score: a reliable descriptor of a complex clinical outcome. Crit Care Med 23:1638–1652
20. Vincent JL, Moreno R, Takala J, et al (1996) The SOFA (Sepsis-related Organ Failure Assessment) score to describe organ dysfunction/failure. Intensive Care Med 22:707–710
21. Piper RD, Cook DJ, Bone RC, Sibbald WJ (1996) Introducing critical appraisal to studies of animal models investigating novel therapies in sepsis. Crit Care Med 24:2059–2070
22. Vincent JL (1997) Dear SIRS, I'm sorry to say that I don't like you. Crit Care Med 25:372–374
23. Rangel-Frausto MS, Pittet D, Costigan M, Hwang T, Davis CS, Wenzel RP (1995) The natural history of the systemic inflammatory response syndrome (SIRS). A prospective study. JAMA 273:117–123
24. Salvo I, de Cian W, Musicco M, et al (1995) The Italian SEPSIS study: preliminary results on the incidence and evolution of SIRS, sepsis, severe sepsis and septic shock. Intensive Care Med 21:S244–S249
25. Sands KE, Bates DW, Lanken PN, et al (1997) Epidemiology of sepsis syndrome in 8 academic medical centers. Academic Medical Center Consortium Sepsis Project Working Group. JAMA 278:234–240
26. Dougnac A, Angus DC, Hernandez G, et al (1996) Severe SIRS in Chile: Natural history and new organ dysfunction scores. Intensive Care Med 22 (suppl 3):321 (Abst)
27. Angus, D. C., Dougnac, A., Hernandez, et al (1996) Sepsis and SIRS: Are we any nearer to consensus? Intensive Care Med 22 (suppl 3):273 (Abst)
28. Bone RC, Grodzin CJ, Balk RA (1997) Sepsis: a new hypothesis for pathogenesis of the disease process. Chest 112:235–243
29. Angus DC (1998) Discourse on method: Measuring the value of new therapies in intensive care. In: Vincent JL (ed), Yearbook of Intensive Care and Emergency Medicine, Springer-Verlag, Berlin, pp 263–279
30. Anonymous (1997) A comparison of reteplase with alteplase for acute myocardial infarction. The Global Use of Strategies to Open Occluded Coronary Arteries (GUSTO III) Investigators. N Engl J Med 337:1118–1123
31. Ware JH, Antman EM (1997) Equivalence trials. N Engl J Med 337:1159–1161
32. The GUSTO Investigators (1993) An international randomized trial comparing four thrombolytic strategies for acute myocardial infarction. N Engl J Med 329:673–682

33. Hornberger J, Wrone E (1997) When to base clinical policies on observational versus randomized trial data. Ann Intern Med 127:697–703
34. Galanos C, Freudenberg MA (1993) Mechanisms of endotoxin shock and endotoxin hypersensitivity. Immunobiology 187:346–356
35. Stewart TE, Meade MO, Cook DJ, et al (1998) Evaluation of a ventilation strategy to prevent barotrauma in patients at high risk for acute respiratory distress syndrome. Pressure- and Volume-Limited Ventilation Strategy Group. N Engl J Med 338:355–361
36. Executive Committee for the Asymptomatic Carotid Atherosclerosis Study (1995) Endarterectomy for asymptomatic carotid artery stenosis. JAMA 273:1421–1428
37. Tu JV, Hannan EL, Anderson GM, et al (1998) The fall and rise of carotid endarterectomy in the United States and Canada. N Engl J Med 339:1441–1447
38. Wennberg DE, Lucas FL, Birkmeyer JD, Bredenberg CE, Fisher ES (1998) Variation in carotid endarterectomy mortality in the Medicare population: trial hospitals, volume, and patient characteristics. JAMA 279:1278–1281
39. Brun-Buisson C (1994) The HA-1A saga: the scientific and ethical dilemma of innovative and costly therapies. Intensive Care Med 20:314–316
40. Greenman RL, Schein RM, Martin MA, et al (1991) A controlled clinical trial of E5 murine monoclonal IgM antibody to endotoxin in the treatment of gram-negative sepsis. JAMA 266:1097–1102
41. Ziegler EJ, Fisher CJ Jr, Sprung CL, et al (1991) Treatment of gram–negative bacteremia and septic shock with HA- 1A human monoclonal antibody against endotoxin. A randomized, double-blind, placebo-controlled trial. N Engl J Med 324:429–436
42. Morris AH, Wallace CJ, Menlove RL, et al (1994) Randomized clinical trial of pressure-controlled inverse ratio ventilation and extracorporeal CO2 removal for adult respiratory distress syndrome. Am J Respir Crit Care Med 149:295–305
43. Willatts SM, Radford S, Leitermann M (1995) Effect of the antiendotoxic agent, taurolidine, in the treatment of sepsis syndrome: a placebo-controlled, double-blind trial. Crit Care Med 23:1033–1039
44. Reinhart K, Wiegand-Lohnert C, Grimminger F, et al (1996) Assessment of the safety and efficacy of the monoclonal anti- tumor necrosis factor antibody-fragment, MAK 195F, in patients with sepsis and septic shock: a multicenter, randomized, placebo- controlled, dose-ranging study. Crit Care Med 24:733–742
45. Chalfin DB, Holbein ME, Fein AM, Carlon G C (1993) Cost-effectiveness of monoclonal antibodies to gram-negative endotoxin in the treatment of gram-negative sepsis in ICU patients. JAMA 269:249–254
46. Knaus WA, Draper E A, Wagner D P, Zimmerman J E (1985) Prognosis in acute organ-system failure. Ann Surg 202:685–693
47. Raffin TA (1989) Intensive care unit survival of patients with systemic illness. Am Rev Respir Dis 140:S28–S35
48. 2nd European Consensus Conference in Intensive Care Medicine (1994) Predicting outcome in ICU patients. Intensive Care Med 20:390–397
49. Weinstein MC, Stason W B (1977) Foundations of cost-effectiveness analysis for health and medical practices. N Engl J Med 296:716–721
50. Ridley SA, Wallace P G (1990) Quality of life after intensive care. Anaesthesia 45:808–813
51. Tarlov AR, Ware JE, Jr, Greenfield S, Nelson EC, Perrin E, Zubkoff M (1989) The Medical Outcomes Study. An application of methods for monitoring the results of medical care. JAMA 262:925–930
52. Visser MC, Fletcher AE, Parr G, Simpson A, Bulpitt CJ (1994) A comparison of three quality of life instruments in subjects with angina pectoris: the Sickness Impact Profile, the Nottingham Health Profile, and the Quality of Well Being Scale. J Clin Epidemiol 47:157–163
53. Kaplan RM, Atkins CJ, Timms R (1984) Validity of a quality of well-being scale as an outcome measure in chronic obstructive pulmonary disease. J Chronic Dis 37:85–95
54. Chelluri L, Grenvik AN, Silverman M (1995) Intensive care for critically ill elderly: mortality, costs, and quality of life. Review of the literature. Arch Intern Med 155:1013–1022

55. Slatyer MA, James OF, Moore PG, Leeder SR (1986) Costs, severity of illness and outcome in intensive care. Anaesth Intensive Care 14:381–389
56. Freemantle N, Drummond M (1997) Should clinical trials with concurrent economic analyses be blinded? JAMA 277:63–64.
57. Weinstein MC, Siegel JE, Gold MR, Kamlet MS, Russell LB, for the Panel on Cost–Effectiveness in Health and Medicine (1996) Recommendations of the panel on cost-effectiveness in health and medicine. JAMA 276:1253–1258
58. Linden PK, Angus D C, Chelluri L, Branch RA (1995) The influence of clinical study design on cost-effectiveness projections for the treatment of gram-negative sepsis with human anti-endotoxin antibody. J Crit Care 10:154–164
59. Russell LB, Gold MR, Siegel JE, Daniels N, Weinstein MC (1996) The role of cost-effectiveness analysis in health and medicine. Panel on Cost–Effectiveness in Health and Medicine. JAMA 276:1172–1177
60. Neonatal Inhaled Nitric Oxide Study Group (1997) Inhaled nitric oxide in full-term and nearly full-term infants with hypoxic respiratory failure. N Engl J Med 336:597–604
61. Roberts MS, Angus DC, Clermont G, and Linde-Zwirble W T (1997) From efficacy to effectiveness: Problems in translating the results of clinical trials into cost effectiveness analyses. Med Decis Making 117:540 (Abst)
62. Davidson TA, Caldwell ES, Curtis JR, Hudson LD, Steinberg KP (1999) Reduced quality of life in survivors of acute respiratory distress syndrome compared with critically ill control patients. JAMA 281:354–360
63. Angus DC, Pinsky MR (1997) Risk prediction: Judging the judges. Intensive Care Med 23:363–365

The Integration of Evidence Based Medicine and Health Services Research in the ICU

D.J. Cook and M.K. Giacomini

Learning Points

- Many health sectors endorse moving toward an evidence-based health system in which decisions made by providers, administrators, policy makers and the public are made, to as large an extent as possible, on the basis of high quality research evidence
- Health services research meets evidence-based medicine (EBM) most decisively at the nexus of what is done compared to what ought to be done
- Evidence shows that the uptake of evidence into practice is not achieved through passive dissemination by publication or education.
- Evidence shows that more active implementation methods are required to change behavior and enhance research uptake, such as educational practice guidelines, individual audit and feedback, academic detailing, opinion leaders, administrative interventions, or computer decision support systems
- The most effective way to integrate valid, beneficial clinical research evidence into practice in the complex, dynamic ICU environment warrants further investigation

During a decade of generating evidence, critically appraising evidence, teaching how to generate evidence, teaching how to critically appraise evidence, writing about how to generate evidence, and writing about how to critically appraise evidence, one of us (DJC) repeatedly asked herself, "What is the point of all of this, if we don't actually use high quality research evidence when we are taking care of our patients?" For example, many studies show that patients with acute myocardial infarction do not consistently receive the 5 drugs which clearly delay mortality. We are just beginning to do similar studies in the intensive care unit (ICU), and the findings are sobering.

Meanwhile, my comrade and wise colleague (MKG) has been advancing our understanding of when and how research evidence can be 'policy relevant' – clinically and at the systems level. We believe that in addition to needing more rigorous basic and clinical research to help improve the outcomes of critically ill patients, another sorely needed source of wisdom is how to ensure optimal evidence uptake and utilization in the ICU. One place we could seek this wisdom is under the umbrella of EBM and health services research.

Introduction: The Emergence of Health Services Research in Critical Care

From the perspective of critical care medicine, health services research has languished in the shadows until recently. Why is this? Health services researchers take as their topic the organizational, cultural, political, and economic structures that undergird health care. They pose system-level questions that may be viewed as abstract and irrelevant at the bedside. Health services research may seem preoccupied with mapping the 'forest' without a close view of the 'trees (i.e., the myriad, complex and immediate clinical decisions facing ICU practitioners daily). Many health services research studies eschew methodological conventions which value controlled experiments to answer specific effectiveness questions; in contrast, health services research draws heavily on observational research designs and often relies on sources such as large administrative databases, surveys, or field observation. Resulting analyses are often complex, and the findings more suggestive than decisive. In summary, clinicians have been slow to recognize and accept the value of health services research, doubting both the relevance of health services research topics to critical care practice and the methodological rigor of health services research studies. These views are now changing.

Meanwhile, ironically, most ICU clinicians and administrators work with insufficient information about the patients they serve, the health workers and services they need to orchestrate appropriate care, and the economics of ICU practice. Our preoccupation with the 'trees' has left us largely unable to track and influence the topography and ecology of the 'forest' on which we ultimately rely. Health care reform and restructuring experiences of the 1980s and 1990s in North America and elsewhere have clarified for intensivists the importance of cultivating a broader analytic view of the health care system and the place of critical care practice within it.

EBM has also influenced critical care practice. EBM involves caring for patients using knowledge, experience, clinical judgment, and current best research evidence, adapted to patient values and each health care setting [1]. As in other countries, the Canadian National Forum on Health has recommended that the health sector should move toward the development of an evidence-based health system in which decisions made by providers, administrators, policy makers and the public are made, to as large an extent as possible, on the basis of high quality research evidence [2].

The notion of 'evidence' embraces a range of questions and study designs beyond effectiveness as determined by a randomized trial. The primacy of rigorous, sufficiently powered randomized trials as the highest form of evidence for issues of prevention or therapy notwithstanding, many other questions are not well addressed by this study architecture. These include issues of prognosis (which require observing the natural history of unselected cohorts rather than highly selected patients entering randomized trials), diagnostic test properties of technologies (which require evaluating the technology in patients who are suspected, and not suspected of having the condition in question), economic analyses of different interventions (which require measuring and/or modeling clinical and economic outcomes), and communication (most suitably advanced with qualitative, interpretive research). Thus, potentially relevant evidence for clinical practice and policy making has many sources, including research from the basic sciences, from patient-centered clinical research (both quantitative and qualitative), and increasingly, from health services research.

EBM sheds light on the decision making process by dissecting how some decisions are strongly, or even exclusively, determined by influences we might generally call 'values' rather than research evidence. For example, the pharmacological management of myocardial infarction is grounded in a robust body of randomized trial evidence (e.g., thrombolytics, anticoagulants, antiplatelet agents, beta blockers, and angiotensin converting enzyme inhibitors). Despite trials showing greater efficacy of tissue plasminogen activator (tPA) compared with streptokinase, streptokinase is the thrombolytic of choice for non-anterior myocardial infarctions in many countries; the main influences of this decision appear to be cost and potential adverse effects. For other drugs, utilization has been shown to be modest across different several health care systems (e.g., beta blockers), yet the influences that determine prescribing remain to be understood. Other critical care interventions upon which strong research evidence bears (e.g., selective digestive decontamination) are heavily influenced by concerns that could be viewed as 'theoretical', and likely, though not yet proven (e.g., the emergence of multiresistant organisms). Thus, different decisions in critical care medicine require considering the risk-benefit and cost-benefit of alternative strategies, as well as diverse patient, professional, system, and/or social values.

Although by definition, EBM concerns primarily medical practice, many decision makers determine the course and outcome of critical care. These include different ICU clinicians (e.g., nurses, housestaff, respiratory therapists, pharmacists, nutritionists, physiotherapists, social services and pastoral care representatives), as well as patients, administrators, and payors. Each of these decision makers brings a different set of interests, objectives and values to critical care practice. Representation of these perspectives to make informed decisions requires obtaining different sorts of evidence. To reflect these more inclusive perspectives, many clinically oriented EBM teaching sessions have endorsed different nomenclature (e.g., 'evidence-based practice' seminars, sessions and workshops). Many journals, interest groups and health care sectors have adapted the lexicon (e.g., 'evidence-based policy making' [3], 'evidence-based editing' [4] and 'evidence based purchasing' [5]).

The Canadian Health Services Research Foundation describes the essential role of health services research: "Health services research is a multidisciplinary enterprise. It picks up where clinical research leaves off, to examine the effectiveness of the organization and delivery of health services in terms of health outcomes and in terms of benefits and costs. The ultimate goal of health services research is to put knowledge to work in ways that significantly improve the health system." (CHSRF website: http://www.chsrf.ca/english/about.html). We suggest that health services research not only picks up where clinical research leaves off, but that health services research principles and perspectives can also help frame the clinical research enterprise and make use of clinical research results. EBM and health services research no longer seem at odds either in their concerns or their methods. Now, health services critical care research is cast in a new and inviting light. Out of the shadows comes a style of investigation that addresses the optimization of health and care, and that offers diverse methodologies for addressing complex systemic questions.

Organizing and delivering optimal critical care requires first understanding, empirically, what care is delivered to whom, by whom, when, with what resources, and to effect what outcomes. In keeping with secular trends in critical care research, most health services research is multidisciplinary and multimethod. The remainder of this chapter will describe a health services research program in the prevention of ventilator-associated pneumonia (VAP). The scope of evidence that will be reviewed and generated demonstrates the blurring boundaries between health services research and EBM.

A Health Services Research Program in VAP Prevention

What is the burden of illness of VAP? In the largest ICU prevalence study conducted to date, VAP accounted for almost half of the infections in ICUs in Europe [6]. Up to 50% of infections in mechanically ventilated patients are caused by VAP [7]. In a Canadian incidence and risk factor study [8], 15% of 1,014 patients mechanically ventilated for >48 hours developed VAP, 9.0±5.9 days after ICU admission. VAP increases the duration of mechanical ventilation and ICU stay among survivors [9], and is associated with an increased attributable mortality [10,11]. The considerable morbidity, mortality and cost associated with this nosocomial infection makes VAP prevention a worthy consideration.

A framework for the integration of health services research and EBM can illuminate a path for health services research that has the potential to bring the best clinical evidence to the care of individual patients and populations of patients. Health services research meets EBM most decisively at the nexus of: what is done compared to what ought to be done. A health services research program in VAP prevention can help to optimize the health of individuals and populations through appropriate and efficient health care delivery, comprised of several steps:

1) critiquing published evidence about effective VAP prevention (considering what *ought to be* done),
2) generating evidence about current VAP prevention practice and its determinants (considering what *is* done),
3) comparing current practice to what is suggested as best practice from the literature (the nexus),
4) using evidence about strategies that change behavior to align current practice with best practice using cognitive (e.g., education), behavioral (e.g., incentives) or administrative (e.g., charting) approaches (considering what *ought to be* done), and
5) re-evaluating practice after introducing these strategies (considering what *is* done).

Semirecumbency for VAP Prevention

Multivariate analysis has identified several independent risk factors for VAP [8,12–14], which include neurologic conditions, acute or chronic lung disease, trauma, burns, prolonged duration of ventilation, reintubation, tracheostomy, frequent circuit changes and patient transport out of the ICU. Other risk factors for VAP relate to the gastrointestinal tract such as enteral nutrition, witnessed aspiration, and supine positioning. When modifiable risk factors for VAP are tested in randomized trials and found to decrease the rate of VAP, these can be considered effective prevention strategies.

Supine positioning is an independent, modifiable VAP risk factor [12] which has been evaluated in 4 trials in which patients were randomized to the supine versus semirecumbent position (45° from the horizontal) [15–18]. The first 3 short-term cross-over trials examined a surrogate outcome for VAP – scintigraphic evidence of aspiration – and found it was lower in patients in the semirecumbent position [15–17]. Recently, Drakulovic and colleagues [18] evaluated the influence of semirecumbency on VAP (not just aspiration) among 86 mechanically ventilated patients, and found the semirecumbent position was associated with lower rates of clinically suspected and microbiologically proven VAP.

In summary, among several VAP prevention strategies tested in randomized trials, nursing patients in the semirecumbent position (at 45° from the horizontal) rather than the supine position (lying flat) is an effective intervention which also appears to be implementable (i.e., has few logistic barriers) and affordable (i.e., requires no purchasing). How might a health services research program be developed to evaluate whether this effective, affordable VAP prevention strategy of semirecumbency is used in practice, when it is used, why it is or is not used, who and what are the determinants of use, and how it might be more consistently and appropriately used? There are several potential health services research models to address these issues; our goal is not to catalog them or suggest a preferred model, but to provide one example of a health services research program in progress on the use of one VAP prevention strategy: the semirecumbent body position (Fig. 1).

Investigative Teams for Health Services Research in Semirecumbency

Health services research is a policy-oriented field that potentially draws on disciplines across the social sciences, health sciences, natural sciences, humanities, law and business [19]. Health services research can provide a vital link between basic disciplinary research and applied health research by adapting theories, methods and concepts from certain disciplines (e.g., sociology) to certain health problems (e.g., changing drug prescribing behavior).

Multidisciplinary health services research typically involves different investigators studying a given health problem from their own disciplinary perspectives; the product is usually multiple discipline-specific analyses that may mesh well with each other, and are usually understood by people within those particular dis-

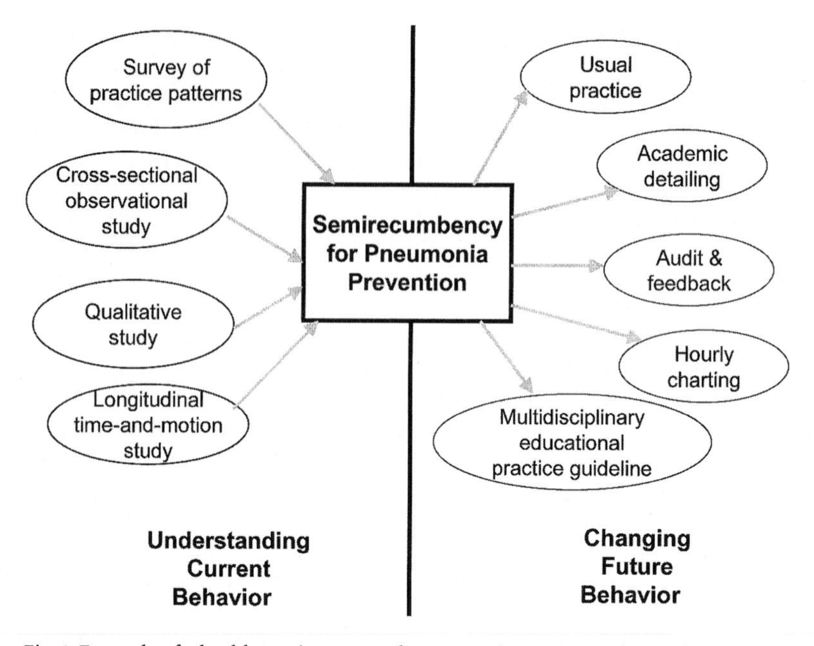

Fig. 1. Example of a health services research program in semirecumbency for mechanically ventilated ICU patients

ciplines. Most critical care health services research is multidisciplinary, involving physicians, biostatisticians, administrators and sometimes economists and others. Interdisciplinary health services research, however, is a more coordinated effort to investigate a given health problem conjointly from several disciplinary perspectives. This research is still discipline-guided, though the process usually yields a hybrid perspective on the same problem. Many critical care health services research programs studying patient activity [20] or health care team behavior are interdisciplinary. Transdisciplinary health services research requires investigators from various disciplines to jointly research a problem and strive to understand it from a common, synthetic framework, as opposed to discrete disciplinary perspectives. This challenging type of critical care health services research is highly suited to sensitive, complex issues such as the process of withdrawal of life support technology [21].

However, different health services research programs and different projects within health services research programs call for different disciplinary representation – not every perspective is relevant to every research question. The investigative team for this health services research program in semirecumbency is represented by medicine, nursing, respiratory therapy, sociology, anthropology, epidemiology, biostatistics and economics. Subgroups of this team are involved in each project, hereafter referred to as the health services research team.

Readers of health services research, just like consumers of other published evidence, need to consider the influence of (and absence of) different disciplinary perspectives on the results of the research they read. For example, given that decisions about semirecumbency are made at the bedside, what would the discipline of economics bring to bear on studying semirecumbency in the ICU? Economists, among other activities, study the costs and cost effectiveness of critical care technologies. Much economic scrutiny of the ICU to date has concerned publicly visible, obviously expensive technologies such as ventilators, dialysis machines, ICU beds and the like [22]. However, health-related technology encompasses the drugs, devices, procedures and organizations used in health care delivery [23]. Thus, semirecumbent positioning is also a technology worthy of economic analysis, with potentially important consequences for health and health resources, even though it is less familiar to the public, has a low 'unit cost' and is not issued through machinery.

Semirecumbency may or may not be a valuable practice when viewed from a broad perspective that takes into account the overall costs of practice in clinical and economic terms. Semirecumbency may involve hidden costs if it makes other daily interventions difficult (e.g., skin care), or if patients dislike it (e.g., they keep sliding out of the bottom of the bed!), etc. On the other hand, economic analysis may demonstrate that semirecumbency indeed costs little in terms of health risks, while lowering VAP and mortality rates and shortening length of ICU stay, thereby saving health resources. If true, such an economic analysis may compel ICU clinicians and managers to invest in the expense of programs to encourage semirecumbent positioning in routine practice. Such a decision may be even more compelling when different (less effective, less readily available, and/or more expensive) VAP prevention strategies are compared with semirecumbency.

Systematic Reviews of VAP Risk Factors and VAP Prevention Strategies

The foundation of responsible research programs is a systematic review of existing published evidence, to build on what is known, and advance our understanding of what is not. A systematic review of risk factors for VAP did not identify supine position as a consistent predictor of VAP [24], although very few risk factor studies measured this independent variable, prohibiting statements about the relative importance of supine positioning compared to other risk factors from observational studies alone. Nevertheless, as described earlier, a relationship between VAP and body position has been strongly suggested by documentation of supine positioning as an independent predictor of VAP in one observational study using multiple regression analysis [12]. This association is augmented by observational data on gastric colonization and subsequent tracheobronchial colonization and VAP [25].

VAP prevention strategies tested in randomized trials have been summarized in several systematic reviews addressing ventilator circuit and secretion management [26], gastrointestinal approaches [27], and pharmacological interventions [28]. Three randomized trials have taken the modifiable risk factor of supine body position and have shown that patients nursed in the supine rather than semirecumbent position had a significantly higher rate of aspiration as demonstrated scintigraphically [15–17]. Torres et al [15] found that after instillation of radioactive technetium sulfur colloid into the stomach, radioactive counts in endobronchial secretions were significantly higher in samples obtained while patients were supine than when they were semirecumbent. In another study [16], scintigraphic evidence of esophageal reflux was found in 81% of patients in the supine position compared to 64% in the semirecumbent position. Orozco and colleagues [17] administered nasogastric technetium sulfur colloid and found that radioactive counts in endobronchial secretions increased over time, but were higher in the supine than the semirecumbent position. A fourth trial evaluated the influence of semirecumbency on VAP itself rather than scintigraphy in mechanically ventilated patients and found that the semirecumbent patients had lower rates of clinically suspected VAP (8% versus 34%, $p=0.003$), and microbiologically confirmed VAP by bronchoalveolar lavage or protected brush catheter (5% versus 23%, $p=0.018$) [18]. In the latter trial, there was an important interaction between supine positioning and enteral nutrition, such that the risk of VAP was significantly higher in supine patients when they were receiving enteral nutrition.

In summary, there is strong physiologic rationale supporting the gastropulmonary route of lung infection in ICU patients, observational evidence suggesting that supine position is a risk factor for VAP, and randomized trial evidence showing that semirecumbency compared to supine positioning lowers the risk of aspiration and VAP in mechanically ventilated patients.

Survey of Practice Patterns

The health services research team began by conducting a survey of ICU directors in France and Canada to determine the utilization of ventilator circuit and secretion management strategies for VAP prevention in critically ill patients in university-affiliated ICUs. We used rigorous questionnaire methodology to develop this instrument, including item generation, item reduction, reliability testing and cross-cultural adaptation, the latter of which is a prerequisite for cross-cultural comparison. Of the French hospitals approached to participate in this study, 72/84 (86%) agreed; of the Canadian hospitals, 31/32 (97%) agreed, representing an overall response rate of 89%. The total number of beds represented was 1,054 in France and 639 in Canada. A full presentation of our findings about ventilator circuit and secretion management is forthcoming; herein, we report only our findings about semirecumbency [29].

French respondents stated that patients were primarily nursed in the semirecumbent position, whereas Canadians reported approximately equal use of the supine and semirecumbent position ($p=0.003$). In terms of decisional responsibility about semirecumbency, Canadians stated more often than French respondents that the intensivists (62% versus 32%, $p=0.008$) and bedside nurses (66% versus 10%, $p<0.0001$) influenced patient positioning, whereas French respondents more often stated that decisional responsibility about semirecumbency was accorded to ICU policy (65% versus 17%, $p<0.0001$).

In this survey, we demonstrated how ventilator circuit and secretion management strategies depend on the decisions of several members of the ICU team, and likely represent different interpretations of the benefits, risks and costs of these interventions. The universal caveat for all self-administered questionnaires still holds; this study is limited in that we recorded practice patterns as stated by ICU directors rather than actually observing them. Direct observation of what actually happens was neither logistically possible nor financially feasible on a binational scale, so we chose a more intense regional study for this purpose (*vide infra*).

Observational Study of Semirecumbency

A 'traditional' health services research project on semirecumbency might carefully examine a large database containing information about the body position of mechanically ventilated ICU patients, relating this position to patient, process, and outcome variables. Data on body position are not collected in our regional database, thus we used a more direct data source and different method for the next phase of this program.

To prospectively observe the body position of mechanically ventilated patients, the health services research team recorded whether patients without contraindications were nursed in the semirecumbent position over 164 patient-ventilator days in four university-affiliated ICUs [30]. All consecutive patients who had been mechanically ventilated for at least 48 hours were eligible over a 5 day period. Patients were excluded if they were post cardiac or neurosurgery, and if they were receiving vasoactive medication other than low dose dopamine. To avoid bias introduced by the observer effect, ICU team members remained unaware of the objectives or hypothesis of this study.

We found no significant differences between the distributions of body position across these four ICUs. The most common body position for all four ICUs was 15-30° from the horizontal. Patients were nursed in a position less than 15° from the horizontal for a range of 15–40% of patient-ventilator days in these four ICUs. During only 5–22% of patient-ventilator days were patients positioned at least 45° from the horizontal. Body position was unrelated to weaning, the presence of a tracheostomy, or the volume or character of endotracheal secretions.

The direct observation of each patient by a single assessor at a consistent time each day, and the multicenter perspective attained were strengths of this study. However, recording body position each hour in each patient would have provided a more continuous and representative 24 hour picture of body position, and represents another project in this program. Blinding of the ICU team to the study objectives to avoid biased ascertainment of practice patterns meant that we could not explore reasons why patients were not in the semirecumbent position. To better understand how body position practice patterns are established and understood by whom, we then embarked on a qualitative study of ICU practitioners.

Qualitative Study of Semirecumbency

Understanding the barriers to using semirecumbency could help to create effective, targeted VAP prevention strategies, which may ultimately decrease the burden of illness of this serious nosocomial infection. The objective of this study is to understand the perspectives of ICU health workers about the potential consequences and determinants of semirecumbent positioning. Since the aim is not to test hypotheses in an experimental setting, naturalistic methods of inquiry are needed [31] to help understand the cognitive, social and systems factors that influence practice patterns.

We are conducting a qualitative study using semistructured interviews and focus groups in two urban ICUs. We are eliciting perceptions of ICU nurses, respiratory therapists, physiotherapists, nutritionists, residents, fellows and attending physicians about why they may or may not use semirecumbency, factors promoting and deterring utilization, and potential policy and health systems changes to encourage semirecumbency. In the pilot phase of this study, we have now analyzed preliminary data from 11 ICU nurse-focused questions framed in five domains: 1) current practice, 2) knowledge assessment, 3) considering research evidence, 4) using semirecumbency in practice, and 5) system support for semirecumbency.

The pilot data generated two insights relevant to our future research on behavioral interventions to encourage semirecumbency. First, lateral positioning was viewed by some nurses as a competing position incompatible with semirecumbency. The implication of this finding is that a practice guideline to encourage semirecumbency will need to squarely address trade-offs against other common body positions. Second, nurses working in an ICU where charting is paperless suggested that the best way to encourage semirecumbency would be to introduce hourly charting by nurses of body position. The implication of this finding is that when we test different strategies to encourage semirecumbency across different ICUs, this simple administrative approach will be included.

Time-in-Motion Study

From the observational study in which we examined body position at one period each day over 164 patient-ventilator days, we learned that semirecumbency was uncommon. However, time-in-motion studies better delineate behavior, multidimensionally and longitudinally [32]. This project will involve case study of selected ICU patients who have no contraindications to semirecumbency (e.g., refractory hypotension) and who are not perceived to require other positions (e.g., prone).

Detailed analysis of the frequency, duration and intensity of actions, interpersonal interactions and latencies will be measured, showing us when and how semirecumbency occurs. Such kinematic data will enlighten us about physical and social activities that influence semirecumbency. In addition to its descriptive merit, this time-in-motion study will generate a typology of forces that compete with the semirecumbent body position.

Summary and Future Plans

Thus far, we have systematically reviewed clinical research supporting the burden of illness of VAP, outlined the rationale for semirecumbency as a VAP prevention strategy, broadly surveyed ICU directors in two countries to learn about stated practice patterns related to body position, prospectively observed body position among mechanically ventilated patients without contraindications in a regional ICU program, and started a local qualitative research project to better understand perceptions about, and barriers to, semirecumbency. We have concluded that:

a) VAP is a nosocomial infection with high morbidity and mortality worth preventing
b) semirecumbency is an implementable and affordable preventive strategy
c) stated and observed practice does not widely endorse semirecumbency for many reasons, and
d) change strategies might require cognitive, behavioral and/or administrative approaches.

A skeptic might say: "Why study semirecumbency? Just do it!" However, research evidence, health care worker habit and preferences, competing alternative body positions, competing alternative VAP prevention strategies, competing alternative activities in the ICU, administrative issues and many other concerns will ultimately determine when and how semirecumbency is used in practice [33]. Better understanding of the scope and determinants of practice variation through quantitative and qualitative research has taught us the importance of approaching this research from several disciplinary perspectives, especially as we move to implement and evaluate strategies to encourage semirecumbency.

Capitalizing on available evidence about effective methods of optimizing practice [34-37], we are now planning to compare different approaches to encourage semirecumbency which have been found to be effective in systematic reviews:

1) an educational practice guideline (cognitive approach)
2) individual audit and feedback to ICU nurses and physicians (behavioral approach), and
3) hourly charting of body position by nurses (administrative approach).

We will use a cluster randomization design.

There are two steps to behavior change: effecting change and sustaining change. Therefore, we will evaluate whether the change is sustained when the interventions are finished (if indeed any change occurs). Endpoints include: process of care variables (e.g., adherence to semirecumbency, utilization of other VAP prevention measures), clinical outcomes (e.g., development of VAP, mortality) and economic outcomes (e.g., duration of mechanical ventilation, duration of ICU stay, resources consumed). Studying semirecumbency with these multiple questions using multiple methods and data sources is a useful model for understanding how to change behavior in the ICU to encourage evidence-based practice.

Conclusion

One might say that as EBM and health services research have matured, they have 'grayed' – that is, the boundaries between them have become grayer and less formidable. Across these disappearing boundaries, more decision makers and academic disciplines are joining in programs of health services research that promise meaningful, useful insights into what optimizes the processes and outcomes of critical care medicine, including applying best evidence at the bedside.

References

1. Cook DJ, Sibbald WJ, Vincent JL, Cerra FB, for the Evidence Based Medicine in Critical Care Group (1996) Evidence based critical care medicine: What is it and what can it do for us? Crit Care Med 24:334–337
2. Watanabe M, Noseworthy T (1997) Creating a culture of evidence-based decision-making in health. Ann Royal Coll Phys Surg Can 30:137–139
3. Ham C, Hunter DJ, Robinson R (1995) Evidence based policymaking. Br Med J 310:71–72
4. Smith R, Rennie D (1995) And now, evidence based editing. Br Med J 311:826
5. Fahey T, Griffiths S, Peters TJ (1995) Evidence based purchasing: Understanding results of clinical trials and systematic reviews. Br Med J 311:1056–1060
6. Vincent JL, Bihari DJ, Suter PM, et al (1995) The prevalence of nosocomial infection in intensive care units in Europe (EPIC). JAMA 274:639–644
7. Alvarez-Lerma F, Palomar M, Martinez-Pellus AE, et al (1997) Aetiology and diagnostic techniques in intensive care-acquired pneumonia: a Spanish multicenter study. Clin Intensive Care 8:164–170
8. Cook DJ, Walter S, Cook RJ, et al (1998) The incidence and risk factors for ventilator-associated pneumonia in critically ill patients. Ann Intern Med 129:433–440
9. Papazian L, Bregeon F, Thirion X, et al (1996) Effect of ventilator associated pneumonia on mortality and morbidity. Am J Respir Crit Care Med 154:91–97
10. Heyland DK, Cook DJ, Griffith LE, et al (1999) The attributable morbidity and mortality of ventilator-associated pneumonia in the critically ill patient. Am J Respir Crit Care Med 159:1249–1256
11. Fagon JY, Chastre J, Vuagnat A, Trouillet JL, Novara A, Gibert C (1996) Nosocomial pneumonia and mortality among patients in intensive care units. JAMA 275:866–869
12. Kollef M (1993) Ventilator-associated pneumonia: A multivariate analysis. JAMA 270: 1965–1970
13. Rello J, Sonora S, Jubert P, Artigas A, Rue M, Valles J (1996) Pneumonia in intubated patients: Role of respiratory airway care. Am J Respir Crit Care Med 154:111–115
14. Kollef MH, Von Harz B, Prentice D, et al (1997) Patient transport from intensive care increases the risk of developing ventilator-associated pneumonia. Chest 112:765–773
15. Torres A, Serra-Batilles J, Ros E, et al (1992) Pulmonary aspiration of gastric contents in patients receiving mechanical ventilation: the effect of body position. Ann Intern Med 116:540–543
16. Ibanez J, Penafiel A, Raurich JM, Marse P, Jorda R, Mata F (1992) Gastroesophageal reflux in intubated patients receiving enteral nutrition: effect of supine and semirecumbent positions. JPEN J Parenter Enteral Nutr 16:419–422
17. Orozco-Levi M, Torres A, Ferrer M, et al (1995) Semirecumbent position protects from pulmonary aspiration but not completely from gastroesophageal reflux in mechanically ventilated patients. Am J Respir Crit Care Med 152:1387–1390
18. Drakulovic MB, Torres A, Bauer TT, et al (1999) Supine body position as a risk factor for nosocomial pneumonia in mechanically ventilated patients: A randomized trial. Lancet 354:1851–1858

19. Hurley J, Barer M, Kephart G, Black C, Cosby J (1999) Integrating health services research into the Canadian Institutes of Health Research. http://www.sshrc.ca/english/programinfo/hidgpapers-html
20. Devlin JW, Boleski G, Mlynarek M, et al (1999) Motor Activity Assessment Scale: A valid and reliable sedation scale for use with mechanically ventilated patients in an adult surgical intensive care unit. Crit Care Med 27:1271–1275
21. Cook DJ, Giacomini M, Johnson N, Willms D, for the Canadian Critical Care Trials Group (1999) Life support technology in the intensive care unit: A qualitative investigation of purposes. Can Med Assoc J 161:1109–1113
22. Cook DJ, Sibbald WJ (1999) The progress, the promise and the paradox of technology assessment in the intensive care unit. Can Med Assoc J 161:1118–1119
23. Battista RN (1989) Innovation and diffusion of health-related technologies: A conceptual framework. Int J Technol Assess Health Care 5:227–248
24. Cook DJ, Kollef M (1998) ICU acquired pneumonia: Assessing risk in critically ill patients. JAMA 279:1605–1606
25. Heyland DK, Mandell LA (1992) Gastric colonization by Gram-negative bacilli and nosocomial pneumonia in the intensive care unit patient: Evidence for causation. Chest 101:87–93
26. Cook DJ, DeJonghe B, Brochard L, Brun-Buisson C (1998) The influence of airway management on ventilation associated pneumonia: Evidence from randomized trials. JAMA 279: 781–787
27. Cook DJ, De Jonghe B, Heyland DK (1997) The relation between nutrition and nosocomial pneumonia: Randomized trials in critically ill patients. Crit Care 1:3–9
28. D'Amico R, Pifferi S, Leonetti C, et al (1998) Effectiveness of antibiotic prophylaxis in critically ill adult patients: Systematic review of randomized controlled trials. Br Med J 316: 1275–1285
29. Cook DJ, Ricard JD, Reeve BK, et al (2000) Ventilator circuit and secretion management: A Franco-Canadian survey. Crit Care Med (in press).
30. Reeve BK, Cook DJ (1999) Semirecumbency among mechanically ventilated ICU patients: A multicenter observational study. Clin Intensive Care 10:241–244
31. Lincoln YS, Guba EG (1985) Naturalistic inquiry. Sage Publications, Newbury Park
32. Thomas DW (1995) Wandering: A proposed definition. J Gerontol Nurs 21:35–41
33. Dowie J (1996) 'Evidence-based', 'cost-effective' and 'preference-driven' medicine: Decision analysis-based medical decision making is the pre-requisite. J Health Serv Res Policy 1:104–113
34. Grimshaw JM, Russell IT (1993) Effect of clinical guidelines on medical practice: A systematic review of rigorous evaluations. Lancet 342:1317–1322
35. Grimshaw J, Freemantle N, Wallace S, et al (1995) Developing and implementing clinical practice guidelines. Qual Health Care 4:55–64
36. Davis DA, Thomson MA, Oxman AD, Haynes RB (1995) Changing physician performance: A systematic review of the effect of continuing medical educational strategies. JAMA 274: 700–705
37. Hunt DL, Haynes RB, Hanna SE, Smith K (1998) Effects of computer-based clinical decision support systems on physician performance and patient outcomes: A systematic review. JAMA 280:1339–1346

Using Systematic Reviews to Inform Decision Makers

D. K. Heyland

Learning Points

To facilitate the incorporation of research findings into the decision making process, decision makers must be aware of the existence and value of systematic reviews.

Systematic reviews:

- are an efficient, practical approach to locating the primary literature and synthesizing what is known about a particular technology or intervention
- provide the best estimate of treatment effect that is generalizable to the broadest range of individuals
- offer informative and illuminating subgroup analysis because of the heterogeneity present and their large sample sizes
- are related to economic evaluations, decision analysis and other forms of integrative research, all of which can be used to inform decision makers about the most recent research findings

As you prepare to attend the monthly business meeting with your intensive care unit (ICU) group, you notice the first item on the agenda is a discussion about capital equipment purchases for the next year. At the beginning of every new fiscal year your group meets to discuss what new technology they want to acquire. Recognizing that the budget is limited, the purpose of today's meeting is to set priorities for expenditure for the next year. With great interest, you note the discussion revolves around the following principles: What are our needs based on the population of patients we serve?(do we have enough patients with acute renal failure to warrant a new continuous hemodialysis machine?); since we train critical care fellows, do we have adequate technology to equip them with the skills and knowledge they need in the future? (do our fellows have enough exposure to non-invasive ventilation?); what kind of technology do our peer hospitals utilize?(the neighboring hospital has a nitric oxide machine, therefore, we should get one too!). Sadly, there was no reference to the 'evidence' that these technologies would improve patient outcomes or were an efficient use of resources. No one referred to or actually requested a systematic review of the literature to support their decisions.

Introduction

This scenario is a representation of current reality in many settings. Whether faced with purchasing new technology, organizing programs of care, or determining the optimal number of beds and human resources to provide care to the critically ill patient, there is little, if any, substantive evidence that decision makers at the local hospital, regional, or system level appeal to the findings of scientific research to guide them in their decision making. In this chapter 'decision makers' refer to those providers and managers concerned about the organization and effect of health care services on individuals and populations. Depending on the context, they may be physicians or may include hospital managers or governmental bureaucrats. Perhaps distinct from the typical provider-patient relationship, these decision makers emphasize the effects and/or provision of services to 'groups' of patients rather than just to an individual patient. This perspective is important to consider when translating the results of research evidence into practice and, as will be discussed later, systematic reviews meet the challenges of this unique perspective.

In this era of information explosion, it would be extremely naive to think that decision makers (or clinicians) can stay current with burgeoning medical literature. The purpose of this article is to suggest that using systematic reviews represents a 'step in the right direction' (not the total solution). Systematic reviews are an efficient, practical approach to locating the primary literature and synthesizing what is known about a particular technology or intervention. In addition, systematic reviews provide the best estimate of treatment effect that is generalizable to the broadest range of individuals. Moreover, because of the heterogeneity present in systematic reviews and their large sample sizes, they offer informative and illuminating subgroup analysis. Finally, systematic reviews are related to economic evaluations, decision analysis and other forms of integrative research, all of which can be used to inform decision makers about the most recent research findings.

Improving Care of the Critically Ill Patient

When considering the challenge to improve the quality of care in the ICU, a simplistic approach to accomplishing this goal would be to stop providing useless or harmful therapies and to provide only those which improve patient outcomes. This simple notion suggests that decision makers are able to easily discern what works and what does not. Clinicians primarily rely on randomized trials and meta-analyses of randomized trials to determine the efficacy of medical interventions. Unfortunately, decision makers often appeal to other kinds of observational research (if they appeal to any research findings at all). One of the barriers to engaging decision makers about 'the evidence' may be the overemphasis on the results of randomized trials. This tends to devalue or denigrate the results of other kinds of evidence that decision makers may be more comfortable with (case studies, anecdotes, etc.). Perhaps a more useful paradigm would view evidence as a continuum of validity rather than as a dichotomous outcome (that evidence is good or bad, present or absent) (Fig. 1). A basic tenet of clinical epidemiology is that good methods of clinical observation lead to correct conclusions (i.e., observations that are relatively free of systematic error and which cannot be easily discounted as arising from chance alone are likely to be correct). On one end of the continuum we have studies that have lots of bias. At the other end of the continuum, we find studies that utilize rigorous methods to limit bias. This paradigm (considering validity as a continuum) enables us to consider (and therefore value!) other forms of research evidence (see Fig. 2).

Each of these methodologies has its strengths, weaknesses and limitations but generally speaking, systematic reviews of randomized trials and individual randomized trials tend to produce more robust results than cohort studies or case control studies. In using other forms of research, though, one gives explicit consideration to the level of evidence and, therefore, the strength of the inference. From studies where there is minimal bias or a low chance of error, we can make strong inferences. Conversely, from studies with a lot of bias or a high chance of error, we can make weak inferences or no inferences at all. Empowered to use a variety of research tools, decision makers are more able to appeal to research findings to inform them in their decision making. While other forms of research methodologies then are allowable, systematic reviews are the best starting place for decision makers.

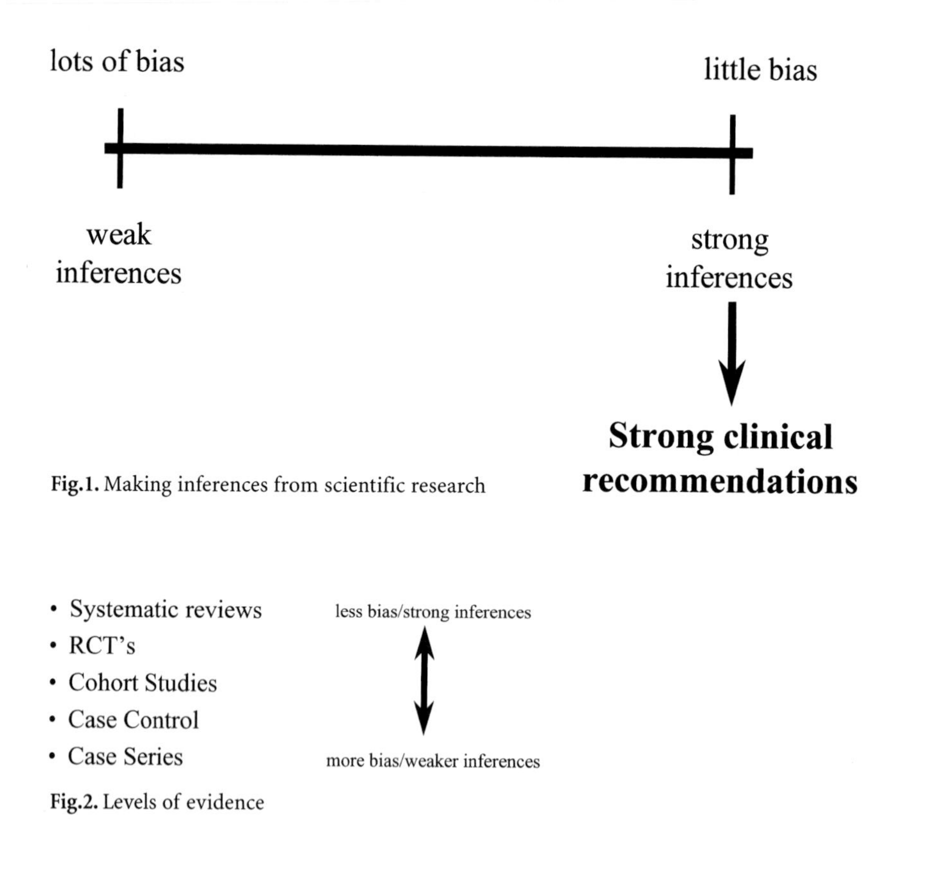

Fig. 1. Making inferences from scientific research

Fig. 2. Levels of evidence

Systematic Reviews

All reviews, narrative and systematic, are retrospective, observational research studies and, therefore, are subject to bias. Systematic reviews differ from narrative reviews in that they employ various methods to limit or minimize bias in the review process. These methods include a comprehensive search of all potentially relevant articles and the use of explicit, reproducible criteria to select articles for inclusion into the review process. The key features of both narrative and systematic reviews are outlined in Table 1. Meta-analyses are a subset of systematic reviews that employ statistical strategies to aggregate the results of individual studies into a numerical estimate of overall treatment effect. Systematic reviews are less likely to be biased, more likely to be up-to-date and more likely to detect small but clinically meaningful treatment effects than narrative reviews [1, 2]. For example it has been shown that narrative reviews may lag behind by more than a decade in endorsing a treatment of proven effectiveness or they may continue to advocate therapy long after it is considered harmful or useless [1].

Controversy Between Randomized Controlled Trials (RCTs) and Meta-Analyses

Recently, meta-analyses have been coming under increasing scrutiny [3]. There has been increasing uncertainty regarding the validity of meta-analyses stemming from comparison of the results of large randomized trials and meta-analyses on the same topic. Such uncertainty likely deters both clinicians and decision makers from incorporating the results of meta-analyses into their decision making. While cautious interpretation of meta-analyses (and randomized trials!) is a good 'rule of thumb', discriminating against meta-analyses is not supported by current evidence, as I will explain below.

LeLorier and colleagues compared the results of 12 large randomized trials (>1000 patients) published in four leading medical journals to 19 meta-analysis previously published [4]. They found significant differences in the results of these comparisons and concluded: "...if there had been no subsequent randomized trial, the meta-analysis would have led to the adoption of an ineffective

Table 1. Systematic and narrative reviews [24]

Feature	Narrative Review	Systematic Review
Question	No specific question, usually broad in scope	Focused clinical question
Search	Not usually specified, potentially biased	Comprehensive, explicit strategy
Selection	Not usually specified, potentially biased	Criterion-based selection
Appraisal	Variable	Rigorous critical appraisal
Synthesis	Qualitative	Qualitative + Quantitative
Inferences	Sometimes evidence-based	Evidence-based

treatment in 32% of cases and rejection of useful treatment in 33% of cases." The person writing the accompanying editorial in the New England Journal of Medicine said: ".. I still prefer conventional narrative reviews" [5]. It is unclear to me why this author would have concluded that narrative reviews are superior to systematic reviews. The argument here is with meta-analysis, the practice of reducing the measure of effect into one number, not with systematic reviews. Subsequent letters to the editor have also refuted the findings of LeLorier and colleagues based on the fact that their methods may have inflated the measure of disagreement [6]. By selecting 12 trials from four leading medical journals, the authors clearly have a non-representative sample of clinical trials. Such journals tend to publish trials whose results disagree with prior evidence. In addition, the authors based their agreement statistics on the presence or absence of a statistically significant p value and ignored the fact that the point estimates may have been similar (although the confidence intervals may be different).Moreover, the credibility of this work is undermined by the fact that the authors seemed to be selective in their choice of comparators. For example, the authors cite discordance between the 1993 EMERAS (Estudio Multicentrico Estreptoquinasa Republicas de America del Sur) trial and a 1985 meta-analysis of thrombolysis for acute myocardial infarction. As suggested by David Naylor, perhaps a more valid comparison would be the ISIS (international study of infarct survival)-2 (a more definitive test of the hypothesis generated from the 1985 meta-analysis), or a 1994 meta-analysis that used individual patient data from all trials of thrombolysis that had more than 1000 patients [7]. Others have challenged the notion that large randomized trials are the gold standard to which the results of meta-analyses should be compared [5]. Potential biases occur in both randomized trials and meta-analyses and neither should be considered the gold standard in the absence of rigorous assessment of the methodologic quality. Finally, it is not surprising that the results of meta-analyses differ from the results of randomized trials; they may be measuring different things. Given the variable characteristics of patients, interventions, outcomes and methods across studies included in a meta-analyses, discrepancies with large trials should be expected (5).

By carefully exploring the discordant results of meta-analyses and randomized trials, one can gain important insights into the treatment effect of the study under investigation. For example, a recent meta-analysis suggested that calcium supplementation may prevent pre-clampsia [8]. A subsequent large, National Institute of Health (NIH)-sponsored, clinical trial concluded that there was no treatment effect in healthy nulliparous women. DerSimonian and Levine [9] explored the heterogeneity across studies in the meta-analysis and the inconsistent results with the large trial. They stratified studies in the meta-analysis on the basis of baseline risk of preeclampsia (event rate in placebo-group). When they divided studies in the meta-analyses into studies of low and high risk patients, it was apparent that there was no treatment effect in low risk patients, consistent with the large randomized trial of low risk women, but there still was a significant treatment effect in the high risk patients.

In summary, bias can exist in both randomized trials and meta-analysis. Previous comparisons of the results of meta-analysis and randomized trials on the same topic have demonstrated concordance in 80–90% of cases [10, 11]. Not surprisingly, on some occasions, discordance is present. By exploring the discrepancy between meta-analyses and randomized trials, one can gain important insights into the effect of interventions.

Validity and Generalizability of Systematic Reviews

While systematic reviews are useful tools to discern whether interventions are efficacious or not, they still need to be evaluated for their methodological quality. Not all systematic reviews (or randomized trials) are created (or completed) equally. What distinguishes a high quality systematic review from a low quality review? A recent publication outlined key criteria that need to be considered when evaluating the strength of review articles [12]. To assess the validity of systematic reviews (or meta-analyses if a quantitative summary is provided), one needs to consider whether a comprehensive search strategy was employed to find all relevant articles, whether the validity of the original articles was appraised, whether study selection, validity assessments and data abstraction were done in a reproducible fashion and whether the results were similar from study to study (statistical homogeneity). Obviously, we can make stronger inferences from studies that employ more rigorous methods (Fig. 3).

One of the weaknesses of randomized trials is their limited generalizability. Because meta-analyses combine many studies with subtle differences in patients, settings, interventions, etc., provided it is clinically reasonable to combine these studies and no statistical heterogeneity is present, the results of meta-analyses have greater generalizability than a single randomized trial. For example, a randomized trial of total parenteral nutrition (TPN) in surgical patients at Veteran Affairs hospitals in the USA (predominantly white males) would have limited generalizability. A meta-analysis of TPN in the critically ill patient combines the results of studies of different patients in different settings and therefore offers the best estimate of treatment effect that is generalizable to a broader range of patients. This is consistent with the perspectives of decision makers who are more concerned with the effects of health care on groups of patients, rather than the individual.

Weaker Inferences ⟷	Stronger Inferences
• Selective search	✓ Comprehensive search
• Small number of trials	✓ Large number of trials
• Weak trial methodology	✓ Strong trial methodology
• Outdated/unmeasured co-interventions	✓ Current/documented co-interventions
• Surrogate endpoints	✓ Clinically important endpoints
• Statistical heterogeneity	✓ Statistical homogeneity

Fig. 3. Making inferences from a meta-analysis of RCTs

Efficiently Locating and Summarizing the Primary Literature

Perhaps one of the reasons why decision makers to not consult the primary evidence is that they do not have the time or knowledge to efficiently locate and retrieve it. For busy clinicians and decision makers, systematic reviews may help. If, for example, a decision maker turned to the primary literature for guidance on utilizing selective decontamination of the digestive tract in their ICU, he or she would find more than one hundred published studies, reviews or commentaries. Even if the search was limited to randomized trials, the decision maker would have to retrieve and synthesize more than 30 studies. Across these numerous studies, populations, interventions, outcome measures and results vary making it difficult to come up with a 'bottom line', which obviously is the primary goal of the decision maker! Fortunately, not one, but several meta-analyses exist. One of the more recent meta-analyses aggregated 33 studies, compared the treatment effect in different populations and interventions, and provided a summary of the previous meta-analyses [13]. Overall, by locating, retrieving, and reading this one paper in an efficient manner, the decision maker is now well informed about the evidence demonstrating that selective decontamination of the digestive tract is associated with a lower rate of pulmonary infections and a small, but clinically important, reduction in mortality.

This example also illustrates the proper role of meta-analyses (and other forms of research evidence). The results of the studies do not make the decision, they inform the decision maker. Decision making is a complex process. The decision maker may appeal to other criteria such as the prevalence of the problems, natural history, costs, values, risk of adverse effects, etc. in making the final decision. A systematic review will not likely address concerns of the effect of selective decontamination of the digestive tract on long-term antibiotic resistance.

Informative Subgroup Analyses

Occasionally, investigators explore the results of various subgroups in the context of randomized trials or meta-analyses. Subgroup analyses are based on differences in baseline patient or treatment characteristics and not events that occur post-randomization [14]. There is considerable debate whether the results of subgroups confirm hypotheses or should be viewed as hypothesis generating exercises. There are several criteria that one can assess to establish the strength of inference from subgroup analysis [15]. Because of the heterogeneity across studies and their typically larger sample size, systematic reviews can provide insights into important subgroup effects. For example, in a recent meta-analysis of TPN in the critically ill patient, there were 26 randomized trials of 2,211 patients that compared the use of TPN to standard care (usual oral diet plus intravenous dextrose) in surgical and critically ill patients [16]. Overall, when the results of these trials were aggregated, there was no difference between the two treatments with respect to mortality (risk ratio= 1.03, 95% confidence intervals, 0.81–1.31). There was a trend to a lower total complication rate in patients who received TPN although this result was not statistically significant (risk ratio = 0.84, 95% confidence intervals, 0.64–1.09). However, heterogeneity across studies precluded strong inferences based on the aggregated estimate and therefore, several *a priori* hypotheses were examined.

Studies including only malnourished patients were associated with lower complication rates but no difference in mortality when compared to studies of non-malnourished patients. Studies published since 1989 and studies with a higher methods score showed no treatment effect while studies published in 1988 or before and studies with a lower methods score demonstrated a significant treatment effect. Complication rates were lower in studies that did not use lipids; however, there was no difference in mortality rates between studies that did not use lipids and those studies that did. Studies limited to critically ill patients demonstrated a significant increase in complication and mortality rates compared to studies of surgical patients.

While the authors had set out to summarize the experimental evidence on the effect of TPN on critically ill patients, only six studies included patients that would routinely be admitted to the ICU as part of their management. Inasmuch as surgical patients and ICU patients have a similar stress response to illness, it was considered to be reasonable to aggregate studies of surgical and critically ill patients. However, the results of the subgroup analysis suggest that both mortality and complication rates may be increased in critically ill patients receiving TPN and these treatment effects may differ from the results in surgical patients. The results of studies evaluating the effect of TPN in surgical patients therefore may not be generalizable to all types of critically ill patients. This leaves a very limited data set from which to base the practice of providing TPN to critically ill patients and the best estimate to date is that TPN may be doing more harm than good. These subgroup findings have important implications for both clinicians and decision makers.

Relationship to Other Forms of Integrative Research

Decision makers often are concerned, not only about efficacy, but about issues of effectiveness and efficiency. Systematic reviews are similar to other forms of integrative or synthetic research, like practice guidelines, economic evaluations and decision analyses. Their unit of study is a primary report in the literature whereas for a clinical trial, the unit of study is the patient. Evidence-based practice guidelines are based on systematic reviews of the evidence. For example, the American College of Physicians guidelines on the management of stroke [17] incorporated the results of a concurrently published systematic review of the literature on the same topic [18]. Economic evaluations examine both the costs and consequences of various interventions. Estimates of the clinical consequences increasingly are derived from systematic reviews. For example, Veenstra and colleagues [19] set out to determine the cost-effectiveness of antiseptic-impregnated central venous catheters for the prevention of catheter-related bloodstream infection. Estimates of baseline risk and risk reduction, which were incorporated into the economic evaluation, came from a meta-analysis of these catheters [20].

Optimizing Use of Systematic Reviews

To facilitate the incorporation of research findings into the decision making process, decision makers must be aware of the existence and value of systematic reviews. To increase the relevance of the review to decision makers, they should be involved early in the research process where they can have an opportunity to influence the content and process of the review. In addition, completed reviews must be readily available and decision makers must have access to the reviews. The Internet and electronic data sources, like the Cochrane Collaboration Library, now and in the future, will likely facilitate ready access to such reviews.

Despite these efforts, barriers will continue to hamper the process of integrating reviews into the decision making process. Each situation may be different and will require an understanding of the barriers and a targeted strategy to overcome them. Moreover, unless the reviews are communicated in a fashion consistent with the language of the decision maker, the reviews will largely remain underutilized. Decision makers tend to be interested in the 'bottom line' only and may not have or take the time necessary to cull the summary points from an extensive review of the literature. The tendencies of decision makers to use anecdotes as a form of communication suggests that strategies to 'package' the results of a systematic review into a narrative story or anecdote may be effective.

Eleanor Chelimsky said: "We use the style of reporting that is most natural to legislative policymakers and their staffs: the anecdote. This may seem somewhat ironic, given that by conducting an evaluation [systematic review] in the first place one has moved deliberately away from the anecdote...to disseminate findings to policymakers it seems that one of the most effective ways to present them is to rediscover the anecdote – but this time an anecdote that represents the broader evaluative evidence." [21]. However, there may be danger of misinterpretation when communicating briefs or summaries to decision makers. A synopsis of the evidence may not allow for an adequate review of quality or validity issues and hence, the strength of inference is lost on those who focus on the bottom line. A good example of this is a recent meta-analysis of albumin supplementation in critical illness [22]. Researchers aggregated 30 randomized studies that evaluated the clinically important benefits of albumin administration in critically ill patients. Most of these individual studies were small and were not thoroughly assessed for quality. A significant proportion of these primary studies were designed to look at physiological endpoints and did not follow patients through the course of the ICU. Finally, some of the studies were very old and therefore contained outdated, and even not measured, co-interventions. While very few study patients died, the overall results showed that albumin administration was associated with an increased risk of death (relative risk of 1.68, 95% confidence interval 1.26 to 2.23). However, given the methodological weaknesses of the primary studies, few or no inferences can be made from the overall estimate of treatment effect (Fig. 3). Yet the synopsis in the published paper [22] said: "The pooled risk of death with albumin was ... 6% (95% confidence intervals 3, 9%) or six additional deaths for every 100 patients treated. We consider that the use of albumin solution in critically ill patients should be urgently reviewed." The synopsis did not reflect the strength of inference (or its validity) and it may be inappropriately applied to all kinds of critically ill patients (although there may be some benefit in some subgroups of critically ill patients). The exaggerated summary statements may be partially to blame for the strong reactions by the medical community and the 'hysterical' response by the lay press about this "killer fluid" [23].

Conclusion

In the last decade, we have seen a proliferation in the number of published systematic reviews (Fig.4). Systematic reviews offer a useful starting place for decision makers to begin to incorporate the results of research findings into their decision making process. Efficiently used, they can access a current synthesis on topics of relevance. Systematic reviews provide the best estimate of treatment effect generalizable to the broadest range of individuals. Moreover, because of the heterogeneity present in systematic reviews and their large sample sizes, they offer informative and illuminating subgroup analysis. Finally, systematic reviews are related to economic evaluations, decision analysis and other forms of integrative research, all of which can be used to inform decision makers about the most recent research findings. As researchers and decision makers begin to participate collaboratively in the review process and as they communicate in the language of decision makers, it is likely that we will be successful in achieving a higher degree of evidence-based decision making.

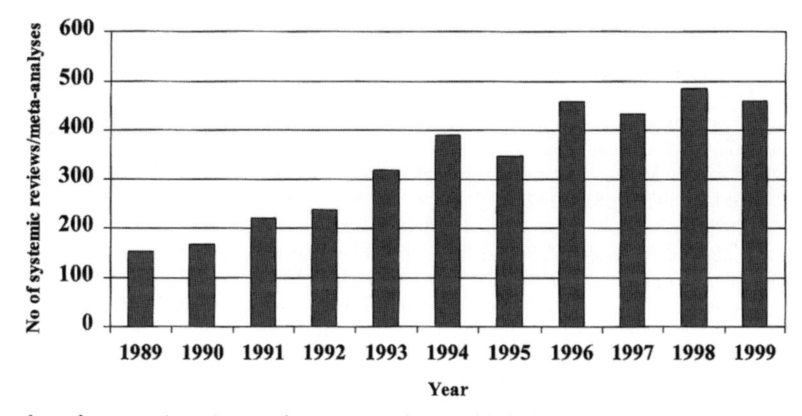

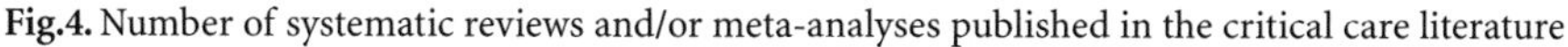

Fig.4. Number of systematic reviews and/or meta-analyses published in the critical care literature

References

1. Antman EM, Lau J, Kupelnick B, Mosteller F, Chalmers TC (1992) A comparison of results of meta-analyses of randomized control trials and recommendations of clinical experts. Treatments for myocardial infarction. JAMA 268:240–248
2. Cooper HM, Rosenthal R (1980) Statistical versus traditional procedures for summarizing research findings. Psychol Bull 87:442–449
3. Anonymous. Meta-analysis under scrutiny. Lancet 1997;350:675.
4. LeLorier J, Gregoire G, Benhaddad A, Lapierre J, Derderian F (1997) Discrepancies between meta-analyses and subsequent large randomized trials. N Engl J Med 337:536–542
5. Bailar JC (1997) The promise and problems of meta-analysis. N Engl J Med 337:559–561
6. Ioannidis JPA, Cappelleri JC, Lau J (1998) Meta-analyses and large randomized trials. N Engl J Med 338:359
7. Naylor D (1997) Meta-analysis and the meta-epidemiology of clinical research. Br Med J 315:617–619
8. Bucher HC, Guyatt GH, Cook RJ, et al (1996) Effect of calcium supplementation on pregnancy-induced hypertension and preeclampsia: a meta-analysis of randomized controlled trials. JAMA 275:1113–1117
9. DerSimonian R, Levine RJ (1999) Resolving discrepancies between a meta-analysis and a subsequent large controlled trial. JAMA 282:664–670
10. Cappelleri JC, Ioannidis JPA, Schmid CH, et al (1996) Large trials vs meta-analysis of smaller trials: How do they compare? JAMA 276:1332–1338
11. Villar J, Carroli G, Belizan JM (1995) Predictive ability of meta-analyses of randomized controlled trials. Lancet 345:772–776
12. Cook DJ, Levy MM, Heyland DK (1998) For the Evidence-Based Medicine in Critical Care Working Group. How to Use a Review Article: Prophylactic endoscopic sclerotherapy for esophageal varices. Crit Care Med 26:692–700
13. D'Amico R, Pifferi S, Leonetti C, et al (1998) Effectiveness of antibiotic prophylaxis in critically ill patients: systematic review of randomized controlled trials. Br Med J 315:1275–1285
14. Yusuf S, Wittes J, Probstfiel J, Tyroler HA (1991) Analysis and interpretation of treatment effects in subgroups of patients in randomized clinical trials. JAMA 266: 93–98
15. Oxman AD, Guyatt GH (1992) Apples, oranges and fish: A consumer's guide to subgroup analyses. Ann Intern Med 116:78–84
16. Heyland DK, MacDonald S, Keefe L, Drover JW (1998) Total parenteral nutrition in the critically ill patient: A meta-analysis. JAMA 280:2013–2019
17. American College of Physicians (1994) Guidelines for medical treatment for stroke prevention. Ann Intern Med 121:54–55
18. Matchar DB, McCrory DC, Barnett HJ, Feussner JR (1994) Medical treatment for stroke prevention. Ann Intern Med 121:41–53
19. Veenstra DL, Saint S, Sullivan SD (1999) Cost-effectiveness of antiseptic-impregnated central venous catheters for the prevention of catheter-related bloodstream infections. JAMA 282:554–560
20. Veenstra DL, Saint S, Saha S, Lumley T, Sullivan SD (1999) Efficacy of antiseptic-impregnated central venous catheters in preventing catheter-related bloodstream infection: A meta-analysis. JAMA 281:261–267
21. Chelimsky E (1995) The politics of dissemination on the hill: what works and what doesn't. In: Sechrest L, Bakker T, Rogers E, Campbell T, Grady M (eds) Effective dissemination of clinical and health information. US Department of Health and Human Services Agency for Health Care Policy and Research, AHCPR, Washington, pp 37–40
22. Cochrane Injuries Group (1998) Human albumin administration in critically ill patients: systematic review of randomized controlled trials. Br Med J 317:235–240
23. Letters to the Editor. Br Med J 317: 882–886
24. Cook DJ, Mulrow C, Haynes RB (1997) Systematic reviews: synthesis of best evidence for clinical decisions. Ann Intern Med 126:376–80

Consensus Methods and Consumer Opinon

J.F. Bion

Learning Points

- Formal consensus methods provide a structured approach to managing uncertainty
- The Nominal Group Technique may substitute for surveys if the composition of the group is representative
- Evidence-based evaluation of the literature should form part of consensus development methods
- Measures of client (patient and staff) satisfaction should be a routine part of benchmarking within an institution

'Quot homines tot sententiae' [So many men, so many opinions].
Publius Terentius Afer (190-159 BC)

Introduction

Opinion is the antithesis of evidence. Our judgement may be clouded by preconceptions, a proprietary attachment to attractive hypotheses, indolence, or the sampling error of personal experience. From the phenomenon of risk-adjustment and the utility of car seat-belts [1] to the unreliability of clinical risk estimation [2], opinion alone provides an insecure foundation on which to construct decisions.

However, there are circumstances in which establishing opinion may be the only basis on which to proceed. The first is when objective evidence is inconclusive or unavailable. There are many examples relevant to intensive care, ranging from uncertainty about the value of the service as a composite entity, through organizational aspects such as nurse staffing ratios or early intervention, to specific technologies such as inhaled nitric oxide or antibiotics for inhalation pneumonitis. Indeed, it is easier to identify uncertainty about the value of many intensive care therapies than it is to ascertain proof of effectiveness. The second area where opinion is important is experiential research evaluating subjective impressions by consumers of a service or intervention. In this instance the views of patients or relatives have as much validity as objective outcomes such as duration of survival, but may be more difficult to measure.

This chapter examines methods of acquiring and evaluating information in circumstances of uncertainty or subjectivity, with particular reference to consensus techniques.

Why are Formal Consensus Methods Needed?

A British prime minister once described consensus as "what you reach when you can't agree". The grain of truth in this statement should not disguise the more important fact that formal consensus techniques offer a method for quantifying the extent of agreement or disagreement in the presence of uncertainty. This is valuable provided that the output of the process does not acquire the status of scientific proof. It should be seen more properly as hypothesis generation, based on collective wisdom or objective data where this exists. Consensus methods facilitate decision-making, and may provide insight into the process of evaluating data, but they do not generate new information, and their conclusions should be subject to further examination.

Consensus development should be based on knowledge, where this exists. Indeed, there would be little need for consensus methods if there were clear answers to every question, but much of medicine has evolved by precedent, individual experience and pragmatism, rather than through scientific method. In consequence, there are often substantial variations in clinical practice, or complex choices available, which make it difficult to decide how best to approach problems such as the organization of a service or the management of individual patients. Few treatment options are free from value judgements. Similarly, in the context of professional self-regulation, medical education, or the development of quality standards, there needs to be some mechanism for obtaining the opinions of the majority of those involved – the 'stakeholders'. Consensus methods facilitate this, using a formal structured approach. Structure is necessary for several reasons: to ensure that opinion is representative; to give weight to the importance of the ideas expressed rather than the importance of the person expressing them; to bring as wide a range of experience to bear on the problem as possible; to clarify reasons for convergence or divergence of opinion; to make it easier to measure agreement or disagreement objectively; and to evaluate the validity of the process and its output. Consensus methods may therefore function as an adjunct to evidence-based medicine (EBM) as well as providing a means for soliciting and structuring the opinions of groups of individuals.

Consensus Methods

There are three main techniques: the Delphi method, nominal groups, and consensus conferences. All three involve aggregating the opinions of groups of individuals according to predetermined criteria or cues, but they differ widely in the way information is obtained or provided, in the way groups interact, in iteration, and in data analysis.

The Delphi method: Named after the Greek oracle, this technique was developed in the 1950s by the RAND corporation as a means of using expert opinion to predict the development of new technologies [3]. It has subsequently become widely used by many professions for consensus development. The method employs iterative questionnaires completed by participants who do not meet together. Large numbers of participants can be surveyed in this way. The process starts with a development phase in which participants are asked to set the agenda for the questionnaire; this is then circulated with a request that participants prioritize the items listed according to the criteria or cues determined during development. The responses are aggregated and then returned to the participants in a format which shows both the group assessments and that particular respondent's assessment for each item. Individuals then have the opportunity to reconsider their assessments which are returned for a second analysis. This process can be repeated, the number of iterations being dependent on the degree of convergence and the participants' enthusiasm.

The advantages of the Delphi method are that it allows individuals to compare their assessments with those of others without incurring the costs and experiencing the potential negative effects of large group meetings. However, the absence of personal interaction is also one of the method's disadvantages, in that it deprives individuals of the opportunity to consider issues in more depth, and to understand the reasons for differences of opinion. An alternative approach which tries to capture the advantages of personal interaction while controlling for the negative aspects is the nominal group technique.

Nominal Groups: The nominal group technique was developed in 1971 [4] as a way of structuring interaction between members of a group, with the aim of facilitating the development of ideas and hypotheses which can then be discussed methodically through the mediating influence of a facilitator. Nominal groups usually have fewer participants than in the Delphi method, around nine to twelve. The process starts with each member of the group developing or evaluating the items or ideas independently; they then meet together to discuss them, the meeting being 'chaired' by a facilitator who ensures balanced treatment of each item. The members then privately reassess or rate each item as soon as its discussion is complete. The individual ratings are subsequently averaged to produce a median value for each item, reflecting the opinion of the group.

Items are rated using the Likert scale from 1 (least important or appropriate) to 9 (most important or appropriate), which allows three categories to be constructed with scores of 1-3, 4-6, and 7-9 indicating low, medium and high priority respectively. The extent to which there is consensus or disagreement within the group can be determined either by indicating the number of group members rating within each band, or by calculating the mean absolute deviation from the median (MADM) values for each item. This allows pre- and post-discussion ratings to be compared to determine the effect of discussion on prioritization and consensus. A reduction in the MADM between first and final ratings therefore indicates an increase in agreement between the participants.

Because the nominal group usually involves a smaller number of participants than the Delphi method, and because personal interaction is an essential element, the membership of the group and the way it is managed are of particular importance. These are considered later. However, both methods are 'closed' in the sense that the participants are usually selected in some way, and information is presented and interpreted in a manner that is not accessible to a wider audience. The perceived need for a more inclusive public forum for open debate prompted the development of the third consensus method, the consensus conference.

Consensus Conferences: This approach to consensus development was introduced by the US National Institutes of Health (NIH) in 1977 for health technology assessment [5]. It has since been taken up by various national groups, and has been used more commonly in intensive care than the other two methods. The format is based on a combination of the scientific conference and the criminal justice jury system. Experts are invited to address specific aspects of a particular issue in open forum and in front of a panel (the jury), the members of which are selected for particular qualities which may not necessarily include expertise in the subject under discussion. There is a chairman for the jury, but no 'judge' in the legal sense. At the end of each expert presentation the audience and the members of the jury may ask questions. At the end of the conference, the jury retires in closed session to consider the evidence and to prepare a consensus statement which is published subsequently in one or more scientific journals. This closed phase of consensus preparation may take place over the course of a weekend (in the model employed by the Société de Réanimation de Langue Française) or overnight in the NIH model.

Consensus conferences have the merit of open debate, but they are costly to set up, and they make two very important assumptions. The first is that the invited speakers have access to, and will present, all relevant evidence, or that if they do not, this will be identified and clarified in public discussion. The second is that the jury has the necessary skills and direction to be able to evaluate the evidence and draw appropriate conclusions from the information presented. Although minority views may be encouraged and presented, there is no formal process such as that used by the nominal group technique for structuring the jury's discussions and for analyzing the output.

Participants, Group Dynamics, and Decision Making

Consensus methods involve aggregating the opinion of groups of individuals. The nominal group technique and consensus conferences involve direct discussions between the participants. The output of these processes is likely to be influenced by the composition of the group, personal bias, interaction between the members, and the quality and presentation of available information.

The participants: The selection of participants in a consensus process should take into account the nature of the question or topic area, the credibility of the output, and practical issues such as cost. It seems reasonable that participants should have some insight into the issues at stake – that they should in some way be 'stakeholders' – and that they should have expertise in the area under investigation, whether as providers, consumers, or managers of health care services. More complex is the issue of how expertise is defined, and how to ensure that those included in the process are representative of the wider community. The approach generally accepted is to seek individuals whose backgrounds (e.g., hospital type, speciality, status) and geographical spread are similar to the majority, though their skills and knowledge may be above average. For small groups, attention may also need to be given to the personalities of the participants. It would appear that if attention is given to these elements, the conclusions of a select group are reasonably representative [6-8]. Heterogeneity within a group may enrich the output if hypothesis generation is one of the tasks, but may impede the development of consensus. Specialist panels tend to rate more investigations or interventions as appropriate within their area of expertise than panels composed of generalists [9,10]. The size of the panel is important in that there is a trade-off between improving reliability with larger numbers [11] while trying to optimize individual participation using smaller groups [12]; the ideal size appears to be between six to twelve individuals.

Group dynamics and role of the facilitator: The tensions within groups and the role of the facilitator have been well described by the psychoanalyst WR Bion, arising from his work in therapeutic military rehabilitation during the Second World War [13]. Similar though less intense problems may appear during consensus development. The facilitator is an important individual whose attitudes and abilities will influence the quality of decision making [14]. The role combines elements of leadership, stimulant, and mediator. It may be necessary to encourage diversity of opinion in order to arrive at consensus, and effective facilitation requires training. In addition to the facilitator, the surroundings in which the meeting is held will influence the participants, for example the use of a round table format to facilitate eye contact, and a level of comfort sufficient to encourage productive thought without inducing sleep.

Provision of information and decision making: The output of consensus development methods is dependent not only on process, but on input – that is, the information on which decisions are to be based, and the way it is presented. Where therapies and interventions are concerned, the gold standard is an evidence-based review of the literature, a major undertaking in its own right. This review should be made available to the participants well before the meeting to allow time for assimilation. The purpose of the meeting is then to determine consensus in areas of uncertainty, and to make judgements over values attached to interventions or outcomes. This will also be influenced by the framework and cues agreed on beforehand, such as the population for whom a treatment is intended. It is uncommon for this level of rigor to be applied to consensus development, reliance usually being placed on the expertise of the participants in conjunction with a limited literature review. Evidence should be evaluated systematically and graded according to standard methods (Table 1).

A key element in the Delphi and nominal group methods is the facility to compare and revise judgements in the light of discussion or feedback of group opinion. Iteration appears to improve consensus modestly using the Delphi method [16], and discussion has a more marked effect using the Nominal Group technique [17]. Factors which influence participants to change their opinions may be normative (based on standards or preferences) or informational (based on objective data).

Table 1. Evaluation of research evidence [15]

Type of study	Level of evidence
Randomized trials with low false-positive and low false-negative rates	1
Randomized trials with high false-positive and high false-negative rates	2
Non-randomized, concurrent cohort studies	3
Non-randomized, historical cohort studies	4
Case series	5

Informational influence is generally stronger. The Delphi technique suffers from the disadvantage that the process of iteration is conducted through the former mechanism, since the process only provides information about group estimates and not the reasons underlying the choices. The introduction of computer-aided analysis and feedback of data in real time may help to streamline the process.

Does the Output from Consensus Methods Influence Clinical Practice?

There have been several reviews of the impact of consensus development on clinical practice. Those examining the output from consensus conferences suggest that they may have relatively little impact on clinical practice [18,19]. A review [20] of ten evaluations of the impact of consensus conferences found that only two had a notable effect on practice, and six had no effect at all. It is likely that translating consensus effectively into sustained changes in practice requires education, reinforcement and feedback within institutions. This would appear to be the mechanism for the reduction in albumin use identified in a study in one hospital [21] following a French-sponsored consensus conference on this subject. More generally, a review [22] of 59 papers reporting the effect of clinical guidelines on practice found that 55 reported a beneficial effect on the process of care, and nine of eleven studies reported improvements in patient outcomes. Guidelines are more likely to influence clinicians if they feel some sense of involvement in their production, and dissemination occurs locally through opinion-leaders as well as the more remote mechanism of publication in peer-reviewed journals. This approach appears to have a beneficial effect on well-defined outcomes such as costs [23, 24].

Applications in Intensive Care

Consensus development methods in intensive care have been applied to specific interventions, technologies and treatments; setting standards and guidelines; hypothesis generation and prioritization of research; and education. The techniques employed have included informal methods such as expert panels and round tables as well as formal methods, of which consensus conferences predominate (Table 2).

Table 2. Examples of consensus methods in intensive care medicine

Topic area	Method	Ref
Critical care medicine	CC	[25]]
Respiratory muscle fatigue	CC	[26]
Sepsis and organ failure definitions	CC	[27]
Acute lung injury definitions	CC	[28]
Acute lung injury management	CC	[29]
Mechanical ventilation	CC	[30]
Cardiopulmonary dysfunction	CC	[31]
Tissue hypoxia	CC	[32]
Catecholamines	CC	[33]
Nitric oxide inhalation	CC	[34]
Pulmonary artery catheterization	CC	[35]
Albumin	CC	[36]
Long term ventilation	CC	[37]
Nutrition	CC	[38]
Sedation	D	[23]
Sedation	S	[24]
Evaluation of fever	EP	[39]
Prediction of outcome	CC	[40]
Research prioritization: UK	S, NG	[8]
Research prioritization: USA nursing	S	[41]
Education: nursing competence	D	[42]
Education: curriculum development	EP	[43]
Education: end-of-life decisions	NG	[44]

CC = consensus conference; D = Delphi method; NG = nominal group; S = survey; EP = expert panel.

The reliance on consensus conferences presumably has an historical basis, as this was the method favored by the NIH [5]. However, other than openness, and a comforting similarity to the usual medical conference format, it seems to have little in particular to recommend it over other methods. Potential weaknesses include dependence on selection of relevant literature by the contributors rather than a formal evidence-based approach, the absence of a rigorous procedure for the subsequent evaluation of the material presented to the jury, and reliance on medical journals for dissemination. In their favor is the provision of guidance to all practitioners from opinion leaders in the field. The output should perhaps best be seen as a form of hypothesis generation requiring subsequent testing. When this approach is adopted, the weaknesses of consensus conferences become apparent [45, 46], including the difficulty of ensuring adequate dissemination even within a single country when ownership of intensive care is split between different speciality groups [47].

There is a strong argument for basing consensus development on objective, formalized methods which ensure equal representation of the main stakeholders.

When this is achieved, provided that the process is transparent, Nominal groups may provide a valid alternative to large surveys [8]. However, whether this approach would hold true across cultures (for example within Europe) needs to be established.

Surveys of Client Satisfaction

An important but sometimes neglected area of medical practice is asking the opinion of the consumer – patient, relative, other members of staff – about the service they have received. Client satisfaction has not received much attention until the last 15 years or so. This may be a consequence of the charitable basis of many public health services obscuring the need for responsiveness to the wishes of patients (or staff on occasion). It is also not so long ago that one of the arguments adduced against Semmelweis' insistence that puerperal fever was spread on the hands of the medical attendants was the impossibility that agents of beneficence (doctors) could do their patients harm.

There are a large number of methods for measuring client satisfaction with care providers, with the outcomes of care, and for measuring staff satisfaction with their work (Table 3). These reflect both the variety of speciality areas, and whether the purpose of measurement is research or organizational audit. The clinical application of these instruments demonstrates the importance to patients of satisfactory clinical outcomes, responsive and listening staff (communication skills), clear explanations, kindness and professional attitudes, involvement in decision making (autonomy), and adequate staffing for the delivery of care [51, 63, 76–79], including intensive care [80]. This is not surprising. Of greater importance is putting in place systems for monitoring the quality of care which do not add substantially to the burden of data collection, which can be linked to other clinical databases, and which become an integral part of improving clinical care. This must be the responsibility of all members of staff within an organization, supported by management, to generate regular reports on a variety of quality measures including patient feedback on the care received [70]. Given good quality care, most survivors of critical illness seem reasonably satisfied with their outcomes [81].

Conclusion

The increasing use of consensus methods in medicine suggests that in the presence of uncertainty, or when value judgements must be made, clinicians prefer to base their practice on agreed norms. Consensus methods provide a structured and verifiable approach to identifying those norms. However, there is a need for greater integration of techniques, in particular with the informal components of consensus conferences. Evidence-based approaches to formal evaluation of the literature should be incorporated more closely into consensus methods. Measures of client (patient and staff) satisfaction should be a routine part of benchmarking within an institution.

Table 3. Instruments for measuring client/job satisfaction

Instrument or scale	Ref
Lifestyle Satisfaction Scale	[48]
Life satisfaction scale	[49]
Multidimensional Assessment of Parental Satisfaction (MAPS) for Children With Special Needs	[50]
Parent Medical Interview Satisfaction Scale (P-MISS)	[51]
Physical Therapy Outpatient Satisfaction Survey (PTOPS)	[52]
Musculo-skeletal care	[53]
Visual analogue scale	[54]
Medical Interview Satisfaction Scale (MISS)	[55]
Consultation Satisfaction Questionnaire (CSQ)	[56]
Gray's Home Care Satisfaction Scale (GHCSS)	[57]
Customer satisfaction questionnaire	[58]
McCloskey/Mueller Satisfaction Scale (MMSS)	[59]
Patients Intentions Questionnaire (PIQ)	[60]
Expectations Met Questionnaire (EMQ)	[60]
Consumer Emergency Care Satisfaction Scale.	[61]
Patient enablement instrument	[62]
Patient nursing satisfaction scale	[63]
La Monica-Oberst Patient Satisfaction Scale (LOPSS) 42 item	[64]
La Monica-Oberst Patient Satisfaction Scale (LOPSS) 28 item	[59]
Verona Expectations for Care Scale (VECS)	[65]
Verona Service Satisfaction Scale (VSSS)	[65]
Physicians' Humanistic Behaviors Questionnaire (PHBQ)	[66]
Dental Visit Satisfaction Scales	[67]
Client satisfaction survey	[68]
Patient Satisfaction Scale	[69]
Patient satisfaction benchmarking	[70]
Brigham and Women's Hospital Patient Satisfaction Survey	[71]
Patient satisfaction survey instrument for use in health maintenance organizations	[72]
Group Health Association of America Consumer Satisfaction Survey	[73]
Organizational Job Satisfaction Scale	[74]
Job Satisfaction Survey	[75]
Organizational Job Satisfaction Scale	[76]

Acknowledgement. An important source reference for this topic is the following review: Murphy MK, Black NA, Lamping DL, McKee CM, Sanderson CFB, Askham J, Marteau T (1998) Consensus development methods, and their use in clinical guideline development. Health Technol Assessment 2: i-iv, 1–88.

References

1. Adams J (1995) Risk. University College London Press, London
2. Christakis NA, Lamont EB (2000) Extent and determinants of error in doctors' prognoses in terminally ill patients: prospective cohort study. Br Med J 320: 469–473
3. Dalkey NC, Helmer O (1963) An experimental application of the Delphi method to the use of experts. Manage Sci 9: 458–467
4. Delbecq A, Van de Ven A (1971) A group process model for problem identification and programme planning. J Appl Behav Sci 7: 467–492
5. Fink A, Kosecoff J, Chassin M, Brook RH (1984) Consensus methods: characteristics and guidelines for use. Am J Publ Health 74: 979–983
6. McKee M, Priest P, Ginzler M, Black N (1991) How representative are members of expert panels? Qual Assur Health Care 3: 89–94
7. Kastein MR, Jacobs M, Van der Hell RH, Luttik K, Touw-Otten FWMM (1993) Delphi, the issue of reliability: a qualitative Delphi study in primary health care in the Netherlands. Technol Forecasting Soc Change 44: 315–323
8. Vella K, Goldfrad C, Rowan K, Bion J, Black N (2000) Use of consensus development to establish national research priorities in critical care. Br Med J 320: 976–980
9. Scott EA, Black N (1991) When does consensus exist in expert panels? J Publ Health Med 13: 35–39
10. 10.Leape LL, Freshour MA, Yntema D, Hsiao W (1992) Small group judgement methods for determining resource based relative values. Med Care 30 (suppl 11): NS28–NS39
11. Richardson FM (1972) Peer review of medical care. Med Care 10: 29–39
12. Shaw ME (1981) Group dynamics. The psychology of small group behaviour. 3rd Edn. McGraw–Hill, New York
13. Bion WR (1961) Experiences in Groups. Tavistock Publications, London
14. Wortman PM, Vinokur A, Sechrest L (1988) Do consensus conferences work? A process evaluation of the NIH consensus development program. J Health Polit Policy Law 13: 469–498
15. Sibbald WJ, Vincent JL (1995) Roundtable Conference on clinical trials for the treatment of sepsis. Intensive Care Med 21: 184–189
16. Woudenberg F (1991) An evaluation of Delphi. Technol Forecasting Soc Change 40: 131–150
17. Kahan JP, Park RE, Leape LL, et al (1996) Variations by specialty in physician ratings of the appropriateness and necessity of indications for procedures. Med Care 34: 512–523
18. Misset B, Artigas A, Bihari D, et al (1996) Short-term impact of the European Consensus Conference on the use of selective decontamination of the digestive tract with antibiotics in ICU patients. Intensive Care Med 22: 981–984
19. Kosecoff J, Kanouse DE, Rogers WH, McCloskey L, Winslow CM, Brook RH (1987) Effects of the National Institutes of Health consensus development program on physician practice. JAMA 258: 2708–2713
20. Lomas J (1991) Words without action? The production, dissemination and impact of consensus recommendations. Annu Rev Publ Health 12: 41–65
21. Durand–Zaleski I, Bonnet F, Rochant H, Bierling P, Lemaire F (1992) Usefulness of consensus conferences: the case of albumin. Lancet 340: 1388–1390
22. Grimshaw JM, Russell IT (1993) Effect of clinical guidelines on medical practice: a systematic review of rigorous evaluations. Lancet 342: 1317–1322
23. Saich C, Manji M, Dyer I, Rosser D (1999) The effect of introducing a sedation guideline on quality and efficiency in intensive care. Br J Anaesth 82: 792a–793 (Abst)
24. Devlin JW, Holbrook AM, Fuller HD (1997) The effect of ICU sedation guidelines and pharmacist interventions on clinical outcomes and drug cost. Ann Pharmacother 31:689–695
25. Parillo JE, Ayres SM (1984) NIH Consensus Development Conference Statement on Critical Care Medicine. Major issues in Critical Care Medicine. Williams & Wilkins, Baltimore
26. Anonymous (1990) NHLBI Workshop summary. Respiratory muscle fatigue. Report of the Respiratory Muscle Fatigue Workshop Group. Am Rev Respir Dis 142: 474–480

27. Bone RC, Balk RA, Cerra FB, et al (1992) Definitions for sepsis and organ failure and guidelines for the use of innovative therapies in sepsis. The ACCP/SCCM Consensus Conference Committee. Chest 101: 1644–1655
28. Bernard GR, Artigas A, Brigham KL, et al (1994) The American–European Consensus Conference on ARDS. Definitions, mechanisms, relevant outcomes and clinical trial coordination. Am J Respir Crit Care Med 149: 818–824
29. Artigas A, Bernard GR, Carlet J, et al (1998) The American–European Consensus Conference on ARDS, Part 2. Ventilatory, pharmacologic, supportive therapy, study design strategies and issues related to recovery and remodelling. Intensive Care Med 24: 378–398
30. Slutsky AS (1994) Consensus conference on mechanical ventilation. Intensive Care Med 20: 64–79
31. Lenfant C (1995) NHLBI Task Force summary. Task Force on Research in Cardiopulmonary Dysfunction in Critical Care Medicine. Am J Respir Crit Care Med 151: 243–248
32. Lemaire F, Apolone G, Blanch L, et al (1996) Tissue hypoxia: How to detect, how to correct, how to prevent? 3rd European Consensus Conference on intensive care organized by the French Language Intensive Care Society with the American Thoracic Society and the European Society of Intensive Care Medicine. Intensive Care Med 22: 1250–1257
33. Anonymous (1997) Consensus Conference: use of catecholamines in septic shock (adults, children). 15th Consensus Conference on intensive care and emergency medicine. Ann Fr Anesth Reanim 16: 205–209
34. Cuthbertson BH, Dellinger P, Dyar OJ, et al (1997) UK guidelines for the use of inhaled nitric oxide therapy in adult ICUs. American-European Consensus Conference on ALI/ARDS. Intensive Care Med 23: 1212–1218
35. Anonymous (1997) Pulmonary Artery Catheter Consensus conference: consensus statement. Crit Care Med 25: 910–925
36. Anonymous (1996) Consensus conference. Use of human albumin solutions in surgical anesthesia and surgical intensive care of adults. Ann Fr Anesth Reanim 15: 407–568
37. Make BJ, Hill NS, Goldberg AI, et al (1998) Mechanical ventilation beyond the intensive care unit. Report of a consensus conference of the American College of Chest Physicians. Chest 113 (suppl 5): 289S–344S
38. Anonymous (1998) Nutrition in the critically ill. Consensus conference. Ann Fr Anesth Reanim 17: 1274–1284
39. O'Grady NP, Barie PS, Bartlett JG, et al (1998) Practice guidelines for evaluating new fever in critically ill adult patients. Task Force of the Society of Critical Care Medicine and the Infectious Diseases Society of America. Clin Infect Dis 26:1042–1059
40. Anonymous (1994) Predicting outcome in ICU patients. 2nd European Consensus Conference in Intensive Care Medicine. Intensive Care Med 20: 390–397
41. Lindquist R, Banasik J, Barnsteiner J, et al (1993) Determining AACN's research priorities for the 90s. Am J Crit Care 2: 110–117
42. Boyle M, Butcher R, Kenney C (1998) Study to validate the outcome goal, competencies and educational objectives for use in intensive care orientation programs. Aust Crit Care 11: 20–24
43. Anonymous (1997) Guidelines for advanced training for physicians in critical care. American College of Critical Care Medicine of the Society of Critical Care Medicine. Crit Care Med 25: 1601–1607
44. Danis M, Federman D, Fins JJ, et al (1999) Incorporating palliative care into critical care education: principles, challenges, and opportunities. Crit Care Med 27: 2005–2013
45. Muckart DJ, Bhagwanjee S (1997) American College of Chest Physicians/Society of Critical Care Medicine Consensus Conference definitions of the systemic inflammatory response syndrome and allied disorders in relation to critically injured patients. Crit Care Med 25: 1789–1795
46. Villar J, Perez-Mendez L, Kacmarek RM (1999) Current definitions of acute lung injury and the acute respiratory distress syndrome do not reflect their true severity and outcome. Intensive Care Med 25: 930–935

47. Loeb T, Kaeffer N, Winckler C (1996) A survey of the diffusion and impact of consensus development conference on infections caused by central venous catheters in an anesthesiologist team. Ann Fr Anesth Reanim 15: 617–622
48. Heal LW, Chadsey-Rusch J (1985) The Lifestyle Satisfaction Scale (LSS): assessing individuals' satisfaction with residence, community setting, and associated services. Appl Res Ment Retard 6: 475–490
49. Kemp BJ, Krause JS (1999) Depression and life satisfaction among people ageing with post-polio and spinal cord injury. Disabil Rehabil 21: 241–249
50. Ireys HT, Perry JJ (1999) Development and evaluation of a satisfaction scale for parents of children with special health care needs. Pediatrics 104: 1182–1191
51. Lewis CC, Scott DE, Pantell RH, Wolf MH (1986) Parent satisfaction with children's medical care. Development, field test, and validation of a questionnaire. Med Care 24: 209–215
52. Roush SE, Sonstroem RJ (1999) Development of the physical therapy outpatient satisfaction survey (PTOPS). Phys Ther 79: 159–170
53. Solomon DH, Bates DW, Horsky J, Burdick E, Schaffer JL, Katz JN (1999) Development and validation of a patient satisfaction scale for musculoskeletal care. Arthritis Care Res 12: 96–100
54. Singer AJ, Thode HC Jr (1998) Determination of the minimal clinically significant difference on a patient visual analog satisfaction scale. Acad Emerg Med 5: 1007–1011
55. Wolf MH, Putnam SM, James SA, Stiles WB (1978) The Medical Interview Satisfaction Scale: development of a scale to measure patient perceptions of physician behavior. J Behav Med 1: 391–401
56. Baker R (1990) Development of a questionnaire to assess patients' satisfaction with consultations in general practice. Br J Gen Pract 40: 487–490
57. Gray YL, Sedhom L (1997) Client satisfaction: traditional care versus cluster care. J Prof Nurs 13: 56–61
58. Andrzejewski N, Lagua RT (1997) Use of a customer satisfaction survey by health care regulators: a tool for total quality management. Public Health Rep 112: 206–210
59. Misener TR, Haddock KS, Gleaton JU, Abu Ajamieh AR (1996) Toward an international measure of job satisfaction. Nurs Res 45: 87–91
60. Williams S, Weinman J, Dale J, Newman S (1995) Patient expectations: what do primary care patients want from the GP and how far does meeting expectations affect patient satisfaction? Fam Pract 12:193–201
61. Davis BA, Bush HA (1995) Developing effective measurement tools: a case study of the Consumer Emergency Care Satisfaction Scale. J Nurs Care Qual 9: 26–35
62. Howie JG, Heaney DJ, Maxwell M, Walker JJ (1998) A comparison of a Patient Enablement Instrument (PEI) against two established satisfaction scales as an outcome measure of primary care consultations. Fam Pract 15:165–171
63. Thomas LH, MacMillan J, McColl E, Priest J, Hale C, Bond S (1995) Obtaining patients' views of nursing care to inform the development of a patient satisfaction scale. Int J Qual Health Care 7: 53–63
64. La Monica EL, Oberst MT, Madea AR, Wolf RM (1986) Development of a patient satisfaction scale. Res Nurs Health 9: 43–50
65. Ruggeri M, Dall'Agnola R (1993) The development and use of the Verona Expectations for Care Scale (VECS) and the Verona Service Satisfaction Scale (VSSS) for measuring expectations and satisfaction with community-based psychiatric services in patients, relatives and professionals. Psychol Med 23: 511–523
66. Weaver MJ, Ow CL, Walker DJ, Degenhardt EF (1993) A questionnaire for patients' evaluations of their physicians' humanistic behaviors J Gen Intern Med 8:135–139
67. Corah NL, O'Shea RM, Pace LF, Seyrek SK (1984) Development of a patient measure of satisfaction with the dentist: the Dental Visit Satisfaction Scale. J Behav Med 7: 367–373
68. Reeder PJ, Chen SP (1990) A client satisfaction survey in home health care. J Nurs Qual Ass 5: 16–24
69. Baradell JG (1995) Clinical outcomes and satisfaction of patients of clinical nurse in psychiatric–mental health nursing. Arch Psychiatr Nurs 9: 240–250

70. Drachman DA (1996) Benchmarking patient satisfaction at academic health centers. Jt Comm J Qual Impr 22: 359–367
71. Hickey ML, Kleefield SF, Pearson SD, et al (1996) Payer-hospital collaboration to improve patient satisfaction with hospital discharge. Jt Comm J Qual Impr 22: 336–344
72. Weiss BD, Senf JH (1990) Patient satisfaction survey instrument for use in health maintenance organizations. Med Care 28: 434–445
73. Jatulis DE, Bundek NI, Legorreta AP (1997) Identifying predictors of satisfaction with access to medical care and quality of care. Am J Med Qual 12: 11–18
74. Sauter MA, Boyle D, Wallace D, et al (1997) Psychometric evaluation of the Organizational Job Satisfaction Scale. J Nurs Meas 5: 53–69
75. Spector PE (1985) Measurement of human service staff satisfaction: development of the Job Satisfaction Survey. Am J Community Psychol 13: 693–713
76. Booth M, Smith DF (1990) Job satisfaction amongst resident medical officers. NZ Med J 103:425–427
77. Kasprow WJ, Frisman L, Rosenheck RA (1999) Homeless veterans' satisfaction with residential treatment. Psychiatr Serv 50:540–545
78. Jatulis DE, Bundek NI, Legorreta AP (1997) Identifying predictors of satisfaction with access to medical care and quality of care. Am J Med Qual 12:11–18
79. Williams S, Weinman J, Dale J, Newman S (1995) Patient expectations: what do primary care patients want from the GP and how far does meeting expectations affect patient satisfaction? Fam Pract 12:193–201
80. Anderson FD, Maloney JP, Beard LW (1998) A descriptive, correlational study of patient satisfaction, provider satisfaction, and provider workload at an army medical center. Mil Med 163:90–94
81. Hurel D, Loirat P, Saulnier F, Nicolas F, Brivet F (1997) Quality of life 6 months after intensive care: results of a prospective multicenter study using a generic health status scale and a satisfaction scale. Intensive Care Med 23:331–337

Benchmarking in the ICU: The Measurement of Costs and Outcome to Analyze Efficiency and Efficacy

H. Burchardi, M. Jegers, M. Goedee, and J. U. Leititis

Learning Points

- Use correct definitions for cost assessment in intensive care medicine
- Beware of difficulties in comparing costs between different health care systems
- Beware of bias in risk adjustment in intensive care medicine
- Start costs assessment and outcome research in your own ICU
- Compare ICU performance only within your own health care system

For some years the German health care authorities have tried to stop the progressive increase in national health care expenditure – with only moderate success. Now the government is planning to create a completely new prospective payment system and for this purpose to adapt and utilize the US-American diagnosis-related groups (DRG) system. What are the risks and the limitations of comparing performance between such different health care systems? Is there evidence that such comparison can be valuable? Anecdotal evidence points to the lack of relevant cost data and economic evaluation studies, a situation which makes such a comparison even more hazardous.

Introduction

Today, intensivists are under increased pressure to curtail expenditure while maintaining high quality patient care. As a result, clinical decisions must often be based upon a simultaneous evaluation of clinical outcome and resource consumption. By regarding intensive care medicine as a process, such evaluations can become an important part of a quality improvement process: evaluation of quality (process / outcome) – assessment of expenditures – improvement of processes and outcome quality – reduction of costs.

Such a process of quality improvement and rationalization should be initiated in one's own department where long-term stable conditions are given and structures are well known.

Benchmarking, i.e., comparison between different ICUs, requires comparable conditions and structures. Such comparisons may be possible and useful within the same country. Between different countries and health care systems, however, conditions are rarely comparable which makes the generalization of benchmarking disputable.

Definitions

Some frequently used terms can be defined as follows (see e.g., [1]):

- Efficacy is the probability of benefit to the patient from a medical intervention for a given medical problem under ideal conditions of use. Efficacy is evaluated only in experimental or quasi-experimental conditions, such as the controlled clinical trial.
- Effectiveness is the probability of benefit to the patient from a medical intervention for a given medical problem under average routine conditions, i.e., in daily practice.
- Efficiency is the effectiveness of an intervention related to the resources used.
- Costs. Resources of various types are used in ICUs: nursing time and physician time, equipment time, disposables, medication, ... An economist would define these resources as 'costs', i.e., the value of something that has to be forgone in order to perform a productive activity [4].
- Cash costs versus accounting costs [5]. When calculating cash costs, only cash outlays are taken into consideration. This method is considered to be unsatisfactory for cost measurement in large and complex organizations. For example, an investment in a building would be recorded as a cost in the fiscal year that the payment is effectively made, with no effect whatsoever on the costs calculated in the subsequent years. Therefore, allocation of the amount invested over the lifetime of the building ('depreciation' or 'amortization') is more appropriate. In fact, this method (resulting in 'accounting costs') is an application of the more general 'accrual principle' in accounting. Its central idea is that costs are allocated to the periods in which the resource paid for is expected to be used. During that period of time the investment is visible on the hospital's financial statement (more specifically on the balance sheet).
- Cost object (or cost center) is the unit of analysis in which the cost is measured. Its choice depends on the research question in hand. Examples are patients, beds, bed-days, diagnoses, activities, the ICU as a unit, ...
- Direct costs are costs fully attributable to a specific cost center.
- Indirect costs are costs shared by more than one cost center. When determining the 'full' cost of the cost object, some part of the indirect costs has to be allocated to the cost object. By definition, this implies some arbitrariness. A specific method is Activity Based Costing (ABC), in which the indirect costs are related to relevant activities ('cost drivers') performed at the cost centers. Note that the notion of cost drivers in ABC is not used with reference to the direct costs. Finally, notice that we use the concept of indirect costs here in an accounting sense, and not in the sense usually understood in health economic analyses: production losses or gains due to illness or its treatment, as a result of absence from work, disability and mortality [20].
- Fixed costs are costs not influenced by the activity level at the cost center. The average fixed cost is the fixed cost divided by the activity level, and therefore decreases when the activity level increases. Fixed costs should not be confused with indirect costs.
- Variable costs are costs influenced by the activity level at the cost center. The variable cost does not decrease when the activity level increases. The average

variable cost is the variable cost divided by the activity level. Frequently, it is assumed to be constant, but this approximation is only valid within a rather narrow range of activity levels. Variable costs should not be confused with direct costs.

- Marginal costs are the costs of producing one extra unit at a given activity level. The marginal cost is not constant by definition. Technically, it can be calculated as the derivative of the (variable) cost with respect to activity.
- Cost-effectiveness. This term is mostly used in an imprecise manner to characterize some relationships between costs and outcome. For health economists, however, 'cost-effectiveness analysis' (CEA) has a very specific meaning: a CEA of a health care intervention or program requires a comparison of alternative methods for patients in a given health condition. This is important especially for new or improved interventions which generally turn out to be more expensive or for situations were restricted resources set limitations for medical services. Cost-effectiveness analyses use a single, summary measure for outcome (e.g., mortality, life-years saved, blood pressure reduction, increased mobility, ...).
- Cost-benefit analysis compares net costs of an intervention (e.g., medical intervention or health care program) with the net cost savings of that intervention entirely expressed in monetary terms.
- Cost-utility analysis compares net costs of an intervention (e.g., medical intervention or health care program) with the net 'utility' gained by that intervention. 'Utility' is a construct of economic theory, reflecting 'the amount of satisfaction one consumer obtains from a certain bundle of commodities' [4]. In health care applications frequently Quality Adjusted Life Years (QALYS) are used as a utility indicator.
- Hospital charges are agreed prices paid in a health care system for a given medical intervention. They should not be confused with costs which are expenses for the hospital. Unfortunately, however, they are frequently used as an indicator of costs.
- Benchmarking means comparison which is involved in the process of continuous quality improvement. In the quality management process the following steps have to be made:
  1) defining a process that requires quality improvement
  2) collecting data that adequately describe the process performance
  3) comparing the performance between institutions
  4) identifying factors that improve performance
  5) adopting these factors
  6) follow-up to confirm the quality improvement and search for further improvement by re-running the quality improvement process.

  The inherent problem of benchmarking, of comparison between different health care systems, is the difficulty of comparability. We know that hospital costs vary considerably between countries, in absolute values and even if adjusted to the gross national product (GNP). We also know that the ratio between ICU costs and total hospital expenditure varies greatly when compared in an international perspective. Can ICUs in different health care systems then be compared, even if the actual costs are adjusted to the GNP?

Data are lacking. International benchmarking for ICUs may be a hopeless illusion.
Nevertheless, it is interesting to realize some similarity between the US prospective payment system and the price relationship for comparable treatments in other countries with adequately developed health care systems.

- Diagnosis-related groups (DRGs). The US DRGs are certainly the most frequently used for international comparisons. These DRGs set fixed prices for the entire hospital treatment including intensive care. In some European countries the adaptation of this typically US prospective payment system is taken into consideration for creating a national system of charges for hospital treatment.
For instance, in Germany some medical procedures are defined in a similar way, the so-called 'Fallpauschalen' (FP) which provides the basis for hospital prices. However, they only cover about 20% of all medical procedures and contain mostly surgical procedures. We compared these FP with DRGs ('all patient DRG' (AP-DRG), New York) and found a remarkably good agreement (Fig. 1). Nevertheless, the usefulness of DRGs to reflect intensive care activities has not been evaluated yet. Furthermore, it must kept in mind that DRGs are charges or 'market prices' for hospital care which should not be confused with costs.
DRGs might be an interesting concept for national health care authorities to look for an adequate price structure in their countries. But, in contrast, hospital and ICU directors have to look at their own expenditures or resource consumption which needs tools for expenditure or cost assessment.

Cost Assessment

As intensive care units (ICUs) are clearly major resource consuming units in the hospital (around 20% of the budget for 5% of the hospital admissions [2]), the

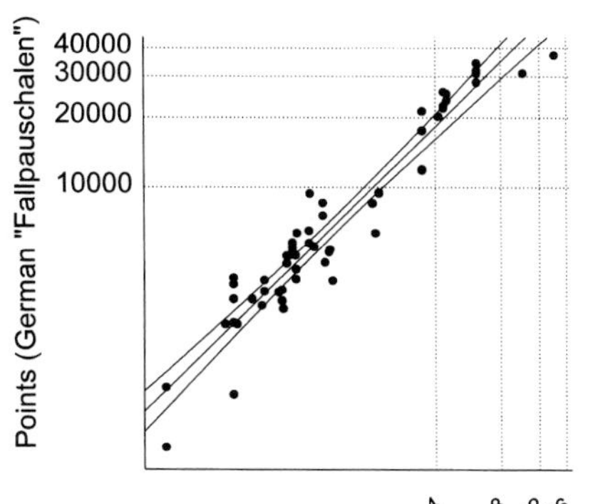

Fig. 1. Comparison between German '*Fallpauschalen*' values (FP, in points, version 1999) and US Diagnosis Related Groups (AP-DRG, New York, version 12.0 3M) (in relative values related to the price of an average case of treatment). Logarithmic plot, 95% confidential interval. Regression: FP = 3654 RV + 2293. Good accordance: $R = 0.93$, $p < 0.001$

problem of accurately calculating ICU costs is an important one, both from a managerial point of view and from a policy standpoint. However, it is obviously difficult to find generally acceptable concepts of ICU costing in Europe. The health care systems differ considerably, but the practice of ICU management a lso varies widely.

In a non-random sample of 88 ICUs in 12 European countries, only 38 ICU directors had knowledge about cost per bed per day of their unit [3]. However, they used their individual cost definitions so that comparability is not given. Only 14 of these ICUs used their own cost accounting system.

From the point of view of intensive care, cost centers can be classified into three broad categories: 1) costs attributed to the department (e.g., personnel, drugs, consumable, devices); 2) costs from interdepartmental services (e.g., laboratory, radiology); and 3) other overhead costs (e.g., estates, capital equipment, housekeeping, laundry) which cannot be influenced by the individual ICU.

Departmental costs are generally defined by the budget for the individual department ('top-down' accounting). Overhead costs can be attributed by the financial department of the hospital; however, allocation of these costs to the ICU is difficult. Costs from interdepartmental services, however, can only be allocated through an internal costing (reflecting, in the ideal situation, real costs borne by these services), which is not generally performed in most European hospitals.

In greater detail, resource consumption can be allocated to different subgroups, so called 'cost blocks'. This offers the possibility of defining a general financial structure for the ICU costs within the hospital. Take as an example the six cost blocks defined by a UK National Working Group: 1) current cost of using capital equipment (e.g., maintenance, depreciation); 2) estates (e.g., building maintenance, energy); 3) non-clinical support services (e.g., administration and management, cleaning); 4) clinical support services (e.g., laboratory, radiology, physiotherapy); 5) consumables (e.g., drugs, fluids, blood and blood products, disposables); 6) staff (e.g., medical, nursing staff, technicians) [6]. A financial evaluation of eleven UK ICUs demonstrated the following distribution of costs (average of financial years 1994 to 1996): 6% equipment, 3% estates, 7% non-clinical support services, 8% clinical support services, 23% consumables, 54% staff [6]. This demonstrates the well-known fact that staff cost is the most important cost block. Nevertheless, there were considerable differences between the various ICUs and hospitals presumably not only caused by differences in case-mix. A similar comparison of cost block structures between different countries and health care systems is still missing. Larger differences might be anticipated if ICUs in different health care systems are compared, e.g., because of different level of staffing or staffing costs. If this is not taken into account, benchmarking studies between different health care systems will be difficult and may even be misleading. Within the same health care system, however, such comparison may be very instructive. Cost containment may stimulate the national authorities or third-party payers to perform such investigations in some selected hospitals which certainly will increase the competition between hospitals in general.

'Top-Down' Versus 'Bottom-Up'

Hospital administrations act in terms of general budgeting and financial control is performed by the 'top-down' principle. An example of this top-down cost assessment in one ICU over a period of three years was published by Singer et al. [7]. Today, when economic pressure also strikes ICUs, one has to know what are the major departmental expenses. Cost containment is only possible with general strategic decisions (e.g., to change the sedation policy or the antibiotic strategy).

An effective way for allocation of direct costs to individual patients using a 'bottom-up' approach is by using a computer-based patient data management system (PDMS). If all prescriptions and actions carried out for the individual patient are recorded by a PDMS, consumables, such as drugs, fluids, nutrition, blood and blood products, disposables (e.g., syringes, catheters, tubes), can easily be assessed. Costs can then be calculated automatically by means of an integrated price-list. Also, clinical support services such as laboratory services, radiology and imaging services can be recorded by the PDMS, but cost assessment can only be done if these services operate with defined prices.

Only this information about direct costs enables the ICU team to identify apparently expensive procedures and strategies and then to look for less costly, but acceptable alternatives. This day-to-day procedure is not a cost-effectiveness analysis, because it is not a well structured trial with alternatives. However, it is perhaps a relevant way of continuing quality improvement in small steps, and with involvement of the whole ICU team.

Activities and Direct Cost Measurement

A remarkable prospective cost accounting analysis was performed by Noseworthy and co-workers [8]. Over one year, all direct costs (e.g., nursing, laboratory, medication, and other supplies as well as procedures) were tracked down to the individual patient by concrete measurement (measuring direct costs and time spent). Indirect costs (e.g., capital resources, nursing management, overtime etc.,) were averaged over all patients on a daily basis. It was found that costs per day and patient were remarkably constant, approximating CAN$ 1,500 /day/patient (1992) with no great variations across different diagnoses. The wide variation of total costs per patient was mainly a result of differences in length of stay. It is evident, however, that this kind of direct cost accounting is highly laborious and virtually unfeasible as a routine procedure.

Another method to estimate direct costs is by quantifying therapeutic activities through the Therapeutic Intervention Scoring System (TISS) [9, 10]. Recently, the TISS scoring procedure has been simplified by Reis Miranda et al. reducing the amount of scoring parameters from 76 to 28 [11]. To date, TISS has repeatedly being used to estimate ICU costs [12, 13]. If data collection conditions remain stable, TISS can at least be used for long-term estimation of treatment activities within one single ICU. Combined with the overall expenditure of the ICU, a monetary value can be attributed to each TISS-point.

Takala and co-workers combined daily TISS scoring with an internal billing system for individual cost accounting. The total expenditures (including personnel costs) of the ICU were divided by the total number of accumulated TISS-points over a 2-year period. They found that a single TISS-point was equivalent to 44.7 US$ in 1993 and to 43.3 US$ in 1994 [15]. In contrast to the above mentioned study of Noseworthy et al. [8], there were considerable differences in costs per admission which were not only due to differences in length of stay, but also due to variations in the different diagnostic groups.

The cost-equivalent per TISS-point is of course very specific for the individual ICU within a certain health care system. TISS-point equivalents from other studies and from other countries differ considerably. Zimmerman and co-workers [16], for example, estimated costs of 300 US$ per TISS-point for 37 US ICUs in 1991. Smithies et al. [17] estimated costs of 27.50 £UK per TISS-point for their ICU (1990).

Patient-related staff services such as nursing time delivered or intensivist and consulting physician time spent on patient treatment, are difficult to assess. Manual timekeeping is extremely time-consuming and can only be done for a short period. The only way is to estimate workload by surrogate markers. TISS has been recommended for estimating nursing workload and nursing costs as well. However, as nursing workload does not directly correlate with the severity of illness and the therapeutic activities for an individual patient, TISS scores tend to underestimate nursing workload. A further simplified system, the Nine Equivalents of Nursing Manpower Use Score (NEMS) needs to be validated for reflecting nursing workload [14]. It has not been used for estimating costs, yet.

As nursing costs account for the major part of ICU costs, this still remains an unsolved basic problem in ICU cost assessment. Estimating costs by TISS scores gives a general information of patient-specific expenditures. However, it does not help us to identify specific cost drivers. This can only be done by direct costs assessment ('bottom-up').

Evaluation of Cost Studies

Criteria

Before comparing costs and performance of different ICUs and evaluating cost studies, there must be a general agreement on definitions and cost concepts. Apparently, there is still a lack of trans-disciplinary collaboration between medical professionals and economists. In numerous studies on ICU costs economists are rarely involved. Therefore, economists could be suspicious about the validity of these papers with respect to a correct definition and application of cost concepts. Below we will develop a list of criteria to be used when evaluating (ICU) cost studies.

Remembering the definition of costs given above, it must be clear that costs are not a concept *per se*. Costs are forgone alternatives for an individual or a specific organization, implying that a cost for one particular cost bearer is not automatically a cost for somebody else [18]. Consider for example the cost of a ventilator in an ICU: from the hospital's point of view, its cost is based on the amount invested and the way it is used. From the insurer's point of view it is the amount paid to the hospital for using the ventilator (no matter how it is determined). From the patient's standpoint his/her costs are the sum of the payments that have to be made as a consequence of being admitted to the ICU and treated with a ventilator. For a sound cost study, it is therefore imperative that the point(s) of view considered should be clearly defined and consistently taken into consideration when calculating costs or, as is frequently done, studying cost containment effects.

Criterion 1a: The cost bearer should be clearly identified

Criterion 1b: Costs should be defined accordingly.

In health care, at least three points of view are possible: the health care provider, the insurer(s), and the patient. In the first case, the cost of resource consumption should be measured. When the insurer's point of view is taken, charges are relevant. For patients, all payments and co-payments should be traced. Therefore, the practice of using charges and microcosting data interchangeably [19] is to be rejected.

The choice of cost centers also has an important bearing on correct cost measurement and must therefore be made clear. It impinges on the distinction between direct and indirect costs. Consider, for example, a hospital bed. If the bed is the unit of analysis, its cost is a direct cost. If, on the other hand, the patient is the object of analysis, the cost of the bed is an indirect cost, to be allocated to all the patients using the bed according to some allocation rule.

In the previous example, the bed is 'direct' for the entire ICU, but there are, at a higher level in the hospital, other costs that are 'indirect' from the ICU's point of view (e.g., hospital management, financial costs, ...). At the first stage, they are to be allocated to the ICU, and then these allocated indirect costs have to be further allocated to the cost centers considered, e.g., the patient.

As allocation rules are always somewhat arbitrary, one could choose only to take direct costs into consideration. Nevertheless, there may be good reasons to be interested in the total (or 'full') cost/unit, defined as the sum of direct and indirect costs per unit. In this case the categories of indirect costs (from the ICU level and from higher levels) concerned should be delineated. In a number of studies, this choice is not explicitly made.

Finally, when including indirect costs, the allocation rules applied should be described and justified.

Criterion 2a: The unit of analysis (cost center; cost object) chosen should be shown to determine the distinction between direct and indirect costs.

Criterion 2b: A choice between direct costs/unit or (direct + some indirect) costs/unit should be made.

Criterion 2c: If indirect costs are included, allocation rules should be described and justified.

As ICU costs are the focus of the present chapter, it seems logical to require that direct ICU cost measurements should be performed at the ICU level instead of being derived from a more aggregate cost figure, such as hospital costs. As logical as this may seem, in a relatively recent review of 20 ICU cost studies, half of them did not meet this requirement [21].

Criterion 3: All direct ICU costs should be measured at the ICU level
Apart from the distinction between direct and indirect costs, the difference between fixed and variable costs is equally important and different in nature. The traditional economic concepts of total costs, average costs, total fixed costs, average fixed costs, total variable costs, average variable costs and marginal costs, cover differing economic contents and mechanisms, and should therefore be used thoughtfully, especially when cost data are used for simulation purposes and ensuing policy recommendations. It is generally known that in the long run all costs are variable. In the present review we consider one year as the relevant time span to make the distinction between fixed and variable costs.

Particularly when indirect methods, such as TISS-based expressions, are applied, the distinction between cost categories can be blurred. Furthermore, in ICU cost studies, fixed costs and indirect costs are frequently, but wrongly, considered to be equivalent concepts [12, 22].

Criterion 4: Fixed, variable and marginal costs should be made explicit and correctly handled.

Finally, once researchers have determined the kind of cost they wish to determine, they should aim at comprehensiveness; all important components of the costs studied should be included in the calculation, and for the others it should be justified why they were left out, the only good reason being their relative unimportance. Difficulties in determining or estimating costs are clearly not a good argument to ignore them (e.g., the physician's costs; frequently when charges are used, say from the point of view of the insurers, fees are not included). In the same vein, the way costs are determined should be made explicit, allowing the reader to assess the quality of the data presented.

Criterion 5a: Costs should be calculated comprehensively. Only immaterial components may be ignored.

Criterion 5b: Determination of each component of costs studied should be made explicit. Furthermore, a sensible methodology should be applied.

It is clear that an assessment of cost studies in respect of Criterion 5b can only be made on an *ad hoc* basis.

Assessment of ICU Cost Studies

Using the above mentioned criteria two of the authors evaluated a randomly selected sample of 23 papers (written in English) in which ICU costs were estimated [7, 8, 12, 16, 19, 22–29] (Table 1). At least 75 of the 103 authors are medical or paramedical professionals demonstrating the lack of involvement of economists. The papers were independently scored on the criteria by assigning a nominal value of 'Yes', 'No' or 'Not applicable'. The overlap in their scores reached 89%. It must be clear that the assessment relates to the way the research was presented in the papers, most of which are published in high standard, scientific journals, and not directly to the way the studies themselves have been performed. Of course, the quality of reporting and research can be expected to be highly correlated.

Table 1. Percentage of papers meeting the quality criteria for ICU cost studies

Criterion	Percentage
1a: Identification of cost bearer	74
1b: Relation cost bearer – cost measured	76
2a: Relation cost centre – direct/indirect costs	38
2b: Choice direct cost versus full cost	50
2c: Description allocation rules for indirect costs	27
3: Measurement of ICU costs at ICU level	91
4: Correct distinction fixed, variable, marginal costs	6
5a: Comprehensive cost calculation	47
5b: Description cost calculation	70

When assessing criterion 1a we have been very lenient, by accepting implicit determinations of cost bearers as shown by a consistent use of cost categories. In a paper using, for example, only charges, we assumed that the authors positioned themselves in the point of view of the insurers, even if they did not mention this explicitly. In spite of this course of action, in about one fourth of the papers the authors fail to make clear who is to bear the costs they calculate, severely limiting the usefulness of their work. Furthermore, in almost another fourth of the papers that meet criterion 1a, the cost definition does not correspond to the designated cost bearer.

The major weaknesses of most papers are to be found in the application of standard cost concepts. In only 38% of cases is the relation between the cost center chosen and the determination of direct and indirect costs explicited (criterion 2a), and even here in a number of cases the indirect costs were wrongfully labeled fixed costs. If these costs were treated as indirect costs, we considered criterion 2a to have been met. Related to this, in only half of the papers did the authors mention whether they were interested in either the direct costs exclusively, or the full costs (direct costs + allocated indirect costs), obscuring the distinction between direct and indirect costs when analyzing the costs described (criterion 2b). The reporting on the procedures applied to allocate the indirect costs is unacceptable, at least for economists, in nearly three-fourths of the cases (criterion 2c). As far as the distinction between fixed, variable and marginal costs is concerned, we must conclude (criterion 4) that in almost none of the papers reviewed here is this distinction made and applied in a correct way, even in the cases where the fixed costs are not mistakenly considered to be the indirect costs.

Comprehensive cost calculations could only be established in about half the cases, although we accepted situations in which it was cogently argued that some cost categories were lacking, either because of their insignificance, or because of data problems (criterion 5a). The presentation of the methodology by which costs were calculated on the contrary seems acceptable in a large majority of cases (criterion 5b).

Contrary to the results obtained by Gyldmark [21], who observed in her study that, in 50% of the papers, reviewed ICU costs were derived from costs at a higher level of aggregation, we found that in almost all cases under the present review, ICU costs were measured at the appropriate level, i.e., the ICU itself (criterion 3).

Measuring Outcome

The value and definition of outcome may be different if defined by patients, healthcare providers, third-party payers, or society. For the patient, survival as well as the resulting quality of life will be most important. The ICU or the hospital director focus more on survival than on long-term morbidity. For third-party payers and for society, however, long-term morbidity and functional status (e.g., activities of daily living) are the most relevant outcome measures because of the long-term monetary consequences.

However, all outcome parameters have their specific problems:

- Mortality is an unambiguous endpoint, but it is a relatively rare event due to the progress in medicine. It is difficult to detect differences in mortality when comparing medical interventions, such as the benefit of different modes of mechanical ventilation for treating acute respiratory failure or the benefit of using continuous renal replacement techniques for treating acute renal failure. ICU mortality closely depends on the admission and discharge policy and is, therefore, significantly influenced by the internal structure of the hospital. Hospital mortality is a preferred endpoint, but it depends also on the quality of the peripheral wards. Using mortality as the only endpoint, other important outcome measures such as functional status, length of stay, resource consumption might be overlooked.
- Functional status of the patient at hospital discharge and at follow-up could be very relevant indications of ICU performance. It is however time consuming and, thus, rarely performed.
- Quality of life (QOL) evaluations are also very difficult to perform and there are only few studies on QOL looking specifically at ICU patients. One recent example is the study by Brooks et al. [40].
- Adverse events and complication rates, such as nosocomial infections, readmission rates, accidental extubations, decubitus ulcer, etc., are useful quality indicators of ICU performance, for instance for quality improvement programs. But if they are used for comparison between different units, the escorting risk factors such as comorbidities, underlying diseases, surgical or medical origin, days on ventilator, must be closely controlled. Again, admission and discharge policies influence complication rates, readmission rates, and the relationship between hospital and ICU mortality.

Predicting Outcome by Scoring Systems

In intensive care medicine insufficient vital functions and acute organ failures are treated. Impairment of vital functions predominantly determines the acute severity of illness. Medical diagnoses, on the other hand, play a minor role in defining the patient's acute situation and predicting survival.

In order to compare patients with different diagnoses and various risks a 'risk adjustment' is required. Severity scoring systems, such as APACHE III, SAPS II, MPM II, are used to quantify the actual severity of illness and to predict probability of survival. These scoring systems can be used for 'standardization' of ICU patients in various situations according to their actual severity of illness. By this method, ICU patients in quite different conditions are made comparable.

To compare the performance of different ICUs or just to look at the performance of your own ICU, the standardized mortality rate (SMR) can be used. SMR is the ratio of actual to predicted mortality. However, there are many potential problems which lead to misinterpretation:

- Differences in patient mix (surgical/medical/trauma patients) may lead to an inadequate calibration. Some diagnoses (e.g., myocardial infarction and cardiopulmonary bypass patients, burns) are even excluded from some scoring systems.
- Problems of 'inter-observer reliability' (i.e., different people collecting data at different times or in different locations obtain the same value for a specific variable in a specific patient). Variables that are subjective, difficult to interpret, or poorly defined may cause poor inter-observer reliability [41].
- 'Lead time bias' (i.e., the effects of variation of treatment before ICU admission, such as emergency service, operations) may create differences in score values in patients even with equal severity of illness.

An overview of the potentials and problems of standardizing patients by severity of illness scores is presented elsewhere in this book.

Comparing Outcomes Among ICUs

The consequences of these above mentioned difficulties are that severity scores and SMR must be used with extreme caution (Table 2). Only if calibration is sufficient, if patient mix and lead time bias (i.e., ICU and hospital system organization) are comparable, and the inter-observer reliability has been minimized, can SMRs can be used to compare the performance of different ICUs. Also, the results of SMRs should be reported together with 95% confidence intervals.

Table 2. Factors that may affect outcomes systematically (modified from [42])

- **What service was provided?**
  e.g., management strategies
- **Who provided the service?**
  e.g., specialists, level of experience, volume of service (overload?)
- **Where was the service provided?**
  e.g., different level of ICUs, of hospitals, of regions
- **When was the service provided?**
  e.g., timing of service, period of the year (seasonal trends)
- **Why was the service provided?**
  e.g., different local practice guidelines, care-paths

A valid use of general prediction models to compare different ICUs requires similarity between the units in age, distribution of severity of illness, and diagnoses. Also the time period should be comparable and sufficiently long to compensate for short term variations.

For a valid comparison the sample size must be large enough. If the outcome is measured as mortality, Randolph et al. [42] recommend, as a rule of thumb, a minimum of a few hundred patients from each ICU (assuming the mortality rate is about 10%). This is not the case in most of the studies.

Other differences may also cause problems for a valid comparison. There are obviously differences between treatment strategies, as preferences for aggressive interventions, even for patients with similar prognosis, vary not only between physicians but also between ICUs. There may be differences of care during transport, in the emergency room, in the operating room, etc., as well as differences in quality of care on peripheral wards. There may also be different lead time bias: correctly, severity scores are calculated as the worst values within the first 24 hrs. But most patients are already on some support on arrival in the ICU or there may have been a transfer among ICUs. In multicenter comparisons significant differences may originate from relatively few ICUs. Thus, it may be useful to perform a multilevel comparison (i.e., not only to look for individual patients within each ICU, but also to look at the characteristics of the different ICUs). All these problems have been described and discussed recently [42, 43].

Even if everything is done well, limitations in the methodology of risk stratification also limit the strength of interference of the results. Only very large and significant differences should be taken into account (e.g., if confidence intervals do not include the average value for the entire sample).

Severity scoring systems provide a risk stratification according to type, severity and physiological derangement of the disease. However, they ignore response to treatment and therapy related factors. Clinical ICU practice varies markedly between countries and healthcare systems. It depends heavily on funding, resource allocation, numbers and level of nursing staff, and medical care. Lamb et al. [44] pointed out that differences in availability of technology, admission and discharge policies (e.g., admission of low risk patients for monitoring), level of health care funding (defined, e.g., by the ratio of the GNP), definition and ratio of ICUs beds, etc., may lead to misinterpretation when comparing ICUs in different health care systems. For correct benchmarking, comparison should only be made within a single homogeneous healthcare and costing system.

Keenan and coworkers [45] tried to assess the efficiency of the admission process to a critical care unit by benchmarking comparison through data from literature. They looked for articles on this topic where the following criteria were fulfilled: 1) critical care patients; 2) cohort study; 3) measurements which allowed identification of patients requiring active critical care versus monitoring alone. From a review of 8 years throughout the available literature, they only found five articles fulfilling all the criteria. However, the differences in preconditions and patient mix did not allow any comparison with each other. They conclude that the current literature does not offer the necessary data for critical care physicians to conduct benchmarking, at least for the admission process.

Nevertheless, outcome analyses can offer some important insights in the impact of the ICU management system. Some interesting studies have demonstrated that intensive care medicine becomes more efficient if the ICU is run by a competent intensivist-directed team [46-50]. A multicenter study of pediatric critical care documented higher survival with on-site, in-house intensivists [46]. The same beneficial effect of a competent team could be shown in adult ICUs; a competent, full-time ICU staff resulted in lower mortality [47] and lower costs [48], or lower mortality from specific diseases but increased charges, which nevertheless was shown to be acceptable (incremental charges of 5,500 US$ for a reduction of mortality from 74% to 57% in patients with septic shock) [49]. A survey from 3,000 ICUs in 1,700 US hospitals concluded that the direct involvement of a medical ICU director reduced length of stay and inappropriate admissions significantly [50].

Combining Costs with Outcome

Thinking in terms of cost-effectiveness means looking at outcome and costs. ICU physicians should endeavor to deliver the most appropriate treatment for their patients at the lowest possible costs.

Cost assessment can be done accurately if adequate tools are available. But this is rarely the case. Computer-assisted patient data management systems in the ICUs make cost assessment easier. Predicting outcome to validate performance, however, is not only inaccurate, it can also be misleading as has been argued above. If we want to compare ICU performance in different countries, this becomes even more discouraging. Often costing is incomparable because of the differences in healthcare systems, in insurance policies, in personnel fees, in drug prices, in hospital administration, and others factors.

Cost Assessment and Performance

Evaluating economic and clinical performance in one's own ICU, however, can be a valuable tool of quality improvement, especially if conducted long-term. Because the structure of the ICU as well as the basic conditions in the hospital (e.g., patient mix, admission and discharge policy, treatment strategies) remain stable within a certain time frame, comparability is provided. For longer periods costs must be adjusted adequately by considering discount rates.

To follow up the economic and clinical performance of the ICU helps to identify potential cost drivers, and to look for containment possibilities. The increased awareness of expenses by the whole team may be even of more importance. Merely strengthening physicians' awareness of cost factors by daily bedside information in a trauma ICU, resulted in significant cost reductions for medications, laboratory tests, chest x-ray films, respiratory therapy, and others, without negative effects on mortality rate [51].

Evaluating costs and outcome is an important tool for analyzing the overall 'process of care', a tool for quality improvement. Before attempting any comparison to other ICUs, an accurate knowledge of the home situation is mandatory. Thus, evaluation of one's own ICU must be the first step.

Effective cost per survivor (ECPS). Smithies et al. [17] developed a model to assess cost performance of ICU care according to patients' severity of illness. Patients were grouped into deciles of risk (APACHE score) and within all risk groups the cost per survivor, the cost per non-survivor, and the ECPS were determined (costs derived as cost per TISS point). The ECPS is the total cost for survivors and non-survivors within one risk group divided by the number of survivors. This provides a useful measure of cost-performance, because ECPS raises considerably with a higher probability of death when more resources are spent for non-survivors. Unfortunately, this study [17] did not clearly define which costs were included.

To give a practical example, in the ICU of the University Hospital of Göttingen we use a PDMS which provides complete data management of all patient-, diagnosis-, and treatment-related data, as well as the administrative and organizational data management. The PDMS is also linked to peripheral work stations, such as to the central laboratory or the pharmacy via the hospital network. By this method, all prescriptions and diagnostic and therapeutic activities for the individual patient are recorded at time of delivery. A detailed price-list enables the cost calculation to be made easily and automatically. Thus, direct patient-related costs for consumables (drugs, fluids, nutrition, blood and blood products, disposables) and services (laboratory, radiology, imaging, bacteriology services, function tests) are individually and completely recorded. In this connection, the direct expenses for the hospital (not charges) are taken into account. For small expenses (e.g., dressings) the amounts and costs were estimated. Staff costs, however, are derived from the hospital administration budget.

In the ICU, 598 mainly surgical patients staying in the unit for 24 hours or more were evaluated (consecutively from May 1997 to February 1998). Hospital mortality was averaged at 12.3% and the mean predicted mortality (SAPS II) was15.5% which corresponds to a mean SMR = 0.79. Direct costs (without personnel) averaged 3,855 DM per admission. Figure 2 shows the distribution of direct costs per survivor, per non-survivor and the ECPS according to the risk-adjusted groups of patients.

Indication for intensive care medicine. Economic evaluations have also been used for analyzing the indications for intensive care medicine. Cohen et al. [52] analyzed retrospectively the incremental charges and benefits of mechanical ventilation (3 days and more) for elderly patients (aged 80 years and older) in a medical-surgical ICU in tertiary-care community teaching hospital. This cost-effectiveness evaluation was performed by assessing incremental hospital charges (= billing records); these charges were then related to years of life saved. A telephone survey was used to follow up hospital survivors for a minimum of 4 years after discharge. Of 45 patients, only 10 survived to leave the hospital. The charge per year of life saved was between US$ 51,854 and US$ 75,090 (1985–1987). These charges increased to US$ 181,308 when the sum of age in years and duration of mechanical ventilation exceeded 100. The authors concluded that cost-effectiveness of prolonged mechanical ventilation in patients aged ≥ 80 years was poor in this subgroup. Unfortunately, the quality of life of the survivors was not been eval-

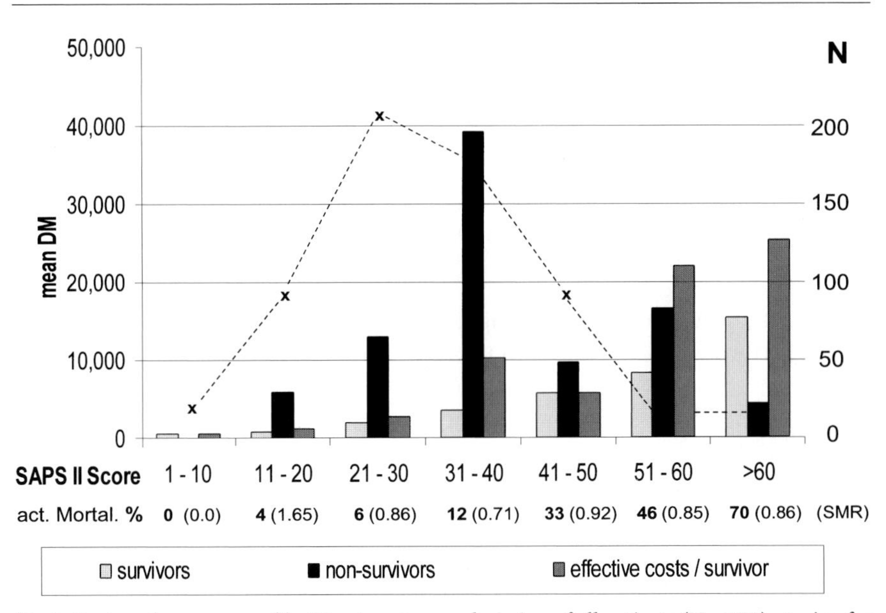

Fig. 2. Cost-performance profile. Direct costs per admission of all patients (N = 598), staying for ≥ 24 hours in our ICU (University Hospital Göttingen) from May 1997 to February 1998. Direct costs (in DM) (without personnel) per admission for survivors, non-survivors and all costs divided by number of survivors (effective costs / survivor). Groups of severity of illness (SAPS II Score) and frequency (x) within these groups. Actual mortality (act. Mortal.) and standardized mortality ratio (SMR)

uated in this study. From an ethical point of view, this analysis raises a serious question: how much is society willing to pay for the survival of elderly patients?

In contrast to that, a recent economic evaluation compared the costs and consequences of a policy of continuing prolonged ICU care with a proposed policy of withdrawing such care [53]. In an adult medical/surgical ICU analyzing the course of 690 consecutive patients, it was found that a considerable proportion of those patients with a prolonged length of stay (> 14 days) in the ICU survived their critical illness (27 of 61 patients survived 12 months). Their long-term quality of life was found to be reasonable. The incremental cost-effectiveness ratio was found to be Can $ 65,219 per life saved or Can $ 4,350 per life-year saved. The authors concluded that even a prolonged ICU stay may represent an efficient use of hospital resources. In this study a sensitivity analysis was performed by varying the key determinants (survival rate and per diem ICU costs) which supported the results.

An alternative approach to assess differences in clinical performance and cost-effectiveness was proposed by Rapoport et al. [34]. By comparing 25 ICUs (3 397 consecutive patients) from US hospitals, a length-of-stay index ('weighted hospital days' (WHD) which weights ICU days more heavily than non-ICU days (first ICU day = 3, each subsequent ICU day = 2, post-ICU days = 1) and the Mortality Probability Model (MPM) were used. Using weighted hospital days as a resource use ('cost') measure, the cost-effectiveness ratio is (WHD)/(number of survivors). The economic performance index was the difference between actual mean resource use and the resource use predicted by a regression including severity of illness and percent of surgical patients. Most of the units studied fell within 1 SD of the mean for both the clinical and the economic indices. This might be an appropriate method to assess the relative performance between ICUs and hospitals. However, several drawbacks have to be considered: the evaluation excluded the days spent before the ICU stay, thus, lead time bias could have had some influence. Further, readmission rates were not taken into account, making comparison between hospitals with different admission and discharge policies disputable. Also, the ratio between ICU days and post-ICU days for calculating resource use may vary in different health care systems. Nevertheless, this approach might be useful for assessing and comparing the overall performance of ICUs within one health care system.

Cost-Effectiveness

Standards for performing cost-effectiveness analysis studies have been described [54, 55]. Recently there have been excellent guides published on how to use articles on economic analysis in medical literature [56, 57].

Accepting these standards, many published studies (75%–80%) on cost-effectiveness analysis were performed inadequately by not fulfilling the required minimal criteria [58]. For a correct cost-effectiveness analysis the following steps are mandatory: 1) description of all choices and alternatives; 2) definition of the perspective (patient, hospital, health care system); 3) determination of costs; 4) determination of effectiveness; 5) stipulation of the time frame; 6) calculation of cost-effectiveness ratios; 7) analyzing sensitivity; 8) identifying cautionary factors [59]. The above mentioned study by Heyland et al. [53] is an example of how to perform a sensitivity analysis on costs and consequences of continuing prolonged ICU care.

The limitation of any generalization is impressively illustrated [60] by the well known GUSTO trial [61]. Here, streptokinase was compared with tissue plasminogen activator (tPA) as thrombolytic strategy for acute myocardial infarction. tPA was found to reduce overall 30-day mortality rates by 0.9%, but increased the risk of disabling stroke by 0.33% compared to streptokinase. Recent additional economic evaluations, using the data of GUSTO, concluded that tPA is cost-effective compared to other alternative therapies [62,63]. However, a further subsequent analysis of the GUSTO data revealed differences in patient management and outcome between the patients treated in the US compared to the groups from other countries [64]. Thus, the results of the economic evaluation may be relevant for the US, but may be of limited value for other countries with different healthcare and costing systems.

These examples show that interpretation of cost-effectiveness evaluations will continue to be difficult, unless reporting of reference case results is standardized [65].

Figure 3 graphically demonstrates the four possible relationships of cost and effectiveness of an intervention compared to its alternatives. For interventions which are more effective and less expensive (i.e., 'dominant', area II) or less effective and more expensive (i.e., 'waste', area IV), decision making is easy. However, areas I and III (i.e., more effective/more expensive and less effective/less expensive) treatment strategies are disputable. This is particularly true for treatment strategies which need a larger amount of resources.

Table 3. User's guide for economic evaluations (modified from [60])

I. Are the results valid?

1) Did the analysis provide a full comparison of effective healthcare strategies?
   i.e., both inputs (costs) and outcomes (consequences) of all alternative interventions must be evaluated
2) Were the costs and outcomes adequately identified, measured and valued?
   i.e., all costs directly attributable to the interventions should be included, according to the perspective chosen (i.e., patient, hospital, third-part payer, society); clinical effectiveness (outcome) must be evident; for correct valuation the differences in timing must adjusted (future costs and consequence discounted? Important for evaluations over 1 year).
3) Was an appropriate allowance made for uncertainties in the analysis?
   i.e., when estimates are used a sensitivity analysis should be performed to determine over what range of assumptions the results remain stable.

II. What are the results?

1) What were the incremental costs and effects of each strategy?
   i.e., calculation of the additional costs and benefits above the baseline.
2) Do incremental costs and effects differ between subgroups?
   i.e., look closely also at the subgroups.

III. Will the results help in caring for my patients?

1) Can my patient expect similar health outcomes?
   i.e., is generalization also allowed for my patients (e.g., different case mix, eligibility criteria?)
2) Can I expect similar costs, or at least, similar levels of resource consumption?
   i.e., is generalization also allowed for my ICU (e.g., different costing, health care system?)
3) Are the treatment benefits worth the harms and costs?

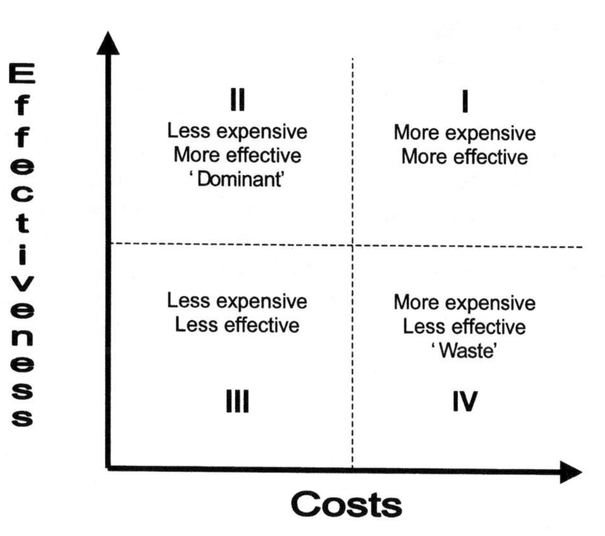

Fig. 3. The cost-effectiveness diagram

It must be kept in mind that the selection of health care strategies is continuously challenged by health care funding. The question is how much society is willing to pay for a benefit in health care. Finally this demands socio-ethical decisions; medicine professionals can only offer the possibilities for improvement and show the alternatives.

Detsky and Naglie [54] concluded: "This type of economic analysis has a very limited role in the care of individual patients by the individual clinicians. ... Individual practitioners cannot be put in the position where they must make these kinds of value judgements; it is probably inappropriate therefore to consider cost-effectiveness considerations in most individual clinical circumstances." And, "Nevertheless, cost-effectiveness analysis demonstrates the consequences of allocation decision. Because clinicians should participate in policy making, they must understand the role of this technique in setting funding priorities."

Thus, medical professionals play an important role in this framework of decision making, partly causing and promoting the development, partly suffering from its consequences, even being blamed for them. Medicine seems to be a captive of its own progress and success; with every advancement into a new area of knowledge and technology, the required resource expenditures increase which might be a further step to the health care system's economic collapse.

Conclusion

As ICUs are major resource consuming units in the hospital, and in the overall health care system, the determination of their costs is an important prerequisite to enhance ICU efficiency defined as maintaining health effects at a lower cost, or increasing health benefits at constant costs. A correct cost calculation must meet some standard criteria of which five were elucidated in the present chapter. In many analyses, errors, inconsistencies, and misconceptions as to the most fundamental cost concepts remain, affecting the quality and usefulness of the results obtained. Direct measurement of patient-related consumption ('bottom-up' cost assessment) can only be easily realized by a patient data management system. Outcome evaluation in intensive care requires risk adjustment which is usually performed by severity of illness scores (SAPS, APACHE). Comparison between different ICUs, however, is often impeded by potentially severe misinterpretations.

Fundamental variations in health care structures and accounting systems in the different countries, lack of standardization of cost assessment, difficulties in risk-adjustment and outcome evaluation, make benchmarking between ICUs in different countries difficult and disputable. However, long-term evaluation of outcome and resource consumption of one's own ICU is a useful tool of continuous quality improvement.

References

1. Frutiger A, Moreno R, Thijs L, Carlet J (1998) A clinician's guide to the use of quality terminology. Working Group on Quality Improvement of the European Society of Intensive Care Medicine. Intensive Care Med 24:860–863

2. Reis Miranda D, Ryan DW, Schaufeli WB, Fidler V (1998) Organisation and management of intensive care. Springer, Heidelberg
3. Jegers M (1997) Cost accounting in ICUs: beneficial for management and research. Intensive Care Med 23:618–619
4. Sher W, Pinola R (1986) Modern micro-economic theory. North Holland, New York
5. Jegers M, Reis Miranda DR (1999) Resource management in the intensive care unit. In: Webb AR, Shapiro M.J, Singer M, Suter PM (eds) Oxford textbook of critical care. Oxford University Press, Oxford, pp 1031–1034
6. Edbrooke D, Hibbert C, Ridley S, Long T, Dickie H (1999) The development of a method for comparative costing of individual intensive care units. Anaesthesia 54:110–120
7. Singer M, Myers S, Hall G, Cohen S, Armstrong R (1994) The cost of intensive care: a comparison on one unit between 1988 and 1991. Intensive Care Med 20:542–549
8. Noseworthy T, Konopad E, Shustack A, Johnston R, Grace M (1996) Cost accounting of adult intensive care: Methods and human and capital inputs. Crit Care Med 24:1168–1172
9. Cullen D, Civetta J, Briggs B, Ferrara L (1974) Therapeutic intervention scoring system: a method for quantitative comparison of patient care. Crit Care Med 2:57–60
10. Keene AR, Cullen DJ (1983) Therapeutic intervention scoring system: Update 1983. Crit Care Med 11:1–3
11. Reis Miranda D, de Rijk A, Schaufeli W (1996) Simplified therapeutic intervention scoring system: The TISS-28 items – Results from a multicenter study. Crit Care Med 24:64–73
12. Dickie H, Vedio A, Dundas R, Treacher DF, Leach RM (1998) Relationship between TISS and ICU cost. Intensive Care Med 24:1009–1017
13. Edbrooke D, Nightingale P (1998) Relationship between TISS and costs in intensive care. Intensive Care Med 24:995–996
14. Reis Miranda D, Moreno R, Iapichino G (1997) Nine equivalents of nursing manpower use score (NEMS). Intensive Care Med 23:760–765
15. Takala J, Ruokonen E (1997) Costs and resource utilization in intensive care. In: Vincent JL (ed) Yearbook of intensive care and emergency medicine. Springer, Heidelberg, pp 885–895
16. Zimmerman J, Shortell S, Knaus W, et al (1993) Value and cost of teaching hospitals: a prospective, multicenter, inception cohort study. Crit Care Med 21:1432–1442
17. Smithies M, Bihari D, Chang R (1994) Scoring systems and the measurement of ICU cost effectiveness. Réanimation Urgences 3:215–221
18. Drummond MF, Stoddart GL, Torrance GW (1987) Methods for the economic evaluation of health care programmes. Oxford Medical Publications, Oxford
19. Brainsky A, Fletcher RH, Glick HA, Lanken PN, Williams SV, Kundel HL (1997) Routine portable chest radiographs in the medical intensive care unit: effects and costs. Crit Care Med 25:801–805
20. Koopmanschap M, Rutten FF (1994) The impact of indirect costs on outcomes of health care programs. Health Economics 3:385–393
21. Gyldmark M (1995) A review of cost studies on intensive care units: Problems with the cost concept. Crit Care Med 23:964–972
22. Gilbertson A, Smith J, Mostafa S (1991) The cost of an intensive care unit: a prospective study. Intensive Care Med 17:204–208
23. Civetta JM, Hudson-Civetta JA, Nelson LD (1990) Evaluation of APACHE II for cost containment and quality assurance. Ann Surg 212:266–274
24. Conti G, Dell'Utri P, Pelaia P, Rosa G, Cocliati AA, Gasparetto A (1998) Do we know the costs that we prescribe ? A study on awareness of the cost of drugs and devices among ICU staff. Intensive Care Med 24:1194–1198
25. Cullen DJ, Keene R, Waternaux C, Kunsman JM, Caldera DL, Peterson H (1984) Results, charges, and benefits of intensive care for critically ill patients: update 1983. Crit Care Med 12:102–106
26. Edbrooke D, Stevens V, Hibbert C, Mann A, Wilson A (1997) A new method of accurately identifying costs of individual patients in intensive care: the initial results. Intensive Care Med 23:645–650

27. Halpern NA, Bettes L, Greenstein R (1994) Federal and nationwide instensive care units and healthcare costs. Crit Care Med 22:2001–2007
28. Norris C, Jacobs P, Rapoport J, Hamilton S (1995) ICU and non–ICU cost per day. Can J Anaesth 42:192–196
29. Parno JR, Teres D, Lemeshow S, Brown RB (1982) Hospital charges and long–term survival of ICU versus non–ICU patients. Crit Care Med 10:569–574
30. Perlstein PH, Atherton HD, Donovan EF, Richardson DK, Kotagal UR (1997) Physician variation and the ancillary costs of neonatal intensive care. Health Services Res 32:299–311
31. Rapoport J, Teres D, Lemeshow S, Avrunin JS, Haber R (1990) Explaining variability of cost using severity-of-illness measure for ICU patients. Med Care 28:338–348
32. Ridley S, Biggam M, Stone P (1991) Cost of intensive therapy. A description of methodology and initial results. Anaesthesia 46:523–530
33. Ridley S, Biggam M, Stone P (1993) A cost–benefit analysis of intensive therapy. Anaesthesia 48:14–19
34. Rapoport J, Teres D, Lemeshow S, Gehlbach S (1994) A method for assessing the clinical performance and cost-effectiveness of intensive care units: A multicenter inception cohort study. Crit Care Med 22:1385–1391
35. Shiell AM, Griffiths RD, Short AI, Spiby J (1990) An evaluation of the costs and outcome of adult intensive care in two units in the UK. Clin Intensive Care 1: 256–262
36. Muñoz E, Josephson J, Tenenbaum N, J. G, Shears AM, al. e (1989) Diagnosis-related groups, costs, and outcome for patients in the intensive care unit. Heart Lung 18:627–633
37. de Keizer NF, Bonsel GJ, Al MJ, Gemke RJ (1998) The relation between TISS and real paediatric ICU costs: a case study with generalizable methodology. Intensive Care Med 24: 1062–1069
38. Holt AW, Bersten AD, Fuller S, Piper RK, Worthley LI, Vedig AE (1994) Intensive care costing methodology: cost benefit analysis of mask continuous positive airway pressure for severe cardiogenic pulmonary oedema. Anaesth Intensive Care 22:170–174
39. Daffurn K (1990) Cost awareness study. Confed Austr Crit Care Nurses J 3:20–23
40. Brooks R, Kerridge R, Hillman K, Bauman A, Daffurn K (1997) Quality of life outcomes after intensive care. Comparison with a community group. Intensive Care Med 23:581–586
41. Féry-Lemonnier E, Landais P, Loirat P, Kleinknecht D, Brivet F (1995) Evaluation of severity scoring systems in ICUs – translation, conversion and definitions ambiguities as a source of inter-observer variability in Apache II, SAPS and OSF. Intensive Care Med 21:356–360
42. Randolph AG, Guyatt GH, Carlet J (1998) Understanding articles comparing outcomes among intensive care units to rate quality of care. Evidence Based Medicine in Critical Care Group. Crit Care Med 26:773–781
43. Randolph AG, Guyatt GH, Calvin JE, Doig G, Richardson WS (1998) Understanding articles describing clinical prediction tools. Evidence Based Medicine in Critical Care Group. Crit Care Med 26:1603–1612
44. Lamb FL, Rhodes A, Bennett ED (1997) Can intensive care units be compared? In: Vincent JL (ed) Yearbook of intensive care and emergency medicine. Springer, Heidelberg, pp 896–905
45. Keenan SP, Doig GS, Martin CM, Inman KJ, Sibbald WJ (1997) Assessing the efficiency of the admission process to a critical care unit: does the literature allow the use of benchmarking? Intensive Care Med 23:574–580
46. Pollack MM, Cuerdon TT, Patel KM, Ruttimann UE, Getson PR, Levetown M (1994) Impact of quality-of-care factors on pediatric intensive care unit mortality. JAMA 272:941–946
47. Li TC, Phillips MC, Shaw L, Cook EF, Natanson C, Goldman L (1984) On-site physician staffing in a community hospital intensive care unit. Impact on test and procedure use and on patient outcome. JAMA 252:2023–2027
48. Brown JJ, Sullivan G (1989) Effect on ICU mortality of a full-time critical care specialist. Chest 96:127–129
49. Reynolds HN, Haupt MT, Thill Baharozian MC, Carlson RW (1988) Impact of critical care physician staffing on patients with septic shock in a university hospital medical intensive care unit. JAMA 260:3446–3450

50. Mallick R, Strosberg M, Lambrinos J, Groeger JS (1995) The intensive care unit medical director as manager. Impact on performance. Med Care 33:611–624
51. Blackstone ME, Miller RS, Hodgson AJ, Cooper SS, Blackhurst DW, Stein MA (1995) Lowering hospital charges in the trauma intensive care unit while maintaining quality of care by increasing resident and attending physician awareness. J Trauma 39:1041–1044
52. Cohen IL, Lambrinos J, Fein IA (1993) Mechanical ventilation for the elderly patient in intensive care. Incremental changes and benefits. JAMA 269:1025–1029
53. Heyland DK, Konopad E, Noseworthy TW, Johnston R, Gafni A (1998) Is it 'worthwhile' to continue treating patients with a prolonged stay (>14 days) in the ICU? An economic evaluation. Chest 114:192–198
54. Detsky A, Naglie I (1990) A clinician's guide to cost-effectiveness analysis. Ann Intern Med 113:147–154
55. Weinstein MC, Siegel JE, Gold MR, Kamlet MS, Russell LB (1996) Recommendations of the Panel on Cost-effectiveness in Health and Medicine. JAMA 276:1253–1258
56. Drummond MF, Richardson WS, O'Brien BJ, Levine M, Heyland D (1997) Users' guides to the medical literature. XIII. How to use an article on economic analysis of clinical practice. A. Are the results of the study valid? Evidence-Based Medicine Working Group. JAMA 277:1552–1557
57. O'Brien BJ, Heyland D, Richardson WS, Levine M, Drummond MF (1997) Users' guides to the medical literature. XIII. How to use an article on economic analysis of clinical practice. B. What are the results and will they help me in caring for my patients? Evidence-Based Medicine Working Group. JAMA 277:1802–1806
58. Udvarhelyi I, Colditz G, Rai A, Epstein A (1992) Cost-effectiveness and cost benefit analyses in the medical literature. Are the methods being used correctly? Ann Intern Med 116: 238–244
59. Chalfin D (1996) Analysis of cost-effectiveness in intensive care: an overview of methods and a review of applications to problems in critcial care medicine. Curr Opin Anaesthesiol 9:129–133
60. Heyland DK, Gafni A, Kernerman P, Keenan S, Chalfin D (1999) How to use the results of an economic evaluation. Crit Care Med 27:1195–1202
61. The GUSTO Investigators G (1993) An international randomized trial comparing four thrombolytic strategies for acute myocardial infarction. The GUSTO investigators. N Engl J Med 329:673–682
62. Mark DB, Hlatky MA, Califf RM, et al. (1995) Cost effectiveness of thrombolytic therapy with tissue plasminogen activator as compared with streptokinase for acute myocardial infarction. N Engl J Med 332:1418–1424
63. Kalish SC, Gurwitz JH, Krumholz HM, Avorn J (1995) A cost-effectiveness model of thrombolytic therapy for acute myocardial infarction. J Gen Intern Med 10:321–330
64. Van de Werf F, Topol EJ, Lee KL, et al. (1995) Variations in patient management and outcomes for acute myocardial infarction in the United States and other countries. Results from the GUSTO trial. Global Utilization of Streptokinase and Tissue Plasminogen Activator for Occluded Coronary Arteries. JAMA 273:1586–1591
65. Siegel JE, Weinstein MC, Russell LB, Gold MR (1996) Recommendations for reporting cost-effectiveness analyses. Panel on Cost-Effectiveness in Health and Medicine. JAMA 276:1339–1341

Assessment of Medical Devices

A.R. Webb

Learning Points

- Health technology assessment is any process of examining and reporting properties of a medical technology used in healthcare
- The priorities against which medical devices are assessed vary between and within countries
- Three questions must be posed for assessment of a medical device: Is it efficacious, is it effective and what is the cost?
- The method of assessment is necessarily different for therapeutic and non-therapeutic devices because outcome benefit is not usually a direct result of using non-therapeutic technology
- Benefits assessment must be thought of in terms of the healthcare system as a whole

Introduction

Health technology assessment is critically important to the development of healthcare as changes are generated by major resource limitations. In most Western societies there is a universal healthcare system funded publicly. Government has a duty to ensure value for money. The costs of healthcare are clearly rising and are not being matched by equivalent increases in resources. In a publicly funded system, revenue is generated by taxing those in work. However, the aging population means there will be less people in work to support those that are retiring. Thus, despite the rising costs, there will, inevitably, be less money to spend on healthcare.

We are beginning to face the problem of how we allocate scarce resources. Questions are being raised about the effectiveness of medical devices that are already in routine use. We have seen important questions raised about pulmonary artery catheters recently [1–4] despite their routine place in many intensive care units (ICUs). When using medical devices we have to ensure that we are making the correct interventions. Health technology assessment seeks to identify the true clinical need and benefit of medical devices.

The ethics of resource allocation dictate that resources have to be allocated to where they have impact. If medical devices are not proved to be of benefit then ethical use of healthcare resources demands that they are not funded. However, this leaves no room for innovation and development. There must be adequate funding of the research required to assess medical devices.

Assessing benefit in terms of health gain is dependent on who is making the assessment. Ultimately, whether a health gain is worthwhile has to be a decision for society.

In most critical care units the problems relating to equipment procurement and use differ considerably from the problems relating to drug procurement and use. Whereas most drugs are given for therapeutic effect, most medical devices depend on a response to information output to generate the appropriate therapy. Even therapeutic devices (e.g., ventilators) provide symptomatic or supportive rather than curative treatment. Randomized controlled trials (RCTs) of one device against another or placebo with mortality outcome measures, in the way drugs are assessed, may not be appropriate to medical devices [5]. In order to understand the assessment process for medical devices we need to understand the developmental process to which health technology assessment applies. Some aspects of that developmental process need to change in the future to ensure devices are brought to market after assessment against appropriate objectives.

The Development of Medical Devices

There are many reasons why a medical device may be developed and procured. However, the final common pathway to development is usually commercial gain by the industry responsible for marketing the product. One of the primary drivers creating the market for technology development is improvement to patient safety. Society is demanding more from its healthcare system and, through Government legislation, standards of patient safety are being raised. New technologies may allow us to intervene in a safer way or provide an intervention that was previously impossible. Other developments may arise from clinicians' wishes to drive the frontiers forward or on the basis of developments in other industries [6] or war [7].

Clinicians have a key role in communicating the need for technology to industry. The clinician acts as the patient advocate but may also communicate needs via governments, health maintenance organizations and hospitals. All of these organizations are influenced by patients (e.g., via pressure groups) or clinicians (as expert advisors). Collectively, these may be considered to be the market for the technology (Fig. 1).

The patient as the consumer does not purchase the product directly. The clinician as the consumer is in a better position to influence choice but, again, does not purchase the product directly. The hospital is usually the direct purchaser of the product but is influenced by patients, clinicians, a health maintenance organization (HMO) and government. Definition of the market is therefore difficult. Furthermore, the fact that it is usually public money spent in procuring the development means the benefits must be tangible in terms of health gain. The viability of the technology from industry's perspective depends on an appropriate mar-

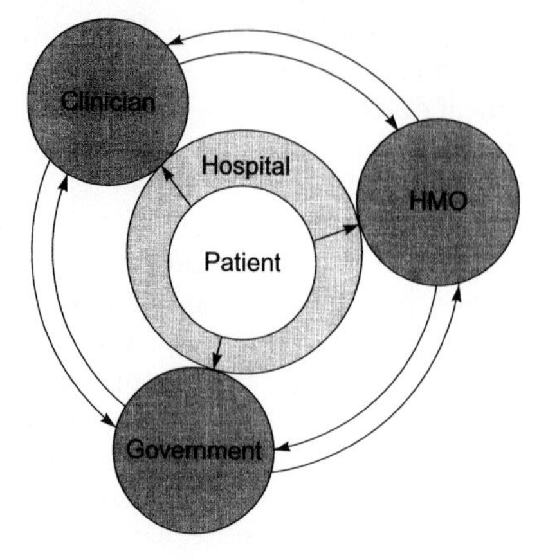

Fig. 1. The market for medical devices and the way its components may influence market decisions. (HMO: health maintenance organization)

ket and the primary assessment tool at this stage is the business case. At this early stage of development the assessment of health gain is rarely possible other than by informed guesswork.

Benefit to society must be considered as an important issue for future industry business cases. Critical care medicine is currently very immature in its definition of benefit. We tend to define benefit in terms of reduced mortality because it is easy to measure. We are just beginning to think about quality of life as an outcome measure [8] but health planners still don't tend to focus on longer term quality of life as a result of using a product at some stage previously in the healthcare system. We must start looking at benefits to the health care system as a whole. Indeed, many technological developments will not affect an easily measurable endpoint, such as mortality, on their own. This is particularly true for a monitoring device. Business cases for monitoring devices are not going to be robust on their own. They must look at how the device fits in with the overall demands of a procedure, the procedure being part of the overall healthcare process. One cannot have a business case for a monitor that will demonstrate benefit in terms of medical outcome. All it can demonstrate is that it does what it says it does safely. In order to obtain a benefit in terms of a medical outcome the business case for a new medical device should consider the device as a part of a process rather than as an individual item.

Health Technology Assessment

Health technology assessment is any process of examining and reporting properties of a medical technology used in healthcare. It should assess the short- and long-term benefits of health technology and, as such, is a form of policy research. Health technology assessment draws on expertise from clinical medicine, epidemiology, biostatistics, engineering, health economics, law and ethics. Table 1 lists the elements of health technology assessment.

The Need for Technology

The questions posed by technology assessment depend on who is asking them. Clinicians will ask very different questions to the health care managers who will ask very different questions to social policy makers. The priorities vary across countries. Even local needs within a country and between various social groups generate different priorities within a country. The priorities to a society cannot be defined globally. The priorities for the hospital cannot be defined locally since different hospitals may be in different sectors of the health care business. Some academic hospitals should be generating hypotheses and perhaps answering the questions that hypotheses pose. Some hospitals simply deliver health care, nothing more nothing less. The questions that they will ask about technologies are clearly quite different to the academic institutes. The questions the health care managers should be asking should really encompass all aspects of the needs of the healthcare system they manage but they often concentrate on financial issues only.

Clinicians need technology assessment because there is little proof of effect for most non-drug technology and most information is gleaned through marketing activities. Because of the economic climate in which we work health systems worldwide are not as tolerant of marketing as an alternative to proper assessment. Three questions must be posed: Is the technology efficacious, is it effective and what is the cost? Efficacious means it works under the best of all possible circumstances. Effectiveness means it will work under the average conditions of use, e.g., late at night when the experts are not around.

Therapeutic Compared with Non-Therapeutic Technology Assessment

The method of technology assessment is necessarily different for therapeutic and non-therapeutic technology because outcome benefit is not usually a direct result of using non-therapeutic technology. Even for therapeutic technology there is a different approach to assessment for drug and non-drug technology. For drugs there is in place, by legislation, a three phase assessment pro-

Table 1. The elements of health technology assessment

- safety
- efficacy
- feasibility
- indications for use
- cost (including the cost effectiveness and the social, economic and ethical costs)
- whether a technology is tenable or untenable

cess. There is little logical reasoning why the lead of the pharmaceutical industry in technology assessment cannot be followed.

Evaluation Against Expectations

There are two early questions that must be answered during the evaluation of a technological development: Does the device do what it is supposed to do and is what it does useful? For a new monitor we may legitimately ask whether the monitor measures what we think it measures. This may be described in terms of accuracy (how close is the measurement to the actual value), precision (how close are repeated measurements of the same quantity to each other), and bias (a fixed error in the measurement from the actual value) [5]. Although accuracy cannot be determined by clinical methods we often assess precision and bias by comparison with another accepted technology [9]. With a new therapeutic device we may ask does it provide the therapeutic support we think it does, again often in comparison with other accepted devices. In this type of evaluation the outcome measure is a simple performance measure of the device itself.

The second question on usefulness can be approached from several directions. For a monitor, the new technology must supply the healthcare worker with information they would not normally have and this information should improve the performance of the healthcare worker. This could be measured by an improved outcome but that depends on the process change resulting from the information gained from the technology. Although a device may provide perfect output to all technical standards the information must be interpreted correctly. In a study of the ability of physicians to interpret the humble electrocardiogram (EKG) 16% of EKGs with ST elevation were incorrectly interpreted as normal [10]. Clearly an outcome assessment of this technology would have been flawed due to poor user performance. The user of the technology is as important in the assessment as the technology itself. Thus technology assessment data may not be truly portable. For a therapeutic device the therapy delivered must be beneficial to the patient resulting in an improvement in mortality or morbidity. Another way of looking at usefulness is based on an advantage to the user although outcome for the patient may be the same. For instance, a monitor may give the clinician some information that does not change a process but enables the clinician to be more confident the process is correct. The outcome for most patients may be the same but the clinician is better informed. For a therapeutic device the development may not alter the therapy but it may allow the clinician to deliver the therapy more easily.

It has been estimated that the healthcare worker does not use 80% of the information that a medical device supplies. However, a technological advance that reduces unnecessary information (if it is not a problem don't tell me about it), presenting only what is needed at the time, could be considered to be useful [11]. Such a strategy of information management allows the healthcare worker to concentrate all efforts on important abnormalities. Although this is a laudable goal there is a danger that reduction in the outward complexity of a process may lead to a reduction in the skill of healthcare personnel [12].

Outcome Assessment

When assessing medical devices it is clear we must be looking for some improvement over what is currently available. Improvement is often defined in terms of patient outcome. However, outcomes can be difficult to define; indeed, what is appropriate evidence can be difficult to define [5]. To most people outcome is synonymous with mortality but this is too hard an endpoint for assessment of most medical devices and totally inappropriate for monitoring technology. On the other hand, reliance on surrogate outcomes does not provide adequate evidence for assessment unless the surrogate is clinically relevant. For instance, postoperative hypertension was demonstrated to be more tightly controlled during the assessment of one closed loop infusion system [13]. What is missing is the evidence that tighter control of blood pressure, over and above the degree of control achieved with standard non-feedback methods, is clinically relevant. In another study closed loop infusion was demonstrated to reduce ICU length of stay [14]. This outcome measure is more relevant clinically.

Clinicians require proof of a meaningful outcome to justify a new technology. Evidence of a meaningful outcome may include effectiveness or cost effectiveness. However, because the ICU is so complex, medical devices may not improve outcome in terms of mortality on their own. Appropriate outcomes for non-drug technology assessment are listed in Table 2.

Assessment of medical devices by determining what would happen if they were removed is a possible mechanism for dealing with existing technology. The effect of removal depends on the outcome measure to which such an assessment is made. Taking away a technology may make no difference to the healthcare system as a whole and this method of assessment may not be applicable practically or ethically. In some cases removing a technology may not impact upon outcome since the technology has already taught us much about the disease process. In a randomized trial involving 20,802 patients comparing the use or no use of pulse oximetry, there was no difference in outcome [15]. We all know the ill effects of hypoxemia and, through the use of pulse oximetry, we have learned how to avoid it. Taking away the pulse oximeter now does not affect outcome for individual patients but the increase in group knowledge having used the device has been a positive outcome in itself. Future generations of clinicians may not avoid hypoxemia if the pulse oximeter was removed since their continuing education would be compromised.

Table 2. Appropriate outcomes for technology assessment of medical devices

- reduced patients in the ICU
- economic outcomes
- improved safety
- improved mortality
- clinician comfort
- patient comfort

Process Research

Since the function of most medical devices is to support a healthcare process it is sensible to consider how the technology affects other steps of the process. This type of research is unfamiliar to clinicians since the outcome is more nebulous than the hard clinical outcomes we are used to. Depending on the technology and the process, the outcome may be improved efficiency in the system as a whole, a change in treatment, or one of the more classical medical outcomes. Efficiency may be measured in terms of cost, ease or speed. Changes to outcome are a result of the change in the process rather than a direct result of the device itself.

Economic Analysis

There are several approaches to economic analysis. A cost minimization approach tests whether the technology can replace an alternative at a lower cost. Cost benefit relates to the number of life years saved by new technologies. Cost effectiveness takes into account life years saved and quality of life, and cost utility is just about quality of life. The difficulty with these analyses relates to the cost side of the equation. In the universal health care system the components of cost are not well defined. Although we may be able to identify the cost of the device, there will be changes to other component costs of the healthcare process in which the device is used.

We rarely evaluate cost against benefit adequately. Where such analyses are done they are against short term benefits that are easily measured. Rarely is the question of benefit to society entertained and therefore an understanding of cost versus benefit in the health care system as a whole is not achieved. In assessing outcome we must focus on longer term health gains in order to understand the impact of technology on society as a whole. This requires longer term follow up studies.

Problems with the Technology Assessment Process

Clinical trials in non-drug technology are rarely as big as their drug technology counterparts. This is for practical reasons since the expense of performing such large trials is beyond the operating budget of most non-drug technology suppliers. The result is that the power of such trials to detect outcome benefits is much reduced. Compounding this problem is the fact that the effect of the technology is rarely pure. For a drug we are dealing with a single effect and few side effects but for non-drug technology there are often artifacts of multiple effects to deal with. Separating out the random noise from true effects requires larger studies.

How Should We Assess Medical Devices?

Medical device assessment should be more structured and should concentrate on the following issues:

Is the Device Safe?

Safety should be studied in two parts including the safety of the device itself and whether it may precipitate a therapeutic action which could be harmful. While the former is often taken care of at an early stage of development, and many analyses are required by legislation, the latter cannot occur until the evaluation phase during clinical trials. Asking whether the device improves patient safety is often part of the usefulness evaluation but asking whether a device is safe to use as part of a process (e.g., is it safe to use a pulmonary artery catheter in the maintenance of hemodynamic stability?) is often either not done at all or done after launch [1]. In general there is a paucity of information on issues of safety in Europe.

Does the Device Complete the Task Claimed of it?

Simple questions asked of a device such as does a ventilator ventilate or is a measured heart rate the heart rate, should be answered against 'gold standards' as part of the evaluation process.

Does the Device's Task have Clinical Utility?

For therapeutic technology the issue of clinical utility covers the procedure in which the technology is used. The technology may allow something to be done that could not be done before and assessment would be based on improved outcome. The technology may improve the process of patient care with assessment based on outcome improvement or cost-efficiency improvement. For monitoring technology the measured variable must have a clinical meaning resulting in a therapeutic decision. It would be the therapeutic process resulting from this decision rather than the technology which may affect outcome or cost-efficiency.

What is the Cost?

Cost should be assessed in both financial and non-financial terms and, in both cases, against benefit. The difficulty with benefit assessment stems from the tendency to think of cost in currency terms and therefore the need to value benefits in currency terms. Benefits are usually assessed as short term, immediate benefits but value to society as a whole must be assessed. Only then can costs be prioritized in the health care system as a whole.

Observational Studies

Much technology development is based on health care workers communicating their needs. If health care workers are asked if they perform a procedure safely they will probably answer 'Yes'. However, observing what doctors and nurses actually do in a clinical environment may demonstrate the need for safety technology in a much more robust way. Observational studies can also provide information on the likely market penetration.

The 'Basket' Approach to the Evaluation of Medical Devices

For individual devices we may assess safety and efficacy but an individual device is usually used as part of a process. The basket of technologies that represent the process (medical devices, procedures, and drugs, collectively known as health technology) should be assessed rather than individual devices. This is particularly true when the assessment requires an outcome change.

Education as an Assessment Goal

Hypothesis generation or knowledge generation should be considered as an important function of technology because some technology is not designed to improve outcome. Thus the use of a monitor may not trigger a therapeutic decision but may simply help our understanding of a process. Such technology may have a limited useful life and, of itself, may not affect a measurable outcome. The knowledge generated may be used to develop therapeutic options but there is potential for new technologies to create the problem for which they are the solution, and hypothesis generation, although important, can actually be taken too far.

Acquiring Technology Assessment Information

Access to Existing Information

Information on existing evidence concerning medical device assessment is available but its whereabouts is not immediately obvious to many. Many technology assessments have been done but there is no single registry or database of current knowledge. If one is about to embark upon a technology assessment it is important to know whether the work has been done before. Similarly, procurement of medical devices requires access to health technology assessment information relating to the device.

Traditional sources of information include bibliographic medical databases such as MEDLINE. In addition to these there are now quality filtered resources such as the Cochrane Library and unfiltered resources such as the Internet [16]. There are Internet sites containing assessments of medical devices that are in current use (e.g., http://nhscrd.york.ac.uk/welcome.html from which a number of other sites can be accessed). Irrespective of the source of the information questions must be focused and filtered to limit the retrieval of inappropriate information [17]. Such focusing should identify the clinical scenario, the device or intervention for which the device is used and a relevant outcome. Filtering the results of a search aims to retrieve information that is best able to answer the question posed. Such filters may be methodological filters [18] or document type filters where an open resource such as the Internet is used. Clearly such filtering is unnecessary in searching a pre-filtered database.

Conclusion

Existing research techniques are sufficiently well developed to deal with the problem of assessing technology and healthcare in its broadest sense. The major problem is the implementation of the methods. We must focus on processes and policy research. We have to look at qualitative research as well. These are not things medical researchers are comfortable with. For health technology assessment to be successful:

- Users and providers of healthcare technology need a better understanding of each other
- Technology benefits are best thought of in terms of the healthcare system
- Objective methods of assessing outcome are necessary but relevant outcome remains difficult to measure
- Measuring outcome by assessing a 'basket of variables' is attractive as a concept, particularly for technology which represents a component of a system but it remains difficult to define appropriate variables
- As the main users of technology, clinicians' input into technology assessment procedures is of great importance.

References

1. Connors AF Jr, Speroff T, Dawson NV, et al (1996) The effectiveness of right heart catheterization in the initial care of critically ill patients. JAMA 276:889–897
2. Prielipp RC, Morell R (1997) Debate: The pulmonary artery catheter, is it safe: To use or not to use. Con: Swan song for the Swan-Ganz? J Clin Monit 13:339–340
3. Tuman KJ (1997) Debate: The pulmonary artery catheter, is it safe? To use or not to use. Pro: A moratorium on PAC is unjustified. J Clin Monit 13:337–338
4. Sprung CL, Eidelman LA (1997) The issue of a U.S. Food and Drug Administration moratorium on the use of the pulmonary artery catheter. New Horiz 5:277–280
5. Society for Critical Care Medicine Coalition for Critical Care Excellence (1995) Standards of evidence for the safety and effectiveness of critical care monitoring devices and related interventions. Crit Care Med 23:1756–1763
6. Hines JW (1996) Medical and surgical applications of space biosensor technology. Acta Astronaut 38:261–267
7. Brewer LA 3rd (1981) A historical account of the "wet lung of trauma" and the introduction of intermittent positive-pressure oxygen therapy in World War II. Ann Thorac Surg 31:386–393
8. Heyland DK, Guyatt G, Cook DJ, et al (1998) Frequency and methodologic rigor of quality-of-life assessments in the critical care literature. Crit Care Med 26:591–598
9. Bland JM, Altman DG (1986) Statistical methods for assessing agreement between two methods of clinical measurement. Lancet 1:307–310
10. Jayes RL Jr, Larsen GC, Behansky JR, D'Agostino RB, Selker HP (1992) Physician electrocardiogram reading in the emergency department: accuracy and effect on triage decisions: findings from a multicentre study. J Gen Intern Med 7:387–392

11. Cook PR, Woods DD, McDonald JS (1991) Evaluating the human engineering of microprocessor-controlled operating room devices. J Clin Monit 7:217–226
12. Jastremski M, Jastremski C, Shepherd M, et al (1995) A model for technology assessment as applied to closed loop infusion systems. Crit Care Med 23:1745–1755
13. Chitwood NR, Cosgrove DM, Lust RM, et al (1992) Multicenter trial of automated nitroprusside infusion for postoperative hypertension. Ann Thorac Surg 54:517–522
14. Sheppard LC, Kouchoukos NT (1977) Automation of measurements and interventions in the systematic care of postoperative cardiac surgical patients. Medical Instrum 11:296–301
15. Moller JT, Pederson T, Rasmussen LS, et al (1993) Randomized evaluation of pulse oximetry in 20,802 patients (parts I and II). Anesthesiology 78:436–453
16. Booth A, O'Rourke AJ (1999) Searching for evidence: principles and practice. ACP J Club 4:133–136
17. O'Rourke AJ, Booth A, Ford N (1999) Another fine MeSH: clinical medicine meets information science. J Inf Sci 24:275–281
18. Haynes RB, Wilczynski N, McKibbon KA, Walker CJ, Sinclair JC (1994) Developing optimal search strategies for detecting clinically sound studies in MEDLINE. J Am Med Inform Assoc 1:447–458

Health Informatics

M. Imhoff

Learning Points

- In health care, information overload is an issue at every level of the continuum of care
- Health informatics provides methods, tools and concepts that help analyze, evaluate, structure, and control health care processes
- Understanding health care means understanding, analyzing and controlling the process of care at the point of care
- Without standardization there cannot be quality control
- Process control is essential to provide better and more cost effective health care

When the machines that men invented over time would now even function: what a pleasant life this would be! (Kurt Tucholsky, German writer and satirist, 1890–1935)

Introduction

Definitions

Health informatics is the development and assessment of methods and systems for the acquisition, processing and interpretation of patient data with the help of knowledge from scientific research.

With a more technical focus, health informatics can be defined as any application of information management technology in health care.

The terminology, especially the distinction between medical informatics and health informatics, is used inconsistently in the literature. For our purposes, we will categorize any of the above mentioned processes under health informatics, thereby focusing on the process and the continuum of care.

Problems

In health care, and especially in intensive care, we are facing a data and information overload, as illustrated by numerous examples:

- An abundance of information is generated during the process of critical care. Much of this information can now be captured and stored using clinical information systems (CIS) that provide for complete medical documentation at the bedside. The clinical usefulness and efficiency of clinical information systems has been proven repeatedly [1-3]. While databases with more than 2,000 individual patient-related variables are now available for further analysis [4], the multitude of variables presented at the bedside even without a CIS precludes medical judgement by humans. A physician may be confronted with more than 200 variables in critically ill patients during typical morning rounds [5]. However, even an experienced physician is often not able to develop a systematic response to any problem involving more than seven variables [6]. Moreover, humans are limited in their ability to estimate the degree of relatedness between only two variables [7]. This problem is most pronounced in the evaluation of the measurable effect of a therapeutic intervention. Personal bias, experience, and a certain expectation toward the respective intervention may distort an objective judgement [8].
- At the level of the hospital enterprise, information overload is an issue, too. In addition to the administrative aspects of such a complex enterprise, new and much more complicated reimbursement and accounting policies lead to an unmatched complexity of data and information [9].
- The volume of scientific literature is growing exponentially. As of 1993, the number of systematic reviews in medicine increased 500 fold over a ten year period [10]. It is impossible for the individual health care professional to keep track of all relevant medical knowledge even in very narrow subspecialities.

Moreover, we know that human errors are unavoidable. They occur infrequently (< 1%), but may compromise patient safety. In the light of the evident information overload they must be regarded as the expression of a systematic fault in the health care delivery system, rather than as an individual shortcoming [11–14].

Health informatics can help solve these problems of information overload. Moehr [15] has given an overview of the potential of health informatics to ameliorate these problems in different areas of health care (Table 1).

To cover the multiple facets of health informatics is far beyond the scope of one chapter in a book. Therefore, we will focus on three aspects with respect to intensive care medicine:

1) Applications of health informatics from the perspective of the health care professional.
2) How can health informatics help understand and evaluate health care processes?
3) How can health informatics help manage and control health care processes?

The Process of Care

Intensive care cannot be seen without the continuum of care. The continuum of care spans the entire process of therapy and care for a patient with one or multiple illnesses (Fig. 1). It encompasses the different treatment and care units, such as the emergency room, operating room, and general ward. Different modalities

Table 1. Problems in health care on different levels of the health process and the potential impact of health informatics methods [15].

Problem	Potential of a health informatics solution	Potential contribution of health informatics
Level of the health care provider		
Deficiency of health sciences	high	Research support
Limited access to scientific results	medium	Expert and factual information systems, evidence-based medicine
Lack of compliance with guidelines and evidence	medium	Assistive systems, education, training, computerized protocols
Limited access to patient specific data	medium	Patient information systems, telehealth
Level of health care management		
Political nature of tasks	unclear	Unclear
Scarcity of resources	medium	Efficiency improvements
Lack of information on health status	medium	Health indices, population health information systems
Inefficiencies of management	medium	Management support systems

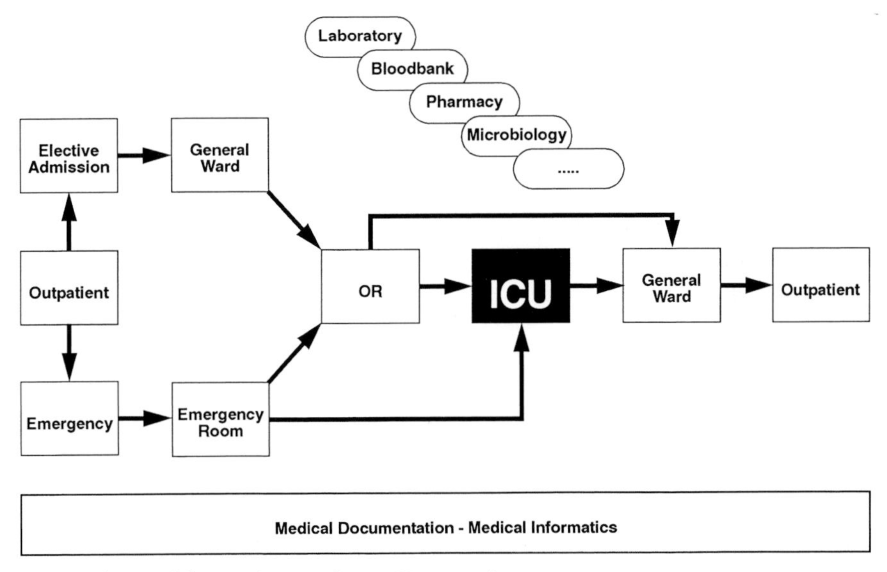

Fig. 1. Schema of the continuum of care. OR: operating room

of diagnostics (laboratory, imaging, etc.) and treatment are available. Medical documentation and ultimately medical informatics provide information and communication throughout and are the formal representation of the continuum of care [16, 17]. Intensive care is only one piece in the process of care, although sometimes a crucial piece. Therefore, it cannot be judged independently, but rather the entire process needs to be analyzed. Many decisions relevant to outcome, acuity, and the cost of caring for the critically ill are made before the patient reaches the ICU. Moreover, pre-ICU decisions and the management of patients, e.g., in high-risk surgery, determine utility or futility, success or failure, and ultimately cost-effectiveness of intensive care. Therefore, any debate regarding cost, efficiency, and outcome in intensive care needs to assess the entire continuum of care, even the entire health care system.

Processes are not only found in health care, but are the focus of any quality, rationalization, and management analysis in the production and service industries. Many people have asked whether we can draw conclusions for health care from the lessons learned in the industry. Table 2 gives an overview of potential analogies between problems noted in the industrial world and those seen in health care.

In a further analogy we can match the three strata of industrial process control to the health care process:

1) The production control level in industrial production translates into the level of hospital administration. Hospital information systems may represent the technological implementation at this level.
2) Conceptually, the process control level in industrial production matches the actual process of care, and the delivery of health care by health care professionals. Therefore, this process control level represents the essence of health

Table 2. The most pressing problems in the industry as identified in a recent survey (Top Business Studie: Peter Diederich, WifoConsult; Prof. Dieter Reckziegel, Delta Management), compared to the problems in hospitals from a business perspective.

Industry	Hospital
Increasing labor costs	Increasing labor costs
Aggressive competition	Increasing competition with other hospitals
Stagnating or falling prices	Managed prices, capitation, etc.
Decreasing profits	Many hospitals in Europe have negative balances
Stagnating market growth	Limitation of potential revenue by state regulation
General economic recession	Little or no budget compensation for inflation
Organizational deficits	Organizational deficits
Stagnating revenues	Stagnating revenues
Increasing customer requirements and demands	Increasing expectations against medical care
Increasing environmental costs	Increasing costs for disposal and energy
(Top) management lacks qualification	Lack of business and management knowledge and experience among health care professionals and administration
Increasing costs for materials and service/maintenance	Maintenance costs increase faster than revenue
Increasing technology costs	Shorter investment cycles for modern therapeutic and diagnostic methods necessary
Short product cycles	Expensive medical devices cannot generate return on investment over their technological life cycle

care. It governs the processes at the point of care, including point-of-care information technology.
3) The field level, i.e., actuators and sensors, in industrial production can be directly matched to the medical instrumentation level, such as patient monitoring, ventilation, and imaging.

For health care we may add another, higher level of information management: The management of scientific and societal information.

In this chapter, the author tries to adhere to this concept and investigate how it can further our understanding of health informatics and information technology in health care.

Goals of Health Informatics

Two principle goals of medical informatics can be distinguished [9]:
1) Provide solutions for problems related to data, information, and knowledge processing.
2) Study general principles of processing data, information, and knowledge in medicine and health care.

The computer should provide advanced services and displays which enhance the convenience, efficiency, and general satisfaction of the user, i.e., the health care professional [18]. Ideally a CIS acquires, distributes and displays patient related data throughout the entire continuum of care.

According to the US Military Health Service: "The mission is to give the right information to the right people at the right time". Quality of data in this respect is critical and, therefore, is a leadership issue. This quality of data is not dependent on the use of computers but on the concepts of data acquisition, data structures, data storage, data distribution and data analysis as they are implemented by the data owners. It will be determined by
1) the accuracy of data,
2) the timeliness of data, and
3) the completeness of data [19].

These three factors are essential to establish information dominance which is important for every information technology approach.

While quality of care and outcome are still high-priority issues in health, the most important aspect today appears to be cost effectiveness. With the ever increasing pressure on health care expenditure the question of cost reduction also rules many information technology decisions. The goal is to reduce the cost and at the same time improve the quality. Information technology may help. Therefore, all concepts and products in health information technology should be evaluated to determine whether they can improve the cost effectiveness of the health care process. Typical cost reduction goals can be:
1) Reduction of staff: A typical example is the obsolescence of manual transcription by electronic order entry systems.

2) Reduction in hospital length of stay: Reduction of the length of stay can either be used to reduce the operating cost of the medical institution or to increase patient numbers to generate higher revenue.
3) Reduction of complications: Reduction of complications improves cost efficiency in two ways: The treatment of complications is costly and complications increase the length of stay. Moreover, good outcome and low complication rates improve the reputation of a medical institution.
4) Better capture of reimbursement items.
5) Better organization: One example for better organization with the help of information technology is the use of activity based costing and management.

Applications of Health Informatics

Health Informatics at Different Levels of the Care Process

Production control level: The production control level focuses on the business administration of a hospital including accounting, billing, and resource management. On this level we find hospital information systems (HIS), which are well developed and widespread. In the US we can even observe a market saturation of these systems.

HIS do not provide detailed information about health care processes. They can provide data about overall structures and resources, including general budgeting, purchasing, customer profiles, e.g., of referring physicians or practices, as well as pooled demographics, diagnostic and therapeutic coding information.

The production control level provides information at an institutional or enterprise level. While this can help to understand the process of care, it provides important information about the institutional framework in which the care processes take place:

1) Resources and resource consumption at the level of institutions and units.
2) Pooled demographics, length of stay, diagnosis and procedure codes.
3) Business administration and costing, although it cannot provide the information needed for activity based costing.

The production control level does not allow control of the individual care processes, albeit, it has a strong influence on the institutional and technical framework of the individual care processes. The production control level handles general resource allocation, e.g., at a departmental level, staff management, and the broad spectrum of standard business administration. While it does not control the care process as such, the production control level manages the entire cash flow of a medical institution or enterprise.

Process control level: The process control level focuses on the processes of care. Therefore, information management at this level has to be located at the point of care. Point-of-care information systems comprise:

- Order entry systems
- Communication systems
- Picture archiving and communication systems (PACS)

- Clinical information systems (CIS)
- Clinical decision support systems (DSS), and
- The electronic patient record (EPR).

The latter is not a uniform system, but rather a transparent information concept that provides the completeness of all patient related information from different information technology systems displayed electronically at the point of care. These systems cover different areas of medical documentation. Ideally, they acquire all patient related data and, therefore, all information about the process of care. In addition to the original medical documentation, they provide essential information for procedure related billing, activity based costing and management (ABC, ABM), decision support and computerized protocols. As they can be used to control and steer the process of care, e.g., by electronic implementation of guidelines, protocols, and clinical pathways, of all information systems they have the most direct effect on the process of care.

Due to their enormous complexity, many of these systems can only cover certain aspects of the process of care, e.g., intelligent order entry, electronic charting, or on-line decision support. Only a minority of medical institutions enjoy the luxury of these information technology systems at the point of care.

At this level, detailed information about the process of care is provided. This includes patient data, process data, process related outcome data, and procedural resource consumption information. Process related information is essential not only to understand how the process is performed, but also to evaluate its quality and, finally, to control the entire process. Therefore, from the health care professional's perspective this level provides the most important application of information technology.

The use of guidelines, protocols, and algorithms in clinical practice can improve patient outcome [13, 20–22]. Numerous studies and reviews have shown this [21]. A large meta-analysis found that the majority of studies showed significant improvements in patient outcome through the implementation of computer-based decision support [23]. It should be noted that none of the investigated systems featured a complete electronic patient record. Even without the use of sophisticated computer systems, protocols can significantly increase improvements in patient care [20].

Point-of-care information systems allow the broadest control over the process of care. Outstanding examples for the control and management of the process control level are computerized protocols (overview in [13]), clinical pathways, and guidelines. Order entry and decision support systems offer a unique opportunity to dramatically improve the quality of care while at the same time reducing overall costs [24, 25].

Recent studies have reported that the incidence of medication errors for hospital inpatients range from 4 to 10% [26]. When a decision support system checked all doctor's orders for drug interaction, of 15,000 daily orders, approximately 400 were changed in a large US institution [27]. It has even been estimated that manual paper-based screening for in-hospital adverse drug effects detects only about 5% of all events that can be detected with computerized systems [28]. In the terminology of total quality management (TQM), an explicit method, e.g., a computerized protocol, is part of the stabilization of the process necessary to improve quality [29,30].

Numerous studies on the impact of clinical pathways in the process of care have been published. Most of these studies span the entire continuum of care, at least during one hospital stay (selection of studies in Table 3). Some studies focus more specifically on intensive care (selection of studies in Table 4).

The studies that focus on intensive care also need to be seen in the perspective of the entire continuum of care. This is most obvious in the study by Back et al. [31] where the largest cost benefit stemmed from preventing ICU admission in the course of elective surgery. This study shows the importance of pre-ICU decisions and treatment for the actual success and cost of intensive care. Simple things that may be part of a pathway such as the testing and replenishing of blood potassium levels prior to cardiac surgery [32], may have a dramatic effect on postoperative intensive care. On the other hand, the early admission of patients to the ICU for hemodynamic optimization may significantly improve outcome and reduce cost [33]. Therefore, it is necessary to develop clinical pathways for the entire continuum of care, as this will have the strongest impact on the overall cost effectiveness and outcome. This approach may also help to limit cases of futile intensive care medicine and make scant ICU beds available for those who will

Table 3. Clinical pathway studies across the continuum of care

Publication	Clinical Setting	N	Efficiency	Outcome
Chang et al, 1999 [46]	Urological surgery	protocol: 1,382 control (historic): 1,279	Hospital LOS: −11% ($p < 0.05$)	Reduction of postoperative complications
Gheiler et al, 1999 [47]	Radical prostatectomy	total: 1,129	Hospital LOS: −34% ($p < 0.05$)	no change
Scranton [48]	Total knee arthroplasty	protocol: 77 control (historic): 52	Hospital LOS: −37% ($p < 0.05$) Hospital charges: −US$1,063	no change
Dzwierzynski et al [49]	Pressure ulcer therapy	protocol: 43 control (historic): 52	Total cost: −23% ($p < 0.05$)	no change
Zehr et al [50]	Esophagectomy	protocol: 96 control (historic): 56	Hospital LOS: −30% ($p < 0.05$) Hospital charges: −34% ($p < 0.05$)	slightly reduced mortality (n.s.)
Zehr et al [50]	Lung resection	protocol: 241 control (historic): 185	Hospital LOS: −20% ($p < 0.05$) Hospital charges: −21% ($p < 0.05$)	no change
Warner et al [51]	Pediatric appendicitis	protocol: 120 control (historic): 122	Hospital LOS: −39% ($p < 0.05$) Hospital costs: −30% ($p < 0.05$)	no change

LOS = length of stay; n.s. = not significant.

Table 4. Clinical pathway studies explicitly involving intensive care

Publication	Clinical Setting	N	Efficiency	Outcome
Price et al [52]	Pediatric cardiac surgery	protocol: 46 control (historic): 58	ICU LOS: –50% ($p < 0.05$) hospital LOS –40% ($p < 0.05$) cost: –49% ($p < 0.05$)	no change
Gandhi et al [53]	Pediatric blunt splenic injury	protocol: 21 control (historic): 28	ICU LOS: –28% (n.s.) hospital LOS: –21% ($p < 0.05$)	no change
Spain et al [54]	Severe head injuries	protocol: 84 control (historic): 49	Vent. days: –21% ($p < 0.05$) ICU LOS: –21% ($p < 0.05$) Hospital LOS: –24% ($p < 0.05$) (only calculated for survivors)	no change in functional outcome or complications, higher mortality through end-of-life decisions by family members
Uzark et al [55]	Pediatric cardiac surgery	protocol: 173 control: 69	Vent days: –40% ($p < 0.05$) Lab tests: –25% Total costs: –20%	no change
Burns et al [56]	Prolonged mechanical ventilation	protocol: 90 control (historic): 124	Vent days: –1.3 days (n.s.) Hospital LOS: –2.1 days (n.s.) Total costs: –US$3,341 per case	no change
Back et al [31]	ICU admissions for carotid endarterectomy	protocol: 63 control (historic): 45	ICU admissions: –70% ($p < 0.05$) Total costs: -41% ($p < 0.05$)	no change
Velasco et al [57]	Adult cardiac surgery	protocol: 114 control (historic): 382	ICU LOS: -46% ($p < 0.05$) Hospital LOS: -31% ($p < 0.05$) Total costs: -US$1,181 ($p < 0.05$)	no change

benefit most. But even on the micro level, clinical pathways provide a tool to improve the quality and cost efficiency of intensive care [34].

The most detailed and explicit algorithms in clinical decision make use of rule-based computer systems [13, 23]. Electronic reminders can significantly improve physicians' compliance with guidelines, reduce the rate of human errors and make physicians more responsive to specific clinical events [35, 36].

There are different levels of clinical decision support. Many systems that implement medical guidelines or clinical pathways are time oriented rather than patient data driven. This contrasts to computerized protocols where actual patient data generates executable instructions (recommendations) on the basis of validated rules [13, 24, 25, 28, 37].

Using data from the most comprehensive singular clinical data repository at the LDS Hospital, Salt Lake City, Utah, USA, Thomsen et al. [38] developed a rule-based decision support system for the mechanical ventilation of the critically ill, which generates, on the basis of actual patient data, explicit, executable and reproducible instructions or recommendations for the next therapeutic step. It was possible to control more than 95% of the ventilation times with these protocols, while intermediate and final clinical outcomes showed a beneficial effect [13].

On the basis of broad clinical experience it can be said that clinical care with bedside computerized protocols is feasible. Moreover, it complies with the ethical imperatives of modern health care [39, 40].

Field level: On the field level, we find all the traditional medical equipment for monitoring, therapy and diagnostics. Typical applications on this level are:
- Patient monitoring
- Life support, e.g., ventilators, IV devices, cardiac assist devices
- Imaging, e.g., magnetic resonance imaging (MRI), computed tomography (CT), ultrasound, etc. Imaging also includes PACS, which in itself bridges the gap between instrumentation and point of care computing.
- Laboratory, both stat lab and hospital lab. Laboratory information systems (LIS) to some extent bridge the gap between this and HIS.

Devices or systems on this level typically provide raw data describing physiological processes. They also provide tools for executing the processes in the continuum of care.

Today, we can see a widespread use of these devices, especially in intensive medicine and emergency care. New developments allow integration of some of the intelligence from the level of process control into these devices. Examples are modern ventilators that allow automatic weaning of 'typical' patients. More intelligent devices like these allow communication to shift from the field level and the process control level to a higher, more 'medical' level. This development has also been observed in the automation industry [41].

These devices monitor, diagnose, or treat individual patients; while they are essential to the execution of the process of care, they provide little information about the process and its underlying rationale. Although medical instrumentation provides tools to enact the process of care, it provides little to control the process of care across the continuum. 'Intelligent' devices at this level can help to optimize micro-processes. In the long run, the micro-processes may even be controlled by decision support systems from the next level up [38, 39]. Despite impressive results, most of the commercially available devices on this level have not been tested for their cost effectiveness in the process of care.

Scientific and Societal Information

The three levels of information management mentioned above are hospital or patient related. They help understand the individual processes of care, but they do not provide the rationale behind these processes.

Scientific and societal information and knowledge provide for the rationale behind the health care processes. Health informatics on this level includes the application of evidence-based medicine (EBM), epidemiology, macro economics, etc. Knowledge in the societal and epidemiologic domains determines the framework of medicine. EBM provides us with methods and concepts to extract and validate the scientific information relevant for the process of care from the vast quantity of scientific literature.

The majority of medical interventions, up to 85% according to some authors, are not supported by clinical data that show that these interventions do more good than harm [13]. Treatments and even guidelines based on uncontrolled clinical experience bear the danger of being widely applied, even if they are useless or harmful [42, 43]. Recent studies suggest that, depending on the country and health care system, up to 50% of hospital care is not clinically warranted [44].

While this level of scientific and societal information does not provide direct control of the process of care, it fulfills two more important tasks:

1) With the help of EBM, it allows the development of guidelines and pathways with strong scientific foundations. It can select concepts that have been proven to do more good than harm.
2) Demographic and epidemiologic data provide information on how to plan health care processes, their goals and their resource allocation.

Implementation of Health Informatics

Production control level: Since this level of information management is essential to run hospitals or other health institutions, technically, in the sense of mere business administration, most institutions in the Western world already have implemented systems of this kind. Therefore, it can be expected that, in many places, at least a rudimentary information infrastructure is present to support the production control level.

Process control level: Today only a few implementations of health informatics at the point of care can be seen. Major impediments to the more rapid spread of information technology to support the medical process control level are:

- lack of a sufficient information infrastructure in the hospital
- lack of communication interfaces between medical devices and information systems

- heterogeneous information systems, and
- a not always sufficiently developed conceptual framework at the medical level.

Field level: On the instrumentation level we see both a broad and deep acceptance of devices. Although more sophisticated devices will replace older ones, for many applications the quantitative demands for devices are satisfied in the developed world.

Scientific and societal information: As EBM is a methodology and a concept rather than a software product, it is very difficult to estimate the degree of penetration in the medical community. While EBM takes place in the head of the physician, health informatics can provide concrete tools for EBM. Other applications, e.g., from the fields of econometric or sociology, are not specific for medicine or are not directly integrated in the process of care.

General Obstacles

But there are even more daring challenges to the implementation of health informatics:
- Changes in the way health care professionals think and act. These may include the standardization of care, the abandonment of personal style, trust in computer systems, etc.
- Major investments in money and manpower, which also include major business risks for medical institutions.
- Substantiation and validation of medical guidelines and common practices.

It must also be kept in mind, that computers do not make (medical) policy, they simply display policy made by clinical leaders [27]. Standard documentation and order entry is no more time consuming with computers than with paper-based documentation [45].

Conclusion

In health care we face information overload on every level of the continuum of care. Health informatics provides methods, tools and concepts that can help analyze, evaluate, structure, and control health care processes. Concepts from the automation industry may help in this development and can be transferred to and modified for health care applications.

The core issues in understanding health care with the help of health informatics are understanding, analyzing and controlling the process of care, gaining information from, and providing information to, the point of care. This process control is essential to provide better and more cost efficient health care.

As the focus is the process of care, health care professionals must assume leadership in health informatics. The following can be considered as key points of action in this field:

- Health care professionals must assume leadership in health informatics.
- Medical guidelines and common practices must be substantiated and validated against scientific evidence.
- Accepted and proven standards must be implemented consistently into common medical practice.

Acknowledgments. The author wishes to thank Mrs. Penelope H. Greco and Mr James Greco, Kittery, Maine, USA, for their critical review of the manuscript.

References

1. Imhoff M (1995) A clinical information system on the intensive care unit: dream or night mare? In: Rubi JAG (ed): Medicina Intensiva 1995, XXX. Congreso SEMIUC. Pictographia, Murcia, pp 17–22
2. Imhoff M (1996) Three years clinical use of the Siemens Emtek System 2000: Efforts and Benefits. Clin Intensive Care 7 (suppl.): 43–44
3. Imhoff M, Lehner JH, Löhlein D (1994) Two years clinical experience with a clinical information system on a surgical ICU. In: Mutz NJ, Koller W, Benzer H (eds) 7th European Congress on Intensive Care Medicine. Monduzi Editore, Bologna, pp 163–166
4. Imhoff M (1998) Clinical Data Acquisition: What and how? Journal für Anästhesie und Intensivmedizin 5: 85–86
5. Morris A, Gardner R (1992) Computer applications. In: Hall J, Schmidt G, Wood L (eds) Principles of Critical Care. McGraw-Hill, New York, pp 500–514
6. Miller G (1956) The magical number seven, plus or minus two: Some limits to our capacity for processing information. Psychol Rev 63: 81–97
7. Jennings D, Amabile T, Ross L (1982) Informal covariation assessments: Data-based versus theory-based judgements. In: Kahnemann D, Slovic P, Tversky A (eds) Judgement under uncertainty: Heuristics and biases. Cambridge University Press, Cambridge, pp 211–230
8. Guyatt GH, Sackett DL, Cook DJ (1993) Users' guides to the medical literature. II. How to use an article about therapy or prevention. A. Are the results of the study valid? Evidence-Based Medicine Working Group. JAMA 270:2598–2601
9. Haux R (1997): Aims and tasks of medical informatics. Int J Med Inf 44: 9–20
10. Chalmers TC, Laus J (1993) Meta-analytic stimulus for changes in clinical trials. Stat Methods Med Res 2: 161–172
11. Abramson NS, Wald KS, Grenvik AN, Robinson D, Snyder JV (1980) Adverse occurrences in intensive care units. JAMA 244:1582–1584
12. Leape L (1994) Error in medicine. JAMA 272: 1851–1857
13. Morris AH (1999) Computerized protocols and beside decision support. Crit Care Clin 15: 523–545
14. Wu AW, Folkman S, McPhee SJ, Lo B (1991) Do house officers learn from their mistakes? JAMA 265: 2089–2094
15. Moehr JR (1998) Informatics in the service of health, a look to the future. Method Inf Med 37: 165–170
16. Gardner RM (1986) Computerized management of intensive care patients. MD Comput 3: 36– 51
17. McDonald CJ, Tierney WM (1988) Computer-stored medical records: Their future role in medical practice. JAMA 259: 3433–3440
18. Metzger J, Teich JM (1994) Designing systems for acceptance by physicians. In: Drazen E (ed): Patient Care Information Systems: Successful Design and Implementation. Springer, New York, pp 83–133
19. Carlson D, Wallace CJ, East TD, Morris AH (1995) Verification & validation algorithms for data used in critical care decision support systems. Proc Annu Symp Comput Appl Med Care: 188–192

20. Grimm RH Jr, Shimoni K, Harlan WR Jr, Estes EH Jr (1975) Evaluation of patient-care protocol use by various providers. N Engl J Med 292:507–511
21. Grimshaw JM, Russell IT (1993) Effect of clinical guidelines on medical practice: a systematic review of rigorous evaluations. Lancet 342:1317–1322
22. Wirtschafter DD, Scalise M, Henke C, Gams RA (1981) Do information systems improve the quality of clinical research? Results of a randomized trial in a cooperative multi-institutional cancer group. Comput Biomed Res 14:78–90
23. Johnston ME, Langton KB, Haynes RB, Mathieu A (1994) Effects of computer-based clinical decision support systems on clinician performance and patient outcome. A critical appraisal of research. Ann Intern Med 120: 135–142
24. Classen DC, Evans RS, Pestotnik SL, Horn SD, Menlove RL, Burke JP (1992) The timing of prophylactic administration of antibiotics and the risk of surgical-wound infection. N Engl J Med 326: 281–286
25. Pestotnik SL, Classen DC, Evans RS, Burke JP (1996) Implementing antibiotic practice guidelines through computer-assisted decision support: clinical and financial outcomes. Ann Intern Med 124: 884–890
26. Lesar TS, Briceland L, Stein DS (1997) Factors related to errors in medication prescribing. JAMA 277: 312–317
27. Teich JM, Glaser JP, Beckley RF, et al (1999) The Brigham integrated computing system (BICS): advanced clinical systems in an academic hospital environment. Int J Med Inf 54: 197–208
28. Classen DC, Pestotnik SL, Evans RS, Lloyd JF, Burke JP (1997) Adverse drug events in hospitalized patients. Excess length of stay, extra costs, and attributable mortality. JAMA 277: 301–306
29. Shewart W (1931) Economic control of quality of manufactured product. D. Van Nostrand, New York
30. Walton M (1986) The Deming management method. Putnam, New York
31. Back MR, Harward TR, Huber TS, Carlton LM, Flynn TC, Seeger JM (1997) Improving the cost-effectiveness of carotid endarterectomy. J Vasc Surg 26:456–462
32. Wahr JA, Parks R, Boisvert D, et al (1999) Preoperative serum potassium levels and perioperative outcomes in cardiac surgery patients. JAMA 281: 2203–2210
33. Wilson J, Woods I, Fawcett J, et al (1999) Reducing the risk of major elective surgery: randomised controlled trial of preoperative optimisation of oxygen delivery. Br Med J 318:1099–1103
34. Marx WH, DeMaintenon NL, Mooney KF, et al (1999) Cost reduction and outcome improvement in the intensive care unit. J Trauma 46: 625–630
35. McDonald CJ (1976) Protocol-based computer reminders, the quality of care and the non-perfectability of man. N Engl J Med 295: 1351–1355
36. McDonald CJ, Wilson GA, McCabe GP Jr (1980) Physician response to computer reminders. JAMA 244: 1579–1581
37. East T (1994) Role of the computer in the delivery of mechanical ventilation. In: Tobin M (ed): Principles and Practice of Mechanical Ventilation. MacGraw-Hill, New York, pp 1005–1038
38. Thomsen GE, Pope D, East TD, et al (1993) Clinical performance of a rule-based decision support system for mechanical ventilation of ARDS patients. Proc Annu Symp Comput Appl Med Care 1993:339–343
39. Morris A (1998) Algorithm-Based Decision-Making. In: Tobin JA, editor: Principles and Practice of Intensive Care Monitoring. McGraw–Hill, New York, pp 1355–1381
40. Sharpe V, Faden A (1998) Medical Harm. Cambridge University Press, Cambridge, UK
41. Polke M (1994) Process Control Engineering. John Wiley & Sons, New York
42. Cook D (1994) Small trials in critical care medicine: What can intensivists learn from them? In: Vincent JL (ed): Yearbook of Intensive and Emergency Medicine. Springer, Berlin, pp 779–785
43. Guyatt G, Drummund M, Feeny D, et al (1986) Guidelines for the clinical and economic evaluation of health care technologies. Soc Sci Med 22: 393–408

44. Axene D, Doyle R (1994) Analysis of medically unnecessary inpatient service. Research Report. Milliman & Robertson, Seattle
45. Teich JM, Spurr CD, Schmiz, JL, O'Conner EM, Thomas D (1995) Enhancement of clinician workflow using computer order entry. J Am Med Informatics Assoc 2 (suppl 5): 459–463
46. Chang PL, Wang TM, Huang ST, Hsieh ML, Tsui KH, Lai RH (1999) Effects of implementation of 18 clinical pathways on costs and quality of care among patients undergoing urological surgery. J Urol 161:1858–1862
47. Gheiler EL, Lovisolo JA, Tiguert R, et al (1999) Results of a clinical care pathway for radical prostatectomy patients in an open hospital - multiphysician system. Eur Urol 35:210–216
48. Scranton PE Jr (1999) The cost effectiveness of streamlined care pathways and product standardization in total knee arthroplasty. J Arthroplasty 14:182–186
49. Dzwierzynski WW, Spitz K, Hartz A, Guse C, Larson DL (1998) Improvement in resource utilization after development of a clinical pathway for patients with pressure ulcers. Plast Reconstr Surg 102:2006–2011
50. Zehr KJ, Dawson PB, Yang SC, Heitmiller RF (1998) Standardized clinical care pathways for major thoracic cases reduce hospital costs. Ann Thorac Surg 66:914–919
51. Warner BW, Kulick RM, Stoops MM, Mehta S, Stephan M, Kotagal UR (1998) An evidenced-based clinical pathway for acute appendicitis decreases hospital duration and cost. J Pediatr Surg 33:1371–1375
52. Price MB, Jones A, Hawkins JA, McGough EC, Lambert L, Dean JM (1999) Critical pathways for postoperative care after simple congenital heart surgery. Am J Manag Care 5:185–92
53. Gandhi RR, Keller MS, Schwab CW, Stafford PW (1999) Pediatric splenic injury: pathway to play? J Pediatr Surg 34:55–58
54. Spain DA, McIlvoy LH, Fix SE, et al (1998) Effect of a clinical pathway for severe traumatic brain injury on resource utilization. J Trauma 45:101–4
55. Uzark K, Frederick C, Lamberti JJ, et al Changing practice patterns for children with heart disease: a clinical pathway approach. Am J Crit Care 7:101–105
56. Burns SM, Marshall M, Burns JE, et al (1998) Design, testing, and results of an outcomes-managed approach to patients requiring prolonged mechanical ventilation. Am J Crit Care 7:45–57
57. Velasco FT, Ko W, Rosengart T, et al (1996) Cost containment in cardiac surgery: results with a critical pathway for coronary bypass surgery at the New York hospital-Cornell Medical Center. Best Pract Benchmarking Healthc 1:21–28

Databases, Registries and Networks

J.L. Vincent and S. Brimioulle

Learning Points

- The use of databases and registries can facilitate comparisons between ICUs at a national and international level
- Many forms of database exist, each with their own strengths and limitations in terms of their applicability, relevance and appropriateness to the question being asked of them
- When selecting or creating a database, it is important to be aware of potential problems including varying quality and uniformity of data collection, incentive or voluntary bias, and possible confounding factors
- Database ownership and decisions regarding data reporting and publications can potentially be the source of problems and need to be addressed and solved by positive dialog
- Closer collaboration through the establishment of international networks will facilitate the conduct of clinical trials and help create a degree of uniformity in ICU organization

"Knowledge is of two kinds. We know a subject ourselves or we know where we can find information upon it" (Samuel Johnson, 1709-1784).

Introduction

Health services research has been defined as "the integration of epidemiologic, sociological, economic, and other analytic sciences in the study of health services. Health services research is usually concerned with relationships between need, demand, supply, use, and outcome of health services. The aim of the research is evaluation, particularly in terms of structure, process, output, and outcome" [1]. In today's climate of rising health care costs, perhaps especially marked in the field of intensive care, physicians are increasingly demanded to explain and account for their actions and expenditure. In order to effectively conduct health services research, to enable comparison between groups of patients, between hospitals, between countries, adequate sources of information are required. Various forms of data collection and storage have been developed and are utilized. Improved computerized accessibility and capabilities, and most recently the Internet, are revolutionizing information acquisition and analysis in this field and will greatly facilitate national and international health services research.

Databases and Registries: Definitions

A research database is a collection of facts and data, usually covering a fairly broad field, which is available for research use and analysis. A research registry is a database focused on a particular disease or intervention, for example organ transplant recipients [2, 3], patients with myocardial infarction [4], trauma patients [5], to name but a few. Databases and registries vary in size, construction, and content, and as such, vary in their degree of relevance and appropriateness to answer any specific health services research question.

Various databases can be described in the intensive care field, and the list below is not intended to be exhaustive but to provide a general overview of database formats.

Local Intensive Care Unit (ICU) Databases

These databases generally gather epidemiological information on the patients admitted to the ICU, i.e., patient age, gender, cause of admission, length of ICU stay, mortality, etc. They can also provide clinical information such as diagnosis, procedures, treatment, etc. They may be useful in evaluating ICU needs in relation to available resources, and could potentially be used to compare ICUs, to assess differences in patient populations between regions and countries, but also to compare ICU performance.

National and International Databases

These gather the same data as ICU databases but on a larger scale, covering many ICUs from various regions, countries and/or continents. Examples of such databases include the Impact database developed in 1996 by the Society of Critical Care Medicine (SCCM) which now has data on over 50,000 patients from 98 ICUs in North America, and the European Consortium which was operated by the European Society of Intensive Care Medicine (ESICM). Such databases are again useful for describing ICU populations and for comparing ICU demographics and performance.

Cohort Databases

These include data gathered by volunteer ICUs on specific groups of patients, for example the SOFA (sequential organ failure assessment) cohort which involved 1,449 patients in 40 ICUs in Europe, Canada, Australia and Brazil [6], the European/North American SAPS II (simplified acute physiology score) database which involved 137 ICUs from 12 countries [7], and the EPIC (European prevalence of infection in intensive care) cohort which involved 1,417 ICUs in Europe and gathered 10,038 case reports [8]. The aim of such cohorts is primarily to validate a scoring system or to evaluate prognostic factors.

Data Registries

As mentioned above, registries are more clearly defined databases, focusing on one disease process, or one specific group of patients. In addition to those listed above, another example of such a registry is the ongoing French acute respiratory distress syndrome (ARDS) registry. The aim of such databases is to provide specific information about one disease process, the patients affected, treatment, outcome, etc.

Multicenter Clinical Trials

While not developed as databases *per se*, the information collected in the course of a multicenter clinical trial may provide excellent database material. Often well-funded by the industry with excellent technical and analytical support, and under strict government regulation, clinical trial data is rigorously collected, detailed and expansive. The aim of a clinical trial and hence the purpose of the data collection is to test the hypothesis that a new diagnostic, monitoring, or therapeutic intervention will prove beneficial to the patients included.

Databases and Registries: Problems

Problems with database information can be related to individual databases, in particular problems with the quality of data collection and ownership rights, or to the comparison of data from different databases.

1) The quality of data collection: Who was responsible for data collection? Were data collectors qualified or trained? Who supervised and verified data collection? Who monitored data input? The database definition and content must be simple enough to allow accurate data collection without being too time consuming or involved. Collection of clinical trial data is generally well-funded, intensively monitored, and controlled by government agencies (for example the FDA [Food and Drug Administration]) at the time of collection and for many years afterwards. However, other types of data collection are often much less regulated, and data collection can become a bit 'hit or miss'. The 'responsible' physician may fell he/she has other priorities and delegate the job to residents or fellows who may lack stimulation as they are unlikely to see any immediate benefit or application from their input. If professional data collectors are involved, problems with payment commonly arise. Institutions, par-

ticularly in Europe, are generally not ready to commit valuable and limited resources to data collection, and unit directors or physicians generally prefer (correctly) to keep limited funding for direct research purposes. Data collection in general lacks immediate patients impact and therefore is placed low on any budget's list of priorities.

2) Accessibility of data: Who has/should have access to the data? Where should the database be stored? What should the data be used for, and what should it not be used for? To whom does the database belong? Who has the right to use the data for publications, and should the original founders of the database be acknowledged in all subsequent publications relating to database-based studies?

3) Lack of harmony in data collection: For example, severity score databases (APACHE, SAPS,.....) use different definitions of organ failure, inconsistent terminology, varying diagnostic criteria, defined levels for variable abnormalities, etc. All these factors can considerably influence the data content and make direct comparison of databases difficult. However, it is important not to attempt to oversimplify data collection. Progress will be stunted rather than promoted by the limitation of definitions and terminology. We will be no closer to solving the sepsis problem if we limit ourselves to any one definition of sepsis. Deciding on a universal definition of liver dysfunction, for example hyperbilirubinemia or altered liver enzymes, will similarly not be useful. Rather we must use information from databases and registries to develop new, better, and more specific definitions.

4) Bias in data collection: In database development various incentives may create a bias in data collection. In clinical trial programs, these incentives can be financial, or due to competitive academic, or even personal, interest. Physicians may want their hospital to be seen to have recruited the largest number of patients, to be able to be included as an author in any publications, or to use material from the database to present at meetings. These incentives may even lead to intentional 'bending' of the rules for inclusion criteria. In other databases, innocent but systematic bias in data collection may occur. For example, the Glasgow coma score (GCS) is difficult to evaluate in sedated patients; different modes of ventilatory support may have an influence on the PaO_2/FiO_2 ratio. Voluntary bias may also occur, for example, if clinical conditions are systematically overevaluated to increase severity scores and hence increase performance rating. Variable physician interest within and among centers may also introduce bias in data collection.

5) Confounders: In comparison of databases, for example, to compare performance of one ICU with another, it is essential to allow for confounders which may bias outcome and influence any comparison. A confounder may be any variable associated with the question being asked, and includes simple parameters such as patient age, diagnosis, treatment, etc. all of which can influence mortality rates. More complex confounders include, for example, the international, north/south gradient in ICU outcome seen across Europe which can be largely explained by smaller ICUs treating sicker patients in Southern Europe [9]. Although the same entry criteria are employed for a particular clinical trial, mortality rates will thus be higher in southern European countries. Such

confounders are difficult to identify, quantify, and adjust for, and a variety of techniques can be employed including patient matching, database stratification, multivariable adjustments including logistic and linear regression techniques, propensity scores, and instrumental variables [10]. It is, however, often impossible to eliminate all confounders and comparison between databases developed in different populations at different times is complex and potentially unreliable.

Databases and Registries: The Future

Database development and use in intensive care is going to become increasingly important as financial pressures increase and health services research comes into its own. Databases must remain simple to facilitate data collection, and a degree of flexibility must be maintained regarding variables to be included. For example, while the decision to utilize just one severity score may appear to make data collection more simple, it would limit progress, damp future research and stifle imagination in this important field. In fact, many scores include the same basic data and can now easily be computed once the primary variables have been entered. Computerized systems certainly represent an important aspect of the future development, analysis, and validation of databases. A lot of basic information, for example, laboratory data, continuous hemodynamic or electrocardiograph (EKG) monitoring can now be collected and entered automatically. Many patient variables, for example the GCS, can be assessed and entered at bedside terminals. For larger national and international databases, data collection and transfer will be facilitated by the development of Internet facilities.

Research Networks and Collaborative Groups

A research network is a group of individuals or centers which have become linked in a collaborative effort to share resources, and enhance data collection and database development in order, ultimately, to improve patient care and ICU performance. Research networks differ in their size, objectives, and structure. Many networks were originally born from the concept of the multicenter clinical trial and their focus was/is to facilitate clinical trial research. Examples of such networks include the Canadian Critical Care Trials Group [11], and the United States Critical Care Clinical Investigation Network [12]. Other research networks were designed primarily to conduct health services outcomes research for specific groups of patients, to continuously monitor and improve quality of care in terms of structure, process and patient outcome [13]. Examples of such networks include the Vermont-Oxford Neonatal Network [14], the Finnish Intensive Care Study Group [15], and the Ontario Adult Cardiac Care Network [16].

National Collaboration

Many important regional and national networks have developed over recent years both to review research proposals and conduct clinical trials, and to perform outcomes research. The Canadian Critical Care Trials Group [11] certainly provides a good example of such a network. First established in 1989, this group now counts a membership of 40, and states their aim is to "foster national collaborative multi-center research into clinically important questions arising in adult intensive care" [17]. As a collaboration, the group develops protocols for clinical trials, using the diverse experience of its members to create studies with scientific precision and clinical relevance, but which are practically and financially feasible. This group has been involved in conducting and publishing critical research in many aspects of intensive care patient management [18–27]. Collaborative groups have formed in many other countries including Italy [28, 29], France [30], and Spain [31], to list just a few examples.

International Collaboration

International collaboration in clinical trials has been excellent. With improvements in communication, particularly email and the Internet, barriers of time and distance have all but disappeared, enabling effective and efficient international networks to be established for clinical trial research. Pressures to perform large randomized trials of new therapies increasingly necessitate multicenter trials and physicians are very keen to contribute and participate. In the recently opened website for the annual Symposium of Intensive Care and Emergency Medicine (http://www.intensive.org), physician visitors to the site who are interested in being involved in future clinical trials are asked to register their details. In less than 6 months, 555 physicians from 49 countries have expressed their interest.

Examples of established international collaboration include the EPIC study which was supported by 1,417 ICUs across Europe [8] without financial incentive. The SOFA study also experienced good international collaboration with 40 ICUs participating again largely in Europe but including a few centers in Australia, Canada and South America [6]. While the EPIC study was conducted over just one day (prevalence study), the SOFA study followed patients throughout their ICU course, creating a much larger and more detailed database. Most recently, a collaborative network of ICUs was established in Western Europe to conduct an epidemiological study of anemia and blood transfusion in the critically ill Europe (the ABC study). This was a voluntary study with a small financial reward to cover administrative costs. The initial aim was to include 3,000 patients, and over 3,500 were in fact enrolled, the organizers having to eliminate some centers and receiving letters from many others expressing their disappointment for not having been included. Many intensivists are not in a position to participate actively in large scale research projects, and the possibility to be part of an international project provides them with an opportunity to be involved in the frontline of clinical medicine. However, differences in the standards and format of intensive care among countries may raise concerns regarding quality assessment in such collaborative studies.

Research Networks and Collaborative Groups: The Future

The future will see more international collaboration. National and regional networks will become part of much larger international networks which will be able to expedite the conduct of multicenter clinical trials, allowing effective therapies to be identified and instituted, and ineffective therapies to be discarded, as rapidly as possible [13]. In addition, attempts to create some degree of uniformity in ICU organization across boundaries will also necessitate collaboration between countries; and economic comparisons in health care finance and resource utilization will increasingly take place across international boundaries. International networks are an established part of modern intensive care. Computerized data collection and electronic communication will facilitate the establishment and maintenance of such networks.

Conclusion

Health services research has become a necessary part of modern intensive care. The optimization of patient care and resource allocation in the light of high financial costs and rapid technological and pharmacological development, demand input from continuous outcomes research. The information sources for outcomes research include databases and registries, developed at both the national and international level. Networks of physicians and centers will make database development and maintenance more simple and rewarding, and will optimize clinical trial conduct. Developments in and access to electronic communication and computer technology will play a vital role in facilitating the large scale collection and comparison of data. The application of the information obtained from such databases and networks will be essential in providing efficient, optimal intensive care organization for the benefit of both staff and patients.

References

1. Dark G (1997) The Online Medical Dictionary. http://www.graylab.ac.uk/cgi-bin/omd
2. Burdelski M, Nolkemper D, Ganschow R, et al (1999) Liver transplantation in children: long-term outcome and quality of life. Eur J Pediatr 158 Suppl 2: S34–S42
3. Brann WM, Bennett LE, Keck BM, Hosenpud JD (1998) Morbidity, functional status, and immunosuppressive therapy after heart transplantation: an analysis of the joint International Society for Heart and Lung Transplantation/United Network for Organ Sharing Thoracic Registry. J Heart Lung Transplant 17: 374–382
4. Becker RC, Burns M, Gore JM, et al (1998) Early assessment and in-hospital management of patients with acute myocardial infarction at increased risk for adverse outcomes: a nationwide perspective of current clinical practice. The National Registry of Myocardial Infarction (NRMI-2) Participants. Am Heart J 135: 786–796

5. Gomberg BF, Gruen GS, Smith WR, Spott M (1999) Outcomes in acute orthopaedic trauma: a review of 130,506 patients by age. Injury 30: 431–437
6. Vincent JL, de Mendonça A, Cantraine F, et al (1998) Use of the SOFA score to assess the incidence of organ dysfunction/failure in intensive care units: Results of a multicentric, prospective study. Crit Care Med 26: 1793–1800
7. Le Gall J-R, Lemeshow S, Saulnier F (1993) A new simplified acute physiology score (SAPS II) based on a European/North American multicenter study. JAMA 270: 2957–2963
8. Vincent JL, Bihari D, Suter PM, et al (1995) The prevalence of nosocomial infection in intensive care units in Europe – The results of the EPIC study. JAMA 274: 639–644
9. Vincent JL, Suter P, Bihari D, Bruining H (1997) Organization of intensive care units in Europe: Lessons from the EPIC study. Intensive Care Med 23: 1181–1184
10. Rubenfeld GD, Angus DC, Pinsky MR, Curtis JR, Connors AFJ, Bernard GR (1999) Outcomes research in critical care: results of the American Thoracic Society Critical Care Assembly Workshop on Outcomes Research. The Members of the Outcomes Research Workshop. Am J Respir Crit Care Med 160: 358–367
11. Cook DJ, Todd RTJ (1997) The Canadian Critical Care Trials Group: A collaborative education organization for the advancement of adult clinical ICU research. Intensive Care World 14: 68–70
12. Calvin JE (1998) Clinical trial networks: a unique opportunity for critical care. Crit Care Med 26: 625–626
13. Keenan SP, Martin CM (1998) Creation of a critical care research network. Curr Opin Crit Care 4: 470–478
14. Horbar JD (1995) The Vermont-Oxford Neonatal Network: integrating research and clinical practice to improve the quality of medical care. Semin Perinatol 19: 124–131
15. Saarela E, Kari A, Nikki P, Rauhala V, Iisalo E, Kaukinen L (1991) Current practice regarding invasive monitoring in intensive care units in Finland. A nationwide study of the uses of arterial, pulmonary artery and central venous catheters and their effect on outcome. The Finnish Intensive Care Study Group. Intensive Care Med 17: 264–271
16. Tu JV, Jaglal SB, Naylor CD (1995) Multicenter validation of a risk index for mortality, intensive care unit stay, and overall hospital length of stay after cardiac surgery. Steering Committee of the Provincial Adult Cardiac Care Network of Ontario. Circulation 91: 677–684
17. Cook DJ (2000) Canadian Critical Care Trials Group. http://critcare.lhsc.on.ca/related/cccs/ ccctg_f.htm
18. Cook DJ, Fuller HD, Guyatt GH, et al (1994) Risk factors for gastrointestinal bleeding in critically ill patients. N Engl J Med 330: 377–381
19. Cook DJ, Guyatt GH, Jaeschke R, et al (1995) Determinants in Canadian health care workers of the decision to withdraw life support from the critically ill. JAMA 273: 703–708
20. Cook DJ, Walter SD, Cook RJ, et al (1998) Incidence of and risk factors for ventilator-associated pneumonia in critically ill patients. Ann Intern Med 129: 433–440
21. Cook D, Guyatt G, Marshall J, et al (1998) A comparison of sucralfate and ranitidine for the prevention of upper gastrointestinal bleeding in patients requiring mechanical ventilation. N Engl J Med 338: 791–797
22. Hebert PC, Wells G, Martin C, et al (1998) A Canadian survey of transfusion practices in critically ill patients. Transfusion Requirements in Critical Care Investigators and the Canadian Critical Care Trials Group. Crit Care Med 26: 482–487
23. Stewart TE, Meade MO, Cook DJ, et al (1998) Evaluation of a ventilation strategy to prevent borotrauma in patients at high risk for acute respiratory distress syndrome. N Engl J Med 338: 355–361
24. Walter SD, Cook DJ, Guyatt GH, et al (1998) Confidence in life-support decisions in the intensive care unit: a survey of healthcare workers. Canadian Critical Care Trials Group. Crit Care Med 26: 44–49
25. Hebert PC, Wells G, Blajchman MA, et al (1999) A multicenter, randomized, controlled clinical trial of transfusion requirements in critical care. N Engl J Med 340: 409–417

26. Heyland DK, Cook DJ, Griffith L, Keenan SP, Brun-Buisson C (1999) The attributable morbidity and mortality of ventilator-associated pneumonia in the critically ill patient. The Canadian Critical Trials Group. Am J Respir Crit Care Med 159: 1249–1256
27. Heyland DK, Cook DJ, Schoenfeld PS, Frietag A, Varon J, Wood G (1999) The effect of acidified enteral feeds on gastric colonization in critically ill patients: results of a multicenter randomized trial. Canadian Critical Care Trials Group. Crit Care Med 27: 2399–2406
28. Gattinoni L, Brazzi L, Pelosi P, et al (1995) A trial of goal-oriented hemodynamic therapy in critically ill patients. N Engl J Med 333: 1025–1032
29. Gattinoni L, Tognoni G, Brazzi L, Latini R (1997) Ventilation in the prone position. The Prone–Supine Study Collaborative Group. Lancet 350: 815
30. Roupie E, Lepage E, Wysocki M, et al (1999) Prevalence, etiologies and outcome of the acute respiratory distress syndrome among hypoxemic ventilated patients. Intensive Care Med 25: 920–929
31. Esteban A, Alia I, Tobin MJ, et al (1999) Effect of spontaneous breathing trial duration on outcome of attempts to discontinue mechanical ventilation. Spanish Lung Failure Collaborative Group. Am J Respir Crit Care Med 159: 512–518

Application and Interpretation: Using Data to Improve Outcomes

Organizational Effects on Outcomes

J. B. Hall

Learning Points

- A wide range of organizations are employed with regard to ICU and intensivist utilization
- As a generalization, smaller hospitals tend to employ multipurpose units with an open ICU approach to physician involvement
- Most studies are consistent with the notion that reorganization of critical care services with senior intensivist oversight improves outcome and/or reduces resource utilization
- Mechanisms underlying any such apparent benefits have not been explored but might include:
  - Protocol implementation
  - Integration of health care team
  - Reduction in complications
  - Physical presence and out of hour coverage
  - Shift from cure to comfort when appropriate to patient management
  - Exploitation of downstream facilities

As in many intensive care units (ICUs) in the United States, intensivists and their non-intensivist colleagues at the University of Chicago debated the virtues of the 'open' and 'closed' unit for many years. This debate centered on the question of whether care was best delivered by consulting intensivists, with primary care responsibilities retained by physicians responsible for care before and after ICU admission ('open' structure), or was care best delivered by transfer of the patient to the care of the intensivist ('closed' structure). While benefits of each system could be imagined, neither system was clearly superior to all participants in this debate and no simple way to compare the approaches in a prospective randomized trial could be conceived.

In 1994, largely because of an increasing shortage of housestaff assigned to various hospital services and because of stipulations as to the amount of time housestaff spend in the learning environment of the ICU, it became necessary to 'close' the ICU with regard to resident coverage and it was deemed necessary to do so with regard to senior staff as well. This transition was recognized as a natural 'experiment' to compare the two structures which was conducted and reported (see reference 19) and forms a part of the database of this chapter's analysis.

The significance of this brief anecdote is that naturally occurring changes in the delivery of health care over time can often provide a vehicle for health outcomes research to analyze the process of health care and, by virtue of analysis of changes longitudinal in time, draw powerful inferences as to the proper organization of services. This is a valuable approach particularly in these arenas that do not necessarily or readily lend themselves to the standard tool of modern clinical science – the randomized prospective clinical trial (RCT).

Introduction

In the US, critical care medicine consumes a disproportionately large share of healthcare resources, with the majority of these resources expended in the ICU. In a survey of data compiled from 1986–1992, it was estimated that while ICU beds comprised <10% of total hospital beds, 22% of total hospital costs were directly related to ICU activity [1]. By other estimates, ICU costs amount to 1% of the gross national product (GNP) in the US – an estimated $80.8 billion in 1997. These estimates likely underpredict current expenditures, since the number of critical care beds is increasing in most facilities and many ICUs are now subserved by 'long term acute care' facilities which continue life-support therapies and provide rehabilitation for survivors of critical illness who cannot receive ongoing care in the nursing home or hospital ward setting but no longer require the minute-to-minute titrated care of the ICU [2].

Despite this high level of activity, some of the most fundamental questions concerning the optimal organization of services to provide critical care remain unanswered, with most institutions having evolved a local approach governed by the historical transition from other forms of care delivery in related but different environments. This chapter will review the nascent literature analyzing the effect of organizational change in the ICU upon outcomes.

The Range of Organizational Approaches

There is a wide range of approaches to the organization of critical care services in the US. Post-operative patients requiring extended critical care are managed under most circumstances by general surgeons, surgical intensivists, or anesthesiologists, while patients with predominantly medical problems are cared for by internists, increasingly with specific critical care training and most often linked to the subspecialty of pulmonary medicine [3]. Some hospitals provide highly integrated and interdisciplinary care, with patients combined in 'medical-surgical' units that do not segregate patients for care, and cared for by surgical and medical intensivists who round together and function without distinction. It appears that economies of scale may drive smaller facilities to such aggregation, while larger facilities may gain both economic and outcome efficiencies by separating patients by problems. This latter strategy often leads to the co-location but separate operation of coronary care, neuro-intensive, medical, surgical, burn, and even bone marrow transplant units.

Prior to the advent of critical care medicine and the creation of associated training programs, critically ill patients were most often cared for by medical or surgical generalists with the aid of organ-system focused subspecialists. This general model of care is still operative in many hospitals, although increasingly individuals with critical care training are involved in patient management. The range of this involvement is broad. In the 'open' ICU, any physician with admitting privileges (conferred by institutional process) admits and directs the care of patients to the ICU, seeking consultation as deemed necessary. In the 'semi-open' ICU, care is directed by the admitting primary care physician but critical care physicians are involved to varying degree, often as requested consultants. In the 'closed' ICU model of care, the critical care physician assumes direct responsibility for the patient and maintains this responsibility until the patient is discharged from the ICU. For the physician practicing in a closed ICU with no history nor experience of this range of options, as is true for many countries and care environments, the consideration of major involvement of physicians without extensive critical care training may seem unwise if not ludicrous, and perhaps an outgrowth of financial and other poorly justifiable motivations. Nonetheless, there are arguments that can be made for ongoing involvement of primary care physicians in the management of the critically ill, most prominently the provision of continuity of care for patient and family when patients are admitted to and discharged from the unit.

A description of the use of these various approaches in the early 1990s has been published [4]. A survey was conducted in 1991 of the 4,233 US hospitals with ICUs; 1,706 hospitals reported data on 2,876 separate ICUs with 32,850 total beds (40% response rate). The smallest hospitals (< 100 beds) tended to have only a single ICU serving multiple patient populations (Fig. 1) while larger hospitals (> 500 beds) usually had a wide range of specialized units (Fig. 2).

Virtually all ICUs had an identified director, and in 63% of units this director had training in internal medicine. Surgeons directed most surgical and neurologic units. Very few units (6%) reported having in-house, 24-hr attending physician coverage. The availability of an in-unit physician or hospital-based critical care

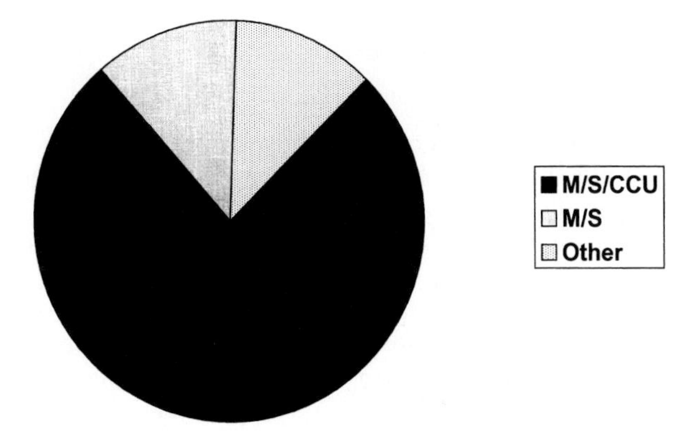

Fig. 1. Distribution of ICU type for hospitals with < 100 beds (M/S/CCU = combined medical, surgical, and coronary care unit; M/S = combined medical-surgical unit. Data from [4])

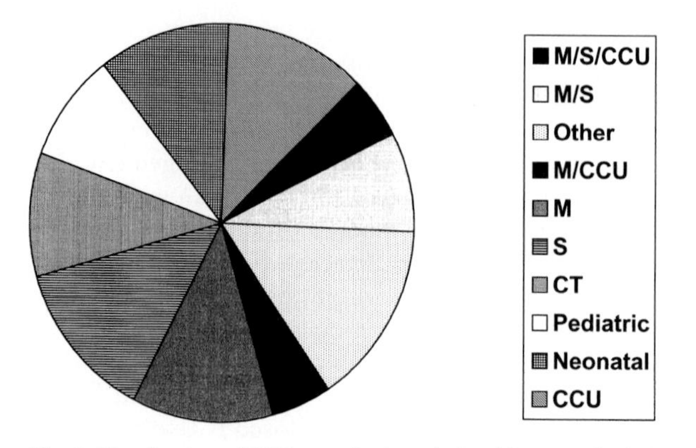

Fig. 2. Distribution of ICU type for hospitals with > 500 beds (M/S/CCU = combined medical-surgical-coronary care unit, M/S = combined medical-surgical unit, M/CCU = combined medical-coronary care unit, M=medical, S=surgical, CT=cardiothoracic, data from [4])

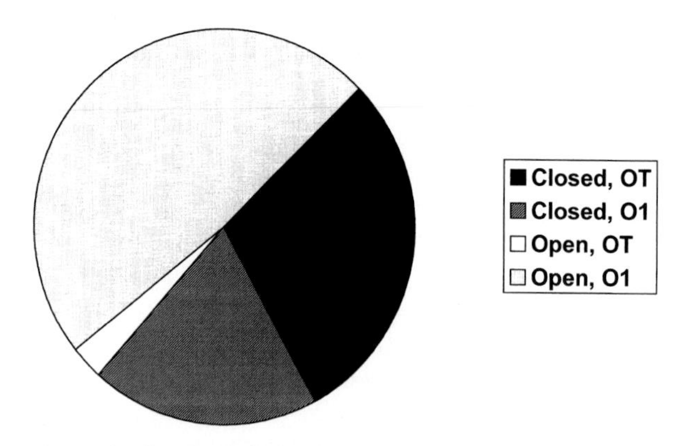

Fig. 3. The distribution of unit policy among medical ICUs (Closed = primary care responsibility transferred to ICU physician, Open = primary care responsibility retained by admitting physician, OT = order writing includes unit physicians, O1 = order writing maintained by admitting physician, data from [4])

specialist varied, not only with hospital size, but also with the type of unit. Neonatal units showed the largest number of full-time attending faculty, with the greatest duration of unit attendance.

The distribution of unit policies as regards an open or closed status can be seen in Figures 3-5. In general, smaller hospitals employing combined ICUs tended to have a higher utilization rate of the open model as compared to specialty units in larger hospitals (compare Figs. 3 and 5). Also, medical units tended to a greater use of the closed model of organization than surgical units (compare Figs. 3 and 4).

While these data provide only a 'snapshot' of the organization of critical care services in the US, which is likely to be a fast moving target, they do make the

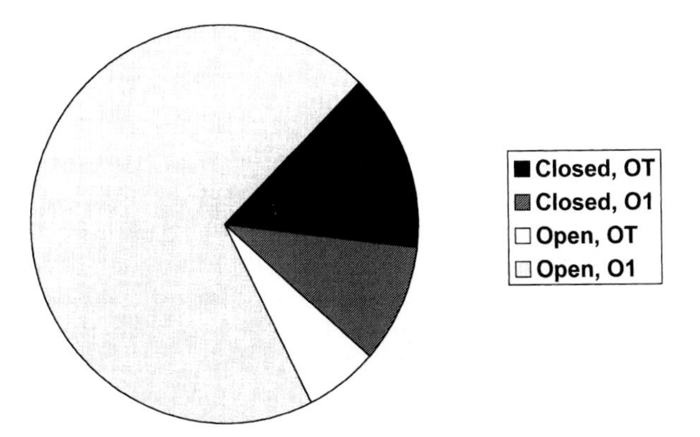

Fig. 4. The distribution of unit policy among surgical ICUs (Closed = primary care responsibility transferred to ICU physician, Open = primary care responsibility retained by admitting physician, OT = order writing includes unit physicians, O1 = order writing maintained by admitting physician, data from reference 4)

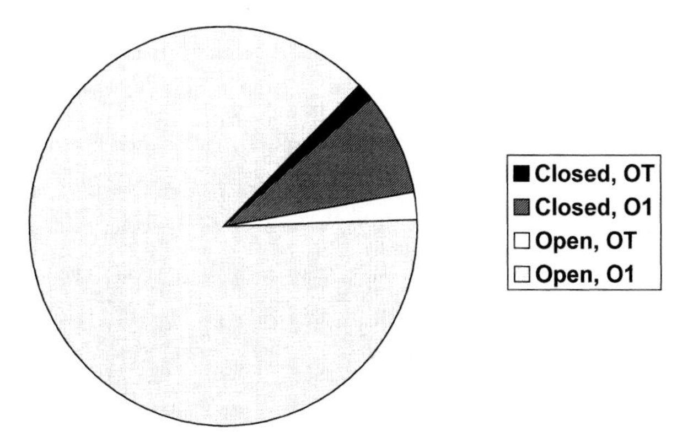

Fig. 5. The distribution of unit policy among combined medical-surgical ICUs. (Closed = primary care responsibility transferred to ICU physician, Open = primary care responsibility retained by admitting physician, OT = order writing includes unit physicians, O1 = order writing maintained by admitting physician, data from [4])

point that very diverse structures of care have been employed in the recent past. It is possible that this diversity necessarily exists because of the exigencies of care in a wide variety of healthcare environments. Alternatively, lack of comparative data has led to a proliferation of approaches that would not occur should sufficient information exist to inform planning of the organization of critical care services. Accordingly, the remainder of this chapter will review existing studies that explore the relationship of organization of critical care to outcomes.

Descriptive Studies Relating Organization to Outcome

Studies Reporting Associations from Multicenter Databases

Some of the earliest studies relating organization of critical care services to outcome measures were provided by the data collection related to the creation of a widely employed tool to assess severity of illness of the critically ill patient, the Acute Physiology and Chronic Health Evaluation or APACHE scoring system [5]. Once a validated tool existed to compare patients across different institutions and healthcare environments, it became possible to describe differences in outcome and to at least speculate if these differences were related to organizational differences. In a comparison of 5,000 ICU patients at 13 tertiary care centers, the creators of the APACHE system described the main characteristic of 'outlier' hospitals with significantly better or worse outcomes as a greater or lesser interaction and coordination of each hospital's ICU staff [6]. This early retrospective observational study was followed by a number of prospective investigations with a larger number and range of institutional characteristics [7–10]. These prospective data collections made a number of observations:

1) there was a substantial variation in mortality and ICU length of stay (LOS) that existed even when appropriate adjustment for severity of illness was performed;
2) risk-adjusted survival was better for a large number of diagnostic categories of critical illness at teaching hospitals, and that at least one characteristic of teaching hospitals was a greater physician activity in the ICU, including a greater physician number, a greater involvement of physician unit directors, and a greater frequency of in-unit or in-hospital night coverage;
3) another possible explanation for improved outcome at teaching hospitals was strong nursing and physician leadership of activities in the ICUs. The lack of an interventional design and the general lack of accepted criteria for success or excellence of critical care services limited the conclusions that could be drawn from these early investigations.

Similar observational reports have been made based upon databases collected for a pediatric risk of mortality (PRISM) score [11–14]; these observations have not been entirely consistent. In an initial investigation [11], it was reported that high-risk pediatric patients had lower mortality when cared for in tertiary care centers as opposed to non-tertiary units, a finding interpreted to imply that greater experience yielded improved outcomes. A follow-up investigation [12] interestingly suggested that presence of a pediatric intensivist conferred benefit of improved survival, although care at a teaching hospital as an independent factor was associated with increased mortality, with the authors speculating that this was the result of increased risk arising from the inexperience of resident trainees. One recent study [14] demonstrated a shorter LOS when pediatric patients were managed in an ICU with a supervising intensivist and resident staff.

Finally, governmental databases have been employed to document the impact of intensivists on postoperative care [15]. In an evaluation of ICU care after aortic surgery in approximately 3,000 patients managed in 19 ICUs in one state between 1994 and 1997, is was observed that absence of a rounding intensivist was independently associated with an increased risk of mortality, and that ICU resource allocation was greatest in ICUs with low nurse:patient staffing ratios and low fractions of critical care certified physicians.

Studies Reporting the Impact of Implementing Care by Intensivists

As critical care physician involvement in ICU care emerged and expanded in the last two decades in the US, a number of 'natural experiments' existed which were exploited by researchers to analyze before and after outcomes. Two early investigations in pediatric [16] and adult [17] patient populations demonstrated that intensivists decreased severity of illness adjusted mortality, reduced admissions with a very low severity of illness [16], and improved survival for patients with the diagnosis of sepsis [17]. In another more recent investigation [18] the introduction of an intensivist to a large community hospital ICU with resident staff resulted in a decrease in mortality from 21 to 16% (with equivalent APACHE II stratification of patients during the periods of comparison), a decrease in ICU LOS from 5 to 3 days, and an improvement in performance on testing for understanding of the pathophysiology of critical illness by resident staff after their rotation in the ICU.

We studied the effect of moving from an open to closed format of care at the University of Chicago in 1994 [19]. Under the open format, primary care attendants admitted patients to the ICU and all patients were followed by an intensivist consultant and housestaff team. With the closed format, care was transferred to the intensivist who followed the patient with a housestaff team whose responsibilities were restricted to the ICU. Thus, while the staff did not change, their organization and relationship to the patient did. With closure of the ICU, the ratio of actual to predicted mortality (using APACHE II adjustment) fell from 0.9 to 0.78. Despite an increase in severity of illness scores during the closed period (average APACHE II scores rising from 15.4 to 20.6 in the transition from open to closed organization), LOS and resource allocation was not different. During the closed ICU study period nurse satisfaction was significantly improved and used of invasive vascular catheters increased. Interruptions in teaching activities were more frequent and extensive in the closed ICU.

Subsequent investigations have yielded similar results. Another study of closing the ICU in a medical unit [20] reported a shorter ICU and hospital LOS and shorter duration of mechanical ventilation after severity of illness adjustment, with no change in mortality. These authors concluded that intensivist-directed care was more efficient without adverse effects on mortality. In a more recent study of closure of a surgical ICU [21], severity of illness adjusted mortality fell when care was directed by surgical intensivists, as did the rate of complications including acute renal failure. Consultation to organ-specific subspecialists fell when care was directed by an intensivist.

Contemporaneous Studies Comparing Closed and Open Formats

No truly randomized studies have been conducted in which patients have been allocated to two different care formats; the evolution of ICU care in a given institution and biases as to the quality of care, as well as the enormous tactical hurdles make it unlikely that such a study could ever be conducted [22]. One recent study [23] compared two patient cohorts admitted to a surgical ICU during the same period of time. Patients were not randomized but according to their attending physician's preference received care via one of two different organizational models. One cohort was cared for by an on-site critical care team of housestaff supervised by an intensivist (CCS), the other by a housestaff team with responsibilities in multiple sites supervised by a general surgeon (NCCS). The primary outcome measures were duration of stay, resource utilization, and complication rate. Despite having a higher mean APACHE II score, the CCS cohort spent less time in the ICU, used fewer resources, had fewer complications, and had lower total hospital charges. The difference between the groups was greatest for the sickest patients. Mortality did not differ between the groups.

Are these results valid? The major defect of the study design was lack of randomization. By APACHE II scores, the CCS cohort had a greater severity of illness, thus potentially biasing the study against benefit of this organizational approach. However, the groups did differ by surgical intervention as recognized by the authors, with a relatively large fraction of patients with esophageal and gastric surgeries in the NCCS cohort. The authors assure us that statistical analysis with removal of these patients did not alter the major findings. Other differences could exist between the groups that were not apparent and would result in bias; imagine that the referral patterns of this hospital have more complex surgeries referred to a cohort of surgeons who are less likely to refer patients to the critical care service. Such a possibility may not be reflected by the single severity of illness score obtained at the time of admission to the ICU and undermines a high level of confidence in these results.

By what Mechanism and to what Degree are these Outcome Changes Effected?

In the aggregate, these studies are rather consistent with the notion that the reorganization of critical care services to include greater oversight by senior intensivists and/or use of teams more geographically focused on the ICU has beneficial effects on patient care and economic outcomes. There is little in this literature to help understand the specific mechanisms by which this occurs or even its full magnitude. Nonetheless, some reasonable speculations can be made.

Does administrative change and protocol implementation make a difference? Some recent studies have suggested that protocols may enhance outcomes and, interestingly, protocols that tend to bypass the physician (at least for day-to-day judgments) may be most beneficial for certain endpoints, such as shortening time to liberation from mechanical ventilation [24]. Protocols may also best implement strategies that are known to be of global benefit to critically ill patients, such as prophylaxis against thromboembolic disease or institution of enteral nutrition. Does the provision of intensivist involvement in the critical care team provide a higher level of integration of physicians with other care providers and hence improved outcome? This intriguing possibility, almost a topic for medical anthropology and not well approached by the methodologies of these studies, is suggested but hardly proved by a number of investigations reviewed here.

Do intensivists reduce complications that lead to morbidity and mortality? Certain complications, such as acquisition of nosocomial infection, are known to dramatically alter outcome for the critically ill [25], and several studies have demonstrated reduced complication rates with intensivist-directed management [15, 23]. Not all studies, however, have observed such reductions in complication rates, our own included [19]. To this point, it is likely that the ability of investigators to prospectively define and identify all significant complications is inadequate.

Is the benefit of intensive care reorganization largely one of 'being there', providing more physicians who are more available to the critically ill patient and with less competition from other clinical responsibilities? The majority of the studies reviewed here were conducted in teaching hospitals, and the reorganization of critical care most often involved attending, fellow, and resident physician deployment to the ICU. If greater presence is essential to derive improved outcome, the implications for non-teaching hospitals, intensivist manpower requirements, and reimbursement requirements would be obvious and enormous. Thus, investigation of approaches which derive the greatest benefit from the wisest deployment of our human resources is urgently needed.

How much benefit is actually quantitated by these studies? The endpoints employed in the majority of these investigations – ICU and hospital mortality, ICU and hospital LOS, estimated cost or number of diagnostic tests and consultations – are crude and do not help us understand the outcomes we are witnessing in the broader context of patients' lives and the entire health care system. As an extreme example, imagine that intensivists help to transform the use of a given ICU, with triage of many patients requiring only monitoring to other hospital environments. They then direct their care toward a large population of patients with complex critical illness but some opportunity for survival. Their excellent care results in a population of patients stabilized and then requiring a more gradual recovery from multi-system organ failure. As well understood by the experienced intensivist, this 'chronic critical care' often need not be conducted in the ICU, particularly with the press of patients requiring this locale for care. Since ongoing care for these patients is beyond the means of the routine ward, transfer to a longterm acute care (LTAC) setting is often effected. This system of care, driven by reimbursement issues as well as care requirements, has grown explosively in a period of time overlapping with many of the studies reviewed here. Short term outcome from the perspective of the ICU or hospital may appear to be salutary, but is incomplete without a further analysis of longterm outcome in the LTAC facility and beyond. Interestingly, one recent study of mechanically ventilated patients sent for LTAC reported a 50% mortality in the LTAC hospital, with only 8% of patients fully functional and living independently at one year [26]. Thus, the success of critical care services as judged by admission hospital outcome, may have significant downsides in longterm follow-up studies. The studies reviewed here do not address how intensivists employ the array of care facilities available to them. Interestingly, other reports have demonstrated an awareness and implementation of withholding and withdrawing care from the hopelessly ill by intensivists that has grown over time [27]. It is conceivable that the reorganization of critical care services by intensivists may more effectively implement a shift of care from 'cure to comfort' when appropriate.

Conclusion

A growing body of literature suggests that reorganization of critical care services impacts on outcomes of critical illness. Not surprisingly, these early studies have been largely descriptive and have attempted to focus on the growing role of the intensivist. These observations, however, are preliminary and rudimentary. We have been biased to believe that the trained intensivist is the vehicle of much of this change, but that idea has not been rigorously tested. Ideally, future studies will include multicenter trials with a diversity of care environments. Measures of longterm benefit beyond crude survival, such as quality of life, must also be assessed [28, 29]. These studies should elaborate the elements of organization that impact outcome, including not only the training and deployment of physician and nursing staff and their organizational relationship to one another, but the use of protocols, care plans, algorithms, networks, and informatics as well.

References

1. Halpern NA, Bettes L, Greenstein R (1994) Federal and nationwide intensive care units and healthcare costs: 1986-1992. Crit Care Med 22:2001–2007
2. Cambell S (1997) HCFA clamping down on long term acute care "hospitals within hospitals." Health Care Strateg Manage 15:12–13
3. Manthous C (1998) In: Hall JB, Schmidt GA, Wood LDH (eds) Principles of Critical Care, 2nd edition. McGraw Hill, New York, pp XXI–XXIV
4. Groeger JS, Strosberg MA, Halperin NA, et al.(1992) Descriptive analysis of critical care units in the United States. Crit Care Med 20:846–863
5. Knaus WA, Draper EA, Wagner DP, et al(1982) Evaluating outcome from intensive care: a preliminary multi-hospital comparison. Crit Care Med 10:491–496
6. Knaus WA, Draper EA, Wagner DP, Zimmerman JE (1986) An evaluation of the outcome of intensive care in major medical centers. Ann Intern Med 104:410–418
7. Knaus WA, Wagner WP, Zimmerman JE, Draper EA (1993) Variations in mortality and length of stay in intensive care units. Ann Intern Med 118:753–761.
8. Zimmerman JE, Shortell SM, Knaus WA, et al (1993) Value and cost of teaching hospitals: A prospective multicenter, inception cohort study. Crit Care Med 21:1432–1442
9. Taylor DH, Whellan DJ, Sloan FA (1999) Effects of admission to a teaching hospital on the cost and quality of care for Medicare beneficiaries. N Engl J Med 340: 293–299
10. Zimmerman JE, Shortell SM, Rousseau DM, et al(1993) Improving intensive care. Observations based on organizational case studies in nine intensive care units: a prospective, multicenter study. Crit Care Med 21: 1443–1451
11. Pollack MM, Getson PR, Ruttimann UE, et al (1987) Efficiency of intensive care. A comparative analysis of eight pediatric intensive care units. JAMA 258:1481–1486.

12. Pollack MM, Alexander SR, Clarke N, et al (1991) Improved outcomes from tertiary center pediatric intensive care; a statewide comparison of tertiary and non-tertiary care facilities. Crit Care Med 19:150–159
13. Pollack MM, Cuerdon TT, Patel KM, et al (1994) Impact of quality-of-care factors on pediatric intensive care unit mortality. JAMA 272:941–946
14. Ruttimann UE, Pollack MM (1996) Variability of duration of stay in pediatric intensive are units: a multi–institutional study. J Pediatr 128:35–44
15. Pronovost P, Jenckes M, Dorman T, et al (1999) Organizational characteristics of intensive care units related to outcomes of abdominal aortic surgery. JAMA 281:1310–1317
16. Pollack MM, Katz RW, Ruttimann UE, et al (1988) Improving the outcome and efficiency of intensive care: the impact of an intensivist. Crit Care Med 16: 11–17
17. Reynolds HN, Haupt MT, Thill-Haharozian MC, et al (1988) Impact of critical care physician staffing on patients with septic shock in a university hospital medical intensive care unit. JAMA 260:3446–3450
18. Manthous CA, Amoateng-Adjepong Y, al-Kharrat T, et al (1997) Effects of a medical intensivist on patient care in a community teaching hospital. Mayo Clin Proc 72:391–399
19. Carson SS, Stocking C, Podsadecki T, et al (1996) Effects of an organizational change in the medical intensive care unit of a teaching hospital: a comparison of 'open' and 'closed' formats. JAMA 276:322–328
20. Multz AS, Chalfin DB, Samson IM, et al (1998) A 'closed' medical intensive care unit (MICU) improves resource utilization when compared with an 'open' MICU. Am J Respir Crit Care 157:1468–1473
21. Ghorra S, Reinert SE, Cioffi W, et al (1999) Analysis of the effect of conversion from open to closed surgical intensive care unit. Ann Surg 229:163–171
22. Hall JB (1999) How and how much can the organization of critical care services influence patient outcomes? J Intensive Care Med 14:251–253
23. Hanson CW, Deutschman CS, Anderson HL, et al (1999) The effect of an organized critical care service on outcomes and resource utilization: a cohort study. Crit Care Med 27:270–274
24. Ely EW, Bennett PA, Bowton DL, Murphy SM, Florance AM, Haponik EF (1999) Large scale implementation of a respiratory therapist-driven protocol for ventilator weaning. Am J Resp Crit Care Med; 159:439–446
25. Pittet D, Tarara D, Wenzel RP (1994) Nosocomial bloodstream infection in critically ill patients. Excess length of stay, extra costs, and attributable mortality. JAMA 271:1598–1601
26. Carson SS, Bach PB, Brzozowski L, Leff A (1999) Outcomes after long-term acute care: an analysis of 133 mechanically ventilated patients. Am J Respir Crit Care Med 159:1568–1573
27. Prendergast TJ, Luce JM (1997) Increasing incidence of withholding and withdrawing of life support from the critically ill. Am J Respir Crit Care Med; 155:15–20.
28. Davidson TA, Caldwell ES, Curtis JR, Hudson LD, Steinberg KP (1999) Reduced quality of life in survivors of acute respiratory distress syndrome compared with critically ill control patients. JAMA 281:354–360
29. Short TG, Buckley TA, Rowbottom MY, Wong E, Oh TE (1999) Long-term outcome and functional health status following intensive care in Hong Kong. Crit Care Med. 27:51–57

Geographical Differences in Outcomes

L.G. Thijs

Learning Points

- There is a significant lack of reliable and un-biased data on intensive care unit (ICU) and hospital outcome in the literature
- From the available data it is clear that marked regional differences exist in crude ICU mortality rate and ICU length of stay
- These differences are in part related to differences in definitions of an ICU and to differences in perceived functions of ICUs
- Regional differences in admission policies, organization of ICUs, type of admissions, severity of illness and source of admission contribute to regional differences in outcome
- Availability of ICU beds related to the total number of ICU beds per country/region population seems to be a crucial factor in regional differences in outcome

Some years ago a tourist from the United States was admitted to our ICU with a life-threatening condition. For obvious reasons, the family was very anxious. They were also worried, not having visited this part of the world before, about the quality of care and the performance of ICUs in this country. The family contacted their private physician in the United States to share their concern. His advice was that all they needed to know was whether the local doctors read the New England Journal of Medicine.

This story demonstrates the fact that people are concerned about regional differences in ICU performance and outcome, even in Western countries. Regional differences in crude mortality rates indeed occur, but do not necessarily reflect differences in quality of care. The quality indicator suggested by the American physician reflected a simplified, albeit original, view on the complexity of the issues involved.

Introduction

The concept of an ICU i.e., a nursing unit within a hospital department or a hospital where comprehensive and specialized care can be provided to critically ill or injured patients was born in the 1950s during an extremely severe poliomyelitis pandemic. In the late 1950s and early 1960s such units, to support severely ill patients with vital organ disturbances, were founded in countries in several continents. These ICUs rapidly evolved, with access to more and more advanced technology. In the last decades a worldwide expansion in the number of ICUs has taken place and acutely injured or severely ill patients are nowadays almost routinely admitted to the ICU. In parallel, intensive care medicine has developed as a multidisciplinary speciality and national, regional and world-wide intensive care organizations have been established [1]. Although from the early days intensive care was a very international enterprise [1], intensive care medicine in individual countries has developed in conjunction with, and influenced by, prevailing medical systems. There are marked national differences in medical heritages with varying health care systems and policies, medical training, legal, financial and insurance systems. These have, to a large extent, shaped intensive care organization and practice in the different countries. The evolution of the ICU to a central hospital faculty where sophisticated monitoring and life-support techniques, specialized nursing and medical knowledge and skills, and comprehensive treatment capabilities are available for critically ill patients has been most impressive. However, this evolution was not made without costs and ICUs are nowadays one of the largest (if not the largest) consumers of hospital resources. It has been estimated that the ICU consumes about 20% of total hospital resources [2]; in the US the figure is even higher [3], but in some countries such as the UK it is significantly lower [4]. Nowadays, nowhere is cost-consciousness more apparent than in the provision of intensive care services [5]. Effectiveness of ICUs has, as a consequence, become a major issue. An essential element herein is clinical outcome, i.e., how the ICU performs. This is an extremely complex issue, but ICU and/or hospital mortality which are clinically highly relevant endpoints and are readily available, are considered a major component of ICU performance assessment.

Since ICUs have developed within, and are embedded in, different national health care systems with differences in funding and health care spending, geographical differences in outcome could be expected. Admission policies, available ICU beds, treatment capabilities and practices, overall population health and age distribution and prevalence of diseases are among the factors that influence ICU outcome and which may differ between countries. This chapter focuses on geographical differences in short term mortality and also on differences in length of ICU stay as an index of cost and resource utilization, limited to adult ICUs.

Geographical Differences in Mortality (Fig. 1)

Europe

A few studies have directly or indirectly addressed differences in mortality in ICUs in various European countries [6-8]. The most in-depth study on the effects of organization and management structures on outcome in European countries is the recently published EURICUS-I study [8]. It has been estimated that there are between 3,000 and 4,000 ICUs in Western Europe [9]. The EPIC study [6], designed

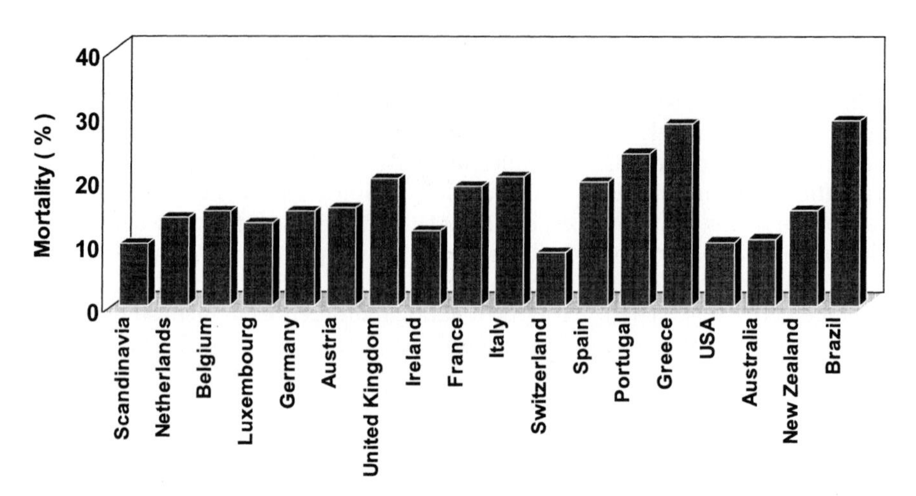

Fig. 1. Geographical differences in ICU outcome. (From [6, 17, 24, 25, 28])

to evaluate the prevalence of ICU-acquired infections, included the largest known sample (n=1,417) from these units in 17 western European countries with a fair distribution between primary, secondary and tertiary centers. Although this study had a 'snapshot' design, i.e., data were collected from 10,038 patients in the ICU during one day, ICU mortality in the following 6 weeks was also registered and is available for 92.4% of the patients (Table 1). The SAPS II study [7] designed to develop and validate a new Simplified Acute Physiology Score, included 9,420 patients enrolled during a 3 month period in 110 ICUs in 10 western European countries and provides data on hospital mortality during a follow-up of 2 months in these countries (Table 1). The EURICUS-I study [8] focused on 89 ICUs in 11 European countries involving 16,059 patients. This study presents both ICU and hospital mortality over a period of 6 months.

The collected data presented in Table 1 show some general trends, although there are differences between the studies. Generally, mortality rates are highest in the southern European countries and in the UK both for ICU mortality and hospital mortality. Of course, these studies have limitations since they, among others, may select the best performing centers. However, as the trend is quite similar in the three studies and this selection may occur in all countries, these data indeed may reflect geographical differences in crude mortality rate. National surveys generally confirm these geographical differences. A study in Portugal including 19 ICUs showed an ICU mortality of 24.5% and a hospital mortality of 32% [10]. Similarly, in Italy a study in which 114 ICUs participated noted a 25.7% ICU mortality [11]. In the Netherlands a survey involving 36 ICUs showed a mean ICU and hospital mortality of 8.1% and 11.9%, respectively [12]. In Finland a 9.9% ICU and a 19.2% mean hospital mortality has been reported in a study which included 25 ICUs [13]. In a recent study [14] involving 17 ICUs in Southwest England, ICU and hospital mortality were 17.8% and 25.9%, respectively, confirming earlier findings in the UK [15, 16].

Table 1. Geographical differences in mortality in Europe

Country/ Region	Number of ICUs EPIC	SAPS II	EURI-CUS-I	ICU mortality % EPIC	EURI-CUS-I	Hospital mortality % SAPS II	EURI-CUS-I
Scandinavia	94	–	–	9.8	–	–	–
Finland	–	7	5	–	8.0	17.6	14.0
Denmark	–	–	6	–	13.0	–	20.0
Netherlands	78	11	7	13.8	10.0	20.0	16.0
Belgium	72	11	6	14.9	7.0	21.7	12.0
Luxembourg	5	–	–	13.0	–	–	–
Germany	268	15*	3	14.9	6.0	15.9	9.0
Austria	75	–	–	15.3	–	–	–
Poland	–	–	10	–	19.0	–	23.0
United Kingdom	194	4	8	19.9	20.0	32.4	31.0
Ireland	15	–	–	11.8	–	–	–
France	264	14	5	18.7	16.0	28.9	22.0
Italy	110	20	7	20.3	18.0	31.3	26.0
Switzerland	49	11	–	8.4	–	13.8	–
Spain	137	17	27	19.4	15.7	27.1	21.0
Portugal	19	–	5	23.9	14.0	–	21.0
Greece	37	–	–	28.5	–	–	–
Total	1.417	110	89	16.8	13.0	22.7	18.0

* including 1 ICU from Austria.

North America

Published data on ICU mortality in the US and in particular in Canada are somewhat limited. A recent large published data base from the US including 37,668 ICU admissions in 285 ICUs in various regions of the country reports on a 12.35% hospital mortality rate [17]. An earlier independent data base from 42 ICUs (16,622 patients) shows a mean ICU and hospital mortality rate of 10% and 16.5%, respectively [18], but included patients with a higher severity of illness [17]. In both studies regional differences in hospital mortality rate were observed, being lowest in western (11.9% and 11.3%) and highest in eastern (21.6% and 14.7%) areas, although paralleling predicted mortality rate [17]. In the older APACHE II database (13 ICUs), ICU and hospital mortality were 11.7% and 19.7%, respectively [19], and in the Mortality Prediction Model (MPM) data base (25 ICUs), hospital mortality was 19.1% [20]. In a recent comprehensive study from Cleveland including 38 ICUs, a 6.3% ICU mortality rate, and a hospital mortality rate of 11.3% was reported [21]. A study including the largest known sample of ICU patients (n=88,050) selected from Massachusetts hospitals showed a hospital mortality rate of 9.7% [22]. A hospital mortality rate of 19.7% was published for the US/Canadian ICUs who took part in the SAPS II study [7].

A Canadian study involving 1,724 patients from two ICUs shows a hospital mortality rate of 24.8% [23]. Although these limited data do not warrant firm conclusions they suggest that the crude hospital mortality of ICU patients is higher in Canada than in the US. They also suggest that mortality rates are somewhat higher in older than in more recent studies. Comparing the data in Table 1 with the results from studies in the US it seems that both crude ICU and hospital mortality rate in the US are generally lower than in many European countries.

Australia / New Zealand

A survey in Australia including 35 ICUs from both rural and metropolitan areas indicates an ICU mortality rate of 10.5% and a hospital mortality of 15.9% [24]. For New South Wales, the most populous state of Australia, these outcome numbers were 10.8% and 16.5%, respectively. Standardized mortality ratios (SMRs) using the APACHE II score show a mean value of 0.78 (0.58 – 1.18), figures which are consistently lower than reported for the US [19]. Less published data are available for New Zealand. For three ICUs including 1,005 patients, an ICU mortality rate of 15% and a hospital mortality rate of 18% (with an APACHE II predicted mortality rate of 19.2%) have been described [25].

Other Countries

Single reports on mortality in ICUs from various other regions have been published. In Japan a study in six ICUs showed a 16.9% crude hospital mortality rate [26]. In Hong Kong, hospital mortality was 36% in 1,573 patients admitted to one 12 bed unit [27]. In Brazil, the mean ICU and hospital mortality of 1,734 patients admitted to 10 ICUs was 29% and 34% respectively [28]. Studies from one Saudi Arabian ICU report on an ICU mortality of 24% and a hospital mortality of 32% [29], whereas in one Tunisian unit ICU mortality was 22.5% [30].

Geographical Differences in Length of ICU Stay (Fig. 2)

Two European comparative studies [7, 8] report on a mean ICU length of stay (LOS) in various European countries (Table 2). The sample size of ICUs of these studies is small (Table 1), and LOS is consistently higher in the older SAPS II study [7], but there is a trend towards a higher LOS in the South of Europe. It is likely that larger centers with more seriously ill patients participated in these studies. National studies with a better balance of types of ICU and a larger number of participating ICUs generally show a shorter LOS. As an example, 3.3 days in Finland [13], 2.94 days in the Netherlands [12], 4.03 days in the UK [14], 8.5 days in Italy [11], and a median of 6 days in Portugal [10]. In the EPIC study, the proportion of patients staying in the ICU for more than 3 weeks was greater than 30% in France, Italy, Spain, Portugal and Greece [9]. These data all indicate a longer LOS in southern than in Northern European countries.

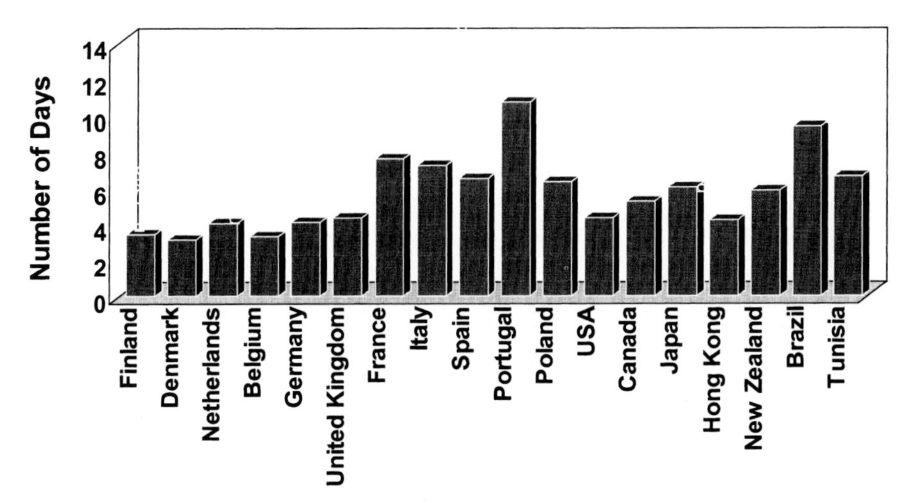

Fig. 2. Geographical differences in LOS. (From [8, 17, 32, 34, 27, 25, 28, 30])

Several large data bases in the US show a similar LOS, ranging from 3.7-4.74 [17, 18, 21, 22]. In the largest published survey on US ICUs nearly 17% of all critical care patients had been in the unit for more than 14 days [31]. This proportion was significantly higher in the large hospitals. In Canada (Ontario), a mean length of stay of 5.2 days has been reported [32] which seems longer than in the US. A comparative study in ICUs in Western Massachusetts and Alberta (Canada) indeed shows that Canadian ICUs had a longer mean length of ICU stay [33]. Reported lengths of stay in other countries include only a few ICUs and are shown in Table 2.

A large number of factors could be responsible for these geographical differences in crude mortality rate and length of ICU stay, including availability of ICU beds, admission policies, type of patients and case-mix, and severity of illness which are not entirely independent variables.

Geographical Differences in Bed Availability

The first European survey in 1986 showed a wide varation in the mean number of beds per ICU in the various countries, ranging from 6 in the UK to 19 in Belgium [35]. More recent comparative studies confirm that there are geographical differences in unit size [8, 9]. In the EPIC study, 57% of ICUs had between six and ten beds, 25% more than ten beds and 18% fewer than six [9]. The proportion of small ICUs was greatest in the UK with 48% having fewer than 6 beds. In general, there is a trend to lower bed availability in southern countries compared with the countries of Northern Europe [8,9,35], the UK being the exception.

The largest published study on ICU organization in the US, involving 2;876 separate ICUs, representing 38.7% of the nation's ICUs, shows that the average ICU size approximates 10 beds and the number of beds per ICU (as well as the

Table 2. Geographical differences in mean length of stay (days)

	ICU	Hospital⁺
Europe: [7,8]	5.2 - 6.6	19.1
Finland [7,8]	3.4 - 4.1	14.0
Denmark [8]	3.1	–
Netherlands [7,8]	4.0 - 5.5	19.3
Belgium [7,8]	3.3 - 6.2	21.5
Germany [7,8]*	4.1 - 6.0	21.0
Poland [8]	6.3	14.8
United Kingdom [7,8]	4.3 - 5.7	18.9
France [7,8]	7.6 - 9.7	18.9
Italy [7,8]	7.2	20.5
Switzerland [7]	4.9	17.6
Spain [7,8]	6.5 - 9.5	22.8
Portugal [8]	10.7	–
USA [17,18,21,22]	3.7 - 4.74	11.6 - 12.0
USA / Canada [7]	5.9	18.2
Canada (Toronto) [32]	5.2	–
New Zealand [25]	5.8	–
Japan [34]	6.0	–
Hong Kong [27]	4.2	–
Brazil [28]	9.4	–
Tunisia [30]	6.6	–

* including one ICU from Austria.

number of ICUs) increases with the increase in hospital size, ranging from 5.6 beds per ICU in the smallest hospitals to 14.3 in the largest hospitals [37]. Studies in Australia indicate an average of 8.7 beds per ICU in New South Wales [24], and in New Zealand the mean number of beds per ICU is 6.4 [38]. In Japan, 38% of ICUs have less than 5 beds, 44.5% between 5 and 8 beds, and 17.5% more than 8 beds [39]. More important, however, is the allocation of hospital beds in the ICU or the number of ICU beds per 100,000 inhabitants. In the 1986 European survey, the number of ICU beds per hospital in 10 western European countries varied from 2.6 in the UK to 4.1 in Denmark [35]. More recent data indicate that indeed there are wide variations in the proportion of hospital beds allocated to the ICU ranging from 1-2% in the UK and Italy [4, 40] to 3.2% in Germany [41]. In the US, a mean of 8.1% of hospital beds is allocated to the ICU [37]. For Canada, this figure is 3% [32,33], for Australia 3% [24], and 2.2% for New Zealand [38].

Estimations of the number of ICU beds per 100,000 inhabitants taken from various sources are presented in Table 3. These numbers, however, largely depend on definitions used to characterize an ICU and on whether coronary care unit (CCU) and pediatric ICU beds are included. Even considering that these numbers

Table 3. ICU beds per 100,000 inhabitants

USA (West Massachusetts) [33]		24.0
Canada:	Ontario [32]	11.2
	Alberta [33]	16.0
Denmark [8]		6.5
Germany [41]		25.0
Netherlands [12]		10.0
United Kingdom [8]		1.8 – 3
Switzerland [42]		11.1
Italy [40]		4 – 9
Australia:	New South Wales [43]	8.0
	Victoria [43]	3.3
	Western Australia [43]	3.0
New Zealand [38]		4.3

are only an indication it is clear that there are major differences. National surveys, however, indicate that there are wide regional differences also within one country. In the Netherlands, as an example, these figures vary from 6 to 17 in different provinces [12], and in Italy they range between 4 and 16 in the various Italian regions [40]. Most of the figures mentioned in this paragraph are not of recent date and probably underestimate the present situation since due to the increasing pressure on ICU beds the number of beds in some countries may have increased.

Geographical Differences in Type of Admission

A number of comparative European studies have classified patients admitted to ICUs as nonoperative/medical, elective or emergency surgery patients [6-8]. Although there are marked differences in study design, the results are remarkably similar (Table 4). Two of these studies [7,8], provide data on these types of admissions in the various countries. In Table 4, the variations in the mean percentage per study and per country are presented. Obviously, there are marked differences between countries, but the reasons for these variations remain obscure. In some countries (e.g., France, Spain) nonoperative patients dominate, their prevalence being markedly higher than the European mean. In contrast, in other countries (e.g., the Netherlands, Germany) postoperative patients are the prevailing type of ICU patient. The ICU sample size per country in these studies, however, is relatively small, and there may be a selection bias. National studies with more participating ICUs are, however, scarce. Studies in the UK report on a proportion of nonoperative patients ranging from a mean of 43.2% to 55.9% [14,15]. In the Netherlands, a national survey showed that 39% of patients could be classified as nonoperative or medical [12]. In Italy, 42% nonoperative patients were identified in a national study [11], and in Portugal 68% [10]. Although these figures are somewhat at variance with the data in Table 4, at least partly, they corroborate the general trend.

In the US, nonoperative patients form the majority of ICU admissions [17, 18, 21, 22]. There are, however, significant differences between the proportion of emergency and elective surgical patients in the various studies (Table 4). Limited data from Canada suggest that about half of the patients are surgical patients and half are medical [23, 33]. Reported data from other countries are too limited to warrant conclusions (Table 4). Taken together, there are differences in the type of patients admitted to ICUs in various countries. These differences may have a bearing on ICU outcome, since several studies have shown that elective surgical patients have by far the lowest mortality rate [16, 18, 22]. Emergency surgical admissions may have a somewhat higher [8, 22], or lower [18], mortality rate than nonoperative admissions (Fig. 3).

Geographical Differences in Location Prior to ICU Admission

Differences in ICU admission practice also influence outcome. Patients admitted directly from the operating room, recovery or emergency room generally have the lowest mortality rate, whereas patients admitted from the hospital wards and particularly from other hospitals exhibit the highest mortality rate [16,18,44] (Fig. 4). This difference remains after controlling for severity of illness and disease category [18, 44]. Patients who are admitted to the ICU several days after hospital

Table 4. Type of patient

	Nonoperative/ Medical (%)	Elective Surgery (%)	Emergency surgery/Trauma (%)
Europe: [6–8]	45 – 54	30 – 32	16 – 23
Finland [7,8]	35 – 46	28 – 45	20 – 26
Denmark [8]	49	25	27
Netherlands [7,8]	29 – 32	46 – 48	19 – 25
Belgium [7,8]	43 – 44	33.5 –48	8 – 15
Germany [7,8]	21 – 25	51 – 57	18 – 28
United Kingdom [7,8]	44 – 48	21 – 24	28 – 36
France [7,8]	79 – 84	7 – 9	9.5 – 12
Italy [7,8]	44 – 53	28 -33	19 – 23
Switzerland [7]	63	22	15
Spain [7,8]	55 – 73	14 – 26	12 – 18
Portugal [8]	50	26	24
Poland [8]	87	7	7
USA [17,18,21,22]	57 – 71.5	15 – 34	6.5 – 23
Canada [23,33]	50 – 53	21	26
New Zealand [25]	76	8	16
Japan [26]	42	52	6
Hong Kong [27]	40	29	31
Brazil [28]	64	23	13

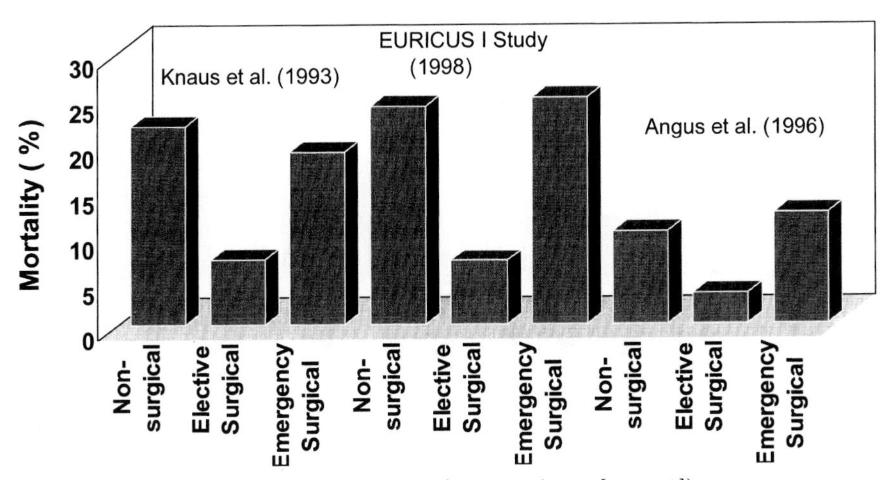

Fig. 3. Differences in outcome related to type of patients. (From [18, 8, 22])

admission and those transferred from another hospital or ICU are more likely to die than those who enter the ICU at the beginning of their hospitalization [45]. This underlines the importance of the functional position of the ICU in the hospital and of both ICU and hospital in the region. In addition, it demonstrates the impact of lead-time bias on outcome [18, 46].

Data from the EURICUS-I study [8], show regional differences in the source of admission to the ICU in Europe, somewhat paralleling the type of patients admitted (Table 5). As pointed out earlier, only a very limited number of ICUs per country participated in this study and the data may, therefore, not be representative. On the other hand, national studies show a surprising similarity with the data presented in Table 5 [12, 14]. An exception is the Italian study [11] showing less patients coming from the operating room (30%) and more from the emergency room (41%) than in the EURICUS-I study.

In Germany, Finland, Belgium and the Netherlands more than half of the patients are admitted to the ICU directly from the operating room or the recovery room. A relatively high proportion of ICU patients come from the emergency room in Belgium, Demark, France, Italy, Spain and Poland. Also in the US, Australia and Brazil a high percentage of patients is admitted to the ICU directly from the emergency room. In the UK, Denmark and Italy, more than 25% of patients are admitted to the ICU from the general hospital wards and a relatively high proportion of ICU patients are transferred from other ICUs or hospitals in France, Italy and Portugal. These data indeed suggests that there are significant geographical differences in admission practice.

Geographical Differences in Severity of Illness

Using the SAPS II scoring system, two comparative studies found the highest severity of illness on admission in the UK among Western European countries

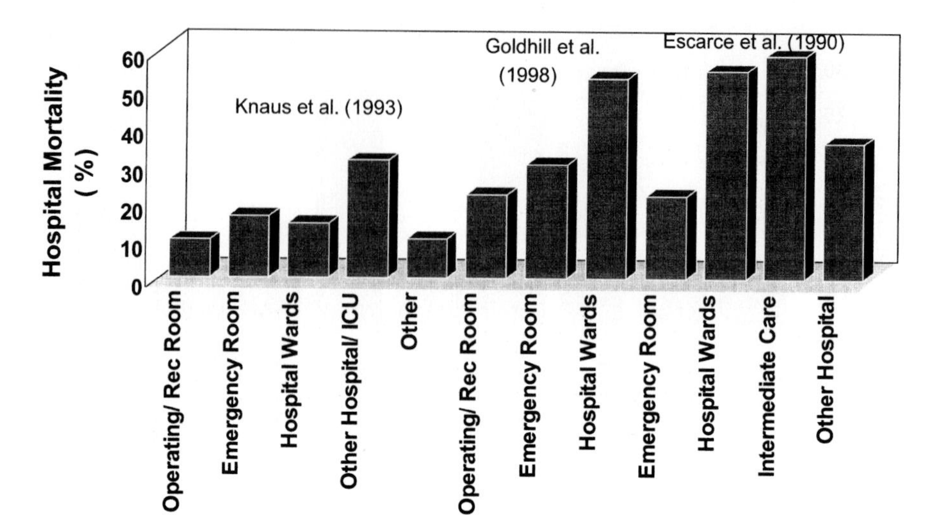

Fig. 4. Differences in outcome related to location prior to ICU admission. (From [18, 16, 44])

Table 5. Location prior to ICU admission

	OR/RR (%)	ER (%)	Hospital ward (%)	Other hospital or ICU (%)	Other (%)
Europe [8]	40.3	30.3	17.0	8.6	3.8
Finland	59.7	20.4	16.8	2.4	0.4
Denmark	41.2	25.2	25.1	6.0	2.5
Netherlands	62.5	16.8	12.5	6.3	1.8
Belgium	52.5	27.5	13.2	5.4	1.3
Germany	67.7	8.9	5.9	6.6	10.9
United Kingdom	45,5	20.1	25.3	5.4	3.7
France	9.1	25.9	19.2	18.7	26.9
Italy	35.4	19.9	25.6	16.8	2.3
Spain	21.8	46.7	17.4	11.2	1.9
Portugal	43.6	20.6	15.3	16.5	3.9
Poland	12.2	60.7	22.6	3.8	0.6
USA [17,18,21,31]	28-43	36-42.5	11-18	5-11	1.5-8
Australia [24]	37	38	20	1	4
New Zealand [25]	18	42	18	15	7
Japan [26]	58	22.5	10	9.5	–
Brazil [28]	35.7	28.2	19.3	14.2	2.6

OR = operating room; RR = recovery room; ER = emergency room.

[7,8]. Southern European ICUs generally had higher SAPS II scores than ICUs in the North of Europe. Similarly, in the EPIC study, between 15 and 20% of ICU patients had an APACHE II score greater than 20 in these countries (including the UK), whereas between 7 and 14% of ICU patients in northern European countries scored such high APACHE II levels. Thus, there seem to be more severely ill patients in the ICUs in Southern countries (and in the UK) than in other geographical areas. This is supported by the finding that in Italy, Portugal, Greece and the UK more than 70% of ICU patients require mechanical ventilation [9, 10], whereas in Northern European countries this is usually less than 60% [9]. In the APACHE II and III data bases in the USA, the mean scores are 14.2 and 45.1-50.0, respectively [17-19]. A recent large study including 116,340 patients from Cleveland, Ohio, calculated a mean APACHE III score of 46.9 [21]. Published mean APACHE II scores in national surveys are 11.4 for the Netherlands [12], 11.7 for Finland [13], 17.9 for the UK and Ireland [15], 19.2 for Portugal [10] and 14.8 (15.3 for New South Wales) for Australia [24$. Comparisons with the APACHE data bases [18,19], show that in Canada [23], the UK [14], New Zealand [25], and Brazil [28], mean severity of illness scores were higher, whereas in Japan [26] they were similar. Although these figures may be global indications for geographical differences in severity of illness among patients admitted to ICUs, selection of participating ICUs, among others, may influence the data, since usually ICUs in the larger and teaching hospitals admit the most sick patients. Studies including a variety of ICU types [10, 12, 13], therefore, best reflect severity of illness.

Geographical Differences in the Organization and Use of ICUs

There are major differences between countries and states in the provision of intensive care services, originating from important distinctions in design and founding of health care services. This is, among other factors, reflected in the organization of ICUs. In the US, the minority of ICUs are open, i.e., admitting physicians have primary responsibility for patient care rather than intensive care physicians with a more specialty-specific designation of ICUs in the larger hospitals [37]. In contrast, in Canada [47] and Australia [24], ICUs, even in larger hospitals, are typically multidisciplinary and intensive care physicians usually have primary responsibility for patient care. In Europe, the majority (74.4%) of ICUs are mixed medical-surgical with no significant differences between countries in this respect [9]. There is a growing trend towards closed units, with more and more trained intensive care physicians involved, particularly in the larger centers, although exact data are missing. In a European survey of 200 ICUs, almost 90% of the units reported that the ICU staff have full responsibility for patient care [48]. This figure, however, most likely represents a selection of larger institutions.

There is evidence that this difference in organization structure has an impact on outcome. Changing from an open to a closed format of care with intensive care physician staffing may result in a decline in mortality rate and LOS [49–54]. In addition to a well-trained intensive care staff, 24 h coverage of ICU-care by a physician is important. In the EPIC study [9], differences were noted in European countries regarding 24 h clinical cover. In 71.7% of ICUs a committed 24 h doctor was on duty, with the highest number of ICUs with such coverage in Italy, France and Spain and the lowest in Finland, Norway and the Netherlands [9].

Interaction and coordination of intensive care staff significantly influences ICU effectiveness. The highest quality of care appears to require a high degree of involvement of both physicians and nurses in ongoing clinical care [19]. A high elementary organizational frame work and organizational commitment lowers mortality [8].

Differences in perceived functions of ICUs in different countries exist which have a bearing on the type of patients admitted with consequences for length of stay and outcome. As an example, ICU utilization in the US is estimated to be more than twice that of Canada [33, 55]. In a comparative study US patients were less severely ill than Canadian patients, who were typically admitted for mechanical ventilation [33]. Even in the same health care system significant differences exist in the utilization of critical care services for cardiac surgery with differences in ICU length of stay [56]. It seems that in the USA and in some northern European countries [12, 41], ICUs also have an extended recovery room function. In addition, there are geographical differences in the percentage of patients admitted for active treatment or only for monitoring.

In the first trans-Atlantic comparison of intensive care, considerably fewer French ICU patients were admitted for monitoring and observation than US patients: 19% versus 34% [57]. A similar difference was found comparing ICUs in Japan (84% active treatment) and in the US (61% active treatment) [26]. These geographical differences in use of ICUs certainly have an impact on ICU outcome, both length of stay and mortality rate

Conclusion

This brief review of the available literature indicates that there are significant geographical differences in the mean mortality rate of ICU patients and differences in mean ICU length of stay. It should be realized that, even within countries, there are larger differences in the mortality rate at the ICU level both in the US [18, 19] and in western Europe [58,59]. A major problem is, however, that the data in the literature are extremely limited, precluding firm conclusions. Moreover the studies providing the data are of different design, including international questionnaires [6, 35], collection of data for the development and validation of scoring systems [7, 17–20], comparisions with US databases in countries outside the US [14, 15, 23, 25-29, 58], collection of data for quality programs [8,21], and national surveys mainly using questionnaires for an inventory of national ICU organization and practice [10–13, 31, 37]. None of these studies provide complete geographical figures, they are often not of recent date which in this fast changing area of medical care limits their significance, and there may be major selection bias since the larger institutions and the best performing ICUs are more likely to participate. National surveys which include the whole spectrum of types of ICU probably best reflect the actual state of affairs. Nevertheless, within these limitations, definite trends coming from various sources can be identified which have been discussed in the previous paragraphs.

The data indeed support that there are geographical differences. A multitude of factors, some of which have been discussed in this chapter, may be responsible for these differences. Among these are ICU bed availability, case-mix and severity of illness, admission policies and use of ICUs. These factors not only affect mortality rate but also length of stay, which increases with severity of illness and is shortest for scheduled surgical patients [8]. Moreover, bed availability, quantity and quality of nursing care in general wards, and the experience of the ICU physicians may affect ICU length of stay [48].

Availability of ICU beds seems to be a crucial factor, which allows for admission of less severely ill patients and for admission for monitoring and postoperative recovery in case beds are available. It can, however, be argued whether such patients should be admitted to the ICU or (other) high-dependency areas.

Intensive care is part of a continuum of progressive patient care and only one component of total care provision. Short term ICU outcome, therefore, is of limited significance due to the relatively short time period over which an overall disease process is assessed [60]. Ultimately, an important part of the value of a critical care delivery system is the effectiveness with which it (either) improves outcome (or decreases costs) for an entire care of disease process [60]. Nevertheless, measurement of clinical outcome in relation to severity of illness is, an important indicator of clinical performance [8]. Evidence has, however, shown that mortality and particularly short-term mortality is a relatively insensitive parameter of performance. There is a need to develop other measures of outcome as well as to continue to improve severity of illness scores [8]. In order to effectively compare different intensive care delivery systems and their outcomes we need first to clarify what constitutes an ICU and, second, to initiate national systems for collecting reliable and complete data on ICU practice and outcome: There is a long way to go.

References

1. Bryan-Brown CW, Crippen DW (1997) International organizations and communications. Crit Care Clin 13: 441–452
2. Reis Miranda D, Gyldmark M (1996) Evaluating and understanding of costs in the intensive care unit. In: Ryand DW (ed) Current Practice in Critical Illness. Chapman & Hall, London, pp 129–149
3. Chalfin DB, Fein AM (1994) Critical care medicine in managed competition and managed care environment. New Horiz 2: 275–282
4. Bion J (1994) Cost containment: The United Kingdom. New Horiz 2: 341–344
5. Osborne M, Evans TW (1994) Allocation of resources in intensive care: a transatlantic perspective. Lancet 343:778–780
6. Vincent JL, Bihari DJ, Suter PM, et al (1995) The prevalence of nosocomial infection in intensive care units in Europe. JAMA 274: 639–644
7. Le Gall JR, Lemeshow S, Saulnier F (1993) A new simplified acute physiology score (SAPS II) based on a European/North American multicenter study. JAMA 270: 2957–2963
8. Reis Miranda D, Ryan DW, Schaufeli WB, Fidler V (1998) Organization and management of intensive care. Springer Verlag, Heidelberg
9. Vincent JL, Suter, P, Bihari D, Bruining H (1997) Organization of intensive care units in Europe: lessons from the EPIC study. Intensive Care Med 23:1181–1184
10. Moreno R, Morais P (1997) Outcome prediction in intensive care: results of a prospective, multicentre, Portuguese study. Intensive Care Med 23:177–186

11. Apolone G, Brazzil Fasiolo S, Japichino G, Melotti R, Serra L (1993) The epidemiology of intensive care in Italy. In: Gullo A (ed) Anaesthesia, Pain, Intensive Care and Emergency Medicine, A.P.I.C.E.: Proceedings of the 12th Postgraduate Course in Critical Care Medicine, Trieste. Springer–Verlag, Heidelberg, pp 709–721
12. Reis Miranda D, Sprangenberg JFA (1992) Quality, efficiency and organization of intensive care units in the Netherlands. Foundation for Research on Intensive Care in Europe, Groningen
13. Niskanen M, Kari A, Halonen P, The Finnish ICU study group (1996) Five-year survival after intensive care. Comparison of 12,180 patients with the general population. Crit Care Med 24:1962–1967
14. Pappachan JV, Millar B, Bennett ED, Smith GB (1999) Comparison of outcome from intensive care admission after adjustment for case mix by the APACHE III prognostic system. Chest 115:802–810
15. Rowan KM, Kerr JH, Major E, McPherson K, Short A, Vessey MP (1993) Intensive Care Society's APACHE II study in Britain and Ireland-I: Variations in case mix of adult admissions to general intensive care units and impact on outcome. Br Med J 307:972–977
16. Goldhill DR, Sumner A (1998) Outcome of intensive care patients in a group of British intensive care units. Crit Care Med 26: 1337–1345
17. Zimmerman JE, Wagner DP, Draper EA, Wright L, Alzola C, Knaus WA (1998) Evaluation of acute physiology and chronic health evaluation III predictions of hospital mortality in an independent database. Crit Care Med 26:1317–1326
18. Knaus WA, Wagner DP, Zimmerman JE, Draper EA (1993) Variations in mortality and length of stay in intensive care units. Ann Intern Med 118: 753–761
19. Knaus WA, Draper EA, Wagner DP, Zimmerman JE (1986) An evaluation of outcome from intensive care in major medical centers. Ann Intern Med 104: 410–418
20. Rapoport J, Teres D, Lemeshow S, Gehlbach S (1994) A method for assessing the clinical performance and cost-effectiveness of intensive care units: A multicenter inception cohort study. Crit Care Med 22:1385–1391
21. Sirio CA, Shepardson LB, Rotondi AJ, et al (1999) Community-wide assessment of intensive care outcomes using a physiologically based prognostic measure. Chest 115:793–801
22. Angus DC, Linde-Zwirble WT, Sirio CA, et al (1996) The effect of managed care on ICU length of stay. JAMA 276:1075–1082
23. Wong DT, Crofts SL, Gomez M, McGuire GP, Byrick RJ (1995) Evaluation of predictive ability of APACHE II system and hospital outcome in Canadian intensive care unit patients. Crit Care Med 23:1177–1181
24. Fisher M, Herkes RG (1995) Intensive care: specially without frontiers In: Parker MM, Shapiro MJ, Porembka IT (eds) Critical Care: State of the Art, vol.15. SCCM, Anaheim, pp 9–27
25. Zimmerman JE, Knaus WA, Judson JA, et al (1988) Patient selection for intensive care: A comparison of New Zealand and United States hospitals. Crit Care Med 16: 318–326
26. Sirio CA, Tajimi K, Tase Ch, et al (1992) An inital comparison of intensive care in Japan and the United States. Crit Care Med 20: 1207–1215
27. Oh TE, Hutchinson R, Short S, Buckley T, Lin E, Leung D (1993) Verification of the acute physiology and chronic health evaluation scoring system in a Hong Kong intensive care unit. Crit Care Med 21:698–705
28. Bastos PG, Sun X, Wagner DP, Knaus WA, Zimmerman JE, The Brazil APACHE III Study Group (1996) Application of the APACHE III prognostic system in Brazilian intensive care units: a prospective multicenter study. Intensive Care Med 22: 564–570
29. Jacobs S, Chang RWS, Lee B, Lee B (1988) Audit of intensive care: a 30 month experience using the Apache II severity of disease classification system. Intensive Care Med 14:567–574
30. Nouira S, Roupie E, EI Atrouss S, et al (1998) Intensive care use in a developing country: a comparison between a Tunesian and a French unit. Intensive Care Med 24: 1144–1151
31. Groeger JS, Guntupalli KK, Strosberg M, et al (1993) Descriptive analysis of critical care units in the United States: Patient characteristics and intensive care unit utilization. Crit Care Med 21: 279–291

32. Sibbald WJ, Singh T (1997) Critical care in Canada, the North American difference. Crit Care Clin 13:347–362
33. Rapoport J, Teres D, Barnett R, et al (1995) A comparison of intensive care unit utilization in Alberta and western Massachusetts. Crit Care Med 23: 1336–1346
34. Tajimi K, Shimada Y, Nishimura S, Sirio CA (1994) Cost containment: the Pacific, Japan. New Horiz 2:404–412
35. Reis Miranda D (1986) ICUs in Europe. In: Reis Miranda D, Langrehr D (eds). The ICU, a cost-benefit analysis Excerpta Medica, Amsterdam, pp 207–219
36. Vincent JL (1990) European attitudes towards ethical problems in intensive care medicine: results of an ethical questionnaire. Intensive Care Med 16:256–264
37. Groeger JS, Strosberg MA, Halpern NA, et al (1992) Descriptive analysis of critical care units in the United States. Crit Care Med 20: 846–863
38. Streat S, Judson JA (1994) Cost-containment: The Pacific, New Zealand. New Horiz 2:392–402
39. Yoshiya I, Baik SW (1997) Critical care in Japan and Korea. Crit Care Clin 13:347–362
40. Apolone G, Melotti R, Repetto, Iapichino G (1994) Cost-containment: Europe, Italy. New Horiz 2:350–356
41. Burchardi H, Schuster, H-P, Zielmann (1994) Cost-containment: Europe, Germany, New Horiz 2:364–374
42. Torrenté A de, Chioléro R, Suter PM (1994) Cost-containment: Europe, Switzerland. New Horiz 2:345–349
43. Dobb GJ (1997) Intensive care in Australia and New Zealand. Crit Care Clin 13:299–316
44. Escarce JJ, Kelley MA (1990) Admission source to the medical intensive care unit predicts hospital death independent of APACHE II score. JAMA 264:2389–2394
45. Rapoport J, Teres D, Lemeshow S, Harris D (1990) Timing of intensive care admission in relation to ICU outcome. Crit Care Med 18:1231–1235
46. Dragsted L, Jörgensen J, Jensen NH, et al (1989) Interhospital comparisons of patient outcome from intensive care: Importance of lead-time bias. Crit Care Med 17:418–422
47. Barnett R, Shustack A (1994) Costcontainment: the Americas, Canada. New Horiz 2:332–335
48. Vincent JL, Thijs LG, Cerny V (1997) Critical care in Europe. Crit Care Clin 13:245–254
49. Brown JJ, Sullivan G (1989) Effect on ICU mortality of a full-time critical care specialist. Chest 96:127–129
50. Reynolds HN, Haupt MT, Thill-Haharozian MC et al (1988) Impact of critical care physician staffing on patients with septic shock in a university hospital medical intensive care unit. JAMA 260:3446–3450
51. Manthous CA, Amoateng-Adjepong Y, al-Kharrat T et al (1997) Effects of a medical intensivist on patient care in a community teaching hospital. Mayo Clin Proc 72:391–399
52. Carson SS, Stocking C, Podsadecki T, et al (1996) Effects of organizational change in the medical intensive care unit of a teaching hospital. JAMA 276: 322–328
53. Multz AS, Chalfin DB, Samson IM et al (1998) A 'closed' medical intensive care unit (MICU) improves resource utilization when compared with an 'open' MICU. Am J Respir Crit Care 157:1468–1473
54. Ghorra S, Reinert SE, Cioffi W et al (1999) Analysis of the effect of conversion from open to closed surgical intensive care unit. Am Surg 229:163–171
55. Jacobs Ph. Noseworthy TW (1990) National estimates of intensive care utilization and costs: Canada and the United States. Crit Care Med 18:1282–1286
56. Mazer CD, Byrick RJ, Sibbald WJ et al (1993) Postoperative utilization of critical care services by cardiac surgery: A multicenter study in the Canadian healthcare system. Crit Care Med 21: 851–859
57. Knaus WA, Le Gall JR, Wagner DP et al (1982) A comparison of intensive care in the USA and France. Lancet ii:642–646
58. Rowan KM, Kerr JH, Major E, McPherson K, Short A, Vessey MP (1993) Intensive Care Society's APACHE II study in Britain and Ireland-II: Outcome comparisons of intensive care units after adjustment for case mix by the American APACHE II method. Br Med J 307:977–981

59. Saarela E, Kari A, Nikki P, Rauhala V, Iisalo E, Kaukinen L (1991) Current practice regarding invasive monitoring in intensive care units in Finland. Intensive Care Med 17:264–271
60. Angus DC, Sirio CA, Clermont G, Bion J (1997) International comparisons of critical care outcome and resource consumption. Crit Care Clin 13:389–407

Disaggregating Data: From Groups to Individuals

J. Carlet, L. Montuclard, and M. Garrouste-Orgeas

Learning Points

- Knowledge derived from large groups of patients is an essential component of quality of care of individuals
- Quality indicators should include items related to equity, humanity, effectiveness and efficiency
- Dynamic assessments of patient status should be used throughout the ICU stay
- Repeated calculation of risk factors (for a given event) can improve therapeutic or preventive decision-making
- Think globally, but act locally and individually

Journalists in France have been using several quality indicators including mortality data to provide a guide of French intensive care units (ICUs) and hospitals. Thus, foreigners who want to plan a visit to France can use not only the "Guide Michelin" for good restaurants, but also "Le guide des Hopitaux: les meilleurs ville par ville". They could then combine the information to build a multiparametric score and select the cities they want to visit!

More seriously, although the three journalists, two of them medical doctors, tried to use 'up to date indicators', including adjusted mortality data, the score was still rather weak, and the publication of the guide induced considerable controversy. We do not know if the guide is used by consumers in order to decide to which hospital they want to be admitted!

Introduction

The literature relating to intensive care outcomes and health services research, in particular using scoring systems to assess severity of illness, has expanded rapidly in the past ten years. Indeed, assessment of severity of illness has been a corner-stone in this process, helping us to understand, and thus to describe, on an international basis the types of patient we are treating in the intensive care unit (ICU). Scoring systems such as the acute physiology, and chronic health evaluation (APACHE, three successive generations) [1, 2], the mortality probability model (MPM) [3] and the simplified acute physiology score (SAPS, I and II) [4, 5], were initially proposed to describe severity of illness and predict the mortality of groups of patients and not to predict the prognosis of a given individual.

APACHE, SAPS and MPM have been extensively used during randomized, controlled trials (RCTs) to be sure that severity of illness was comparable in compared groups. Similar scores have been described in children (the pediatric risk of mortality, PRISM [6] and the pediatric index of mortality, PIM [7]) and in neonates (the clinical risk index for babies, CRIB [8]).

Additional scores, based on the number of organ system failures have also been described, including the organ system failure (OSF) score initially described by Knaus et al. [9], the multiple organ dysfunction score (MODS) [10], the sequential organ failure assessment (SOFA) score [11] and the logistic organ dysfunction (LOD) score [12]. As the concept of quality assessment in the ICU became more and more popular, these different scores were proposed by their progenitors as valuable instruments for this purpose [13–15]. In addition, several authors suggested using the scores for assessment of individual patients. Quality indicators established for groups of patients can be used in this way, but only in part, as individual patients do not often fit neatly into 'evidence-based' methodology. Thus, 'evidence-based medicine' should always be combined with 'individual' or 'anecdotal' based medicine.

Assessing Severity of Groups of Patients for Research Purposes

Severity scoring systems have been widely used during RCTs, cohort studies using multivariate analysis, and case control studies, in order to be sure that the severity of illness was comparable in the studied groups or to adjust data for admission severity. However, many studies assess severity only on admission, since most of the available scoring systems have not been validated over time. It is very likely that trends in severity during the first few days would be far more helpful in predicting mortality than just the admission score, and several studies have now been performed in this field [16–19].

In addition, these scores only partly take the underlying condition of the patients into account. In many studies, for example during sepsis [20], both the SAPS II (which includes minimal information on the underlying condition), the number of organ system failures (OSF), and the McCabe and Jackson Score (underlying condition of the patient) are independent predictors for mortality, suggesting that SAPS II alone is not robust enough to describe severity of illness and the underlying condition of critically ill patients.

Finally, and even more importantly, severity scores can predict mortality only in very large groups of patients, with a case mix close to the one of the database used to create the score. They cannot be relied on in small groups of several hundred patients.

Using Severity Scores to Assess Quality of Care in the ICU: A Dangerous Exercise

This encompasses the comparison of actual ICU length of stay (LOS) or mortality to that predicted by severity scoring systems. The ratio of the observed/predicted mortality defines the standardized mortality ratio (SMR). An SMR of greater than 1 indicates that the unit performs 'worse' than predicted, below 1, 'better' than predicted. Knaus and colleagues have been the most active in defending the feasibility of such comparisons, provided that an appropriate scoring system, properly customized for the given case mix, is used [13–15]. Indeed studying a large group of patients is a prerequisite for this type of exercise.

Many authors emphasize that these comparisons are difficult and potentially dangerous, mainly because the case mix of a given unit is likely to be very different from the case mix of the large data base (usually 10,000 to 20,000 patients) used to validate and calibrate the score [21–26]. The score often needs to be customized for specific subpopulations of patients like patients with sepsis or septic shock [27].

Mortality is a very provocative endpoint, both for patients and consumers, for health care workers who need to know how they are performing, and for health care managers who want to know where they put their money. Thus, the way such comparisons of performance are planned and utilized will determine whether the results of the exercise are helpful or harmful [28–31].

A first necessity is to avoid the assumption that there is an '*a priori*' relationship between SMR and quality (or performance) of the units which are studied. The usefulness of the comparison is to detect outliers (using a 95 %, or 99 % confidence interval), either with very low or very high SMRs, and to understand why these units look different. The reason for a high SMR, could indeed be a poor performance by the unit, but could also be due to a specific case mix or specific policies to admit or discharge patients. Case mix issues are of paramount importance. In particular, immunosuppressed patients, or patients transferred from another ward or another ICU (lead time bias) will increase observed mortality and SMR. On the contrary, patients with certain acute medical conditions, e.g., acute intoxications, acidosis, acute asthma, have very good prognoses and will decrease SMR as compared to patients with severe sepsis or septic shock, acute renal failure and acute respiratory distress syndrome (ARDS).

For a given unit with a high SMR, it is very important to make collective efforts to understand why this could be occurring. In addition to case mix issues, specific discharge procedures (leaving a dying patient on the ICU as opposed to discharging to other wards) could explain high SMRs if we use ICU mortality; it may thus be more appropriate to use hospital or 3 to 6 month mortality. Admission and discharge policies are known to be very different from one country to the next (see chapter by L.G. Thijs, pp 292–308). If, after a very careful assessment of the case mix of the unit, no explanation other than poor quality of care can be found, then, and only then, should an extensive analysis of all the components of quality be made, including structures and processes of care, in order to explain the poor performance.

It is equally important to understand a low SMR. Before patting oneself on the back and concluding that the quality of care must be excellent, the case mix on such a unit should also be assessed. Just verifying that severity indexes are comparable over time is not enough to ascertain stability in case mix (Table 1). Other information is needed, including the number of patients coming from the emergency room, the number of patients transferred from other wards, hospitals and ICUs, as well as the LOS. Unexpected re-admissions and the proportion of patients dying with do-not-resuscitate (DNR) orders must also be checked. Considering the example given in Table 1, although mean SAPS II was unchanged over time, the case mix altered significantly in the last 2 years with a decrease in the LOS, and a higher proportion of patients coming from the community, in particular from the emergency room. These factors could, thus, very well explain the decrease in SMR in our unit without jumping immediately to the conclusion that it must be due to an improvement in the quality of care (which, of course, remains a possibility!).

When national or international comparisons are attempted [32-36], these case mix issues have to be taken into account, before concluding that the quality of care in a given unit is better than predicted, because it is then mandatory in the networking and benchmarking philosophy, to describe what this unit is doing which could explain this good performance, and which could be helpful to other units and patients. It may well be that this unit has very specific and 'creative' protocols and clinical pathways, or different 'official' guidelines; these differences should be explored and described carefully.

The principle of benchmarking is to provide people with information helping them to do better, not to check that everybody is doing the same, using the same processes of care. However, there are other ways to use the information which could be far more dangerous; for example, it could be used to lobby health care deciders that the amount of resources available for the ICUs in a given hospital, health maintenance organization (HMO), city, or even country [37] is too low, hence the high SMR. It can also be used by managers to close ICUs in hospitals because their SMR is too high. Journalists could also decide to use such data to provide a 'Michelin guide' of ICUs in a country or continent. This has been tried in France.

Table 1. Evolution of SMRs over years in Saint-Joseph Hospital ICU

	1995	1996	1997	1998	1999
Mortality	22 %	22,4 %	22,8 %	19 %	17 %
SMR	0,92	0,91	0,82	0,78	0,67
SAPS II	35	36	39	38	37
LOS	10,3	12,1	11,2	9,8	7,8

SMR: standardized mortality ratio; LOS: length of stay.

Applying Prognostic Models and Quality Indicators from 'Groups' of Patients to Individuals

Patients who have to choose a health care insurance system, an HMO, or the hospital in which they will have their surgical procedure performed may wish to have access to information on quality indicators from a particular HMO or hospital, in order to help them make a good choice. Different components of the quality in health care will be considered to reach a decision: equity, humanity, effectiveness, and as a citizen, efficiency of care [28]. Patients like to feel they will be admitted to the right unit at any time of the day, including the ICU if needed, and that they will benefit from the best therapies during their stay including preventive measures. They want to be treated with humanity and compassion and to be discharged at the right time. They would probably also like, at least in theory, that the team treating them will try to avoid embarking on futile therapies and be able to provide palliative and terminal care when necessary, this being decided after extensive, honest and transparent discussions with them and their relatives.

In addition, patients may also wonder what information is available from outcome research built on groups of patients to help health care practitioners take the most appropriate decisions during their ICU stay, including triage specific preventive measures, and the withholding and withdrawing of supportive therapies.

The Role of Triage Policies

Triage is a very important step in the ICU process and a very important part of our job. Patients would be very concerned by triage policies, in particular in countries in which the number of ICU beds is limited [38]. Triage should not be made by untrained personnel, and triage policies should be precise and stable over time. Severity scoring systems cannot be used arbitrarily to accept or refuse patients for admission to the ICU [39], although, in combination with other available information, can be used as part of the decision process.

Finally, it is essential that studies are conducted to follow patients who are not admitted to the ICU either because their severity of illness is too low or too high, because their underlying condition is too poor, or because of a lack of available ICU beds [40].

Quality Indicators in the ICU Available to Individuals or their Relatives

Since most patients do not plan to be admitted to the ICU, SMRs are not very appropriate information for them, or for their relatives. On the contrary, they may very well ask for information on other quality indicators either related to structures (e.g., the nurse to bed ratio), to processes of care (e.g., triage policies, hygiene precautions or antibiotic protocols), or to results (e.g., unplanned readmissions, rates of nosocomial infections, errors or iatrogenic events happening in the ICU, or in the hospital) [41, 42] (Table 2).

Table 2. The quality assessment checklist in the ICU [41]

- ⇒ Assessment of the structures: ICU design, organization, education, equipment, personnel ratios
- ⇒ Assessment of the process: objectives of the unit; admission, triage and discharge policies; communication issues; do-not-resuscitate and withdrawal policies; guidelines, clinical pathways, compliance with and implementation of guidelines; relations with other services; implementation of quality improvement activities
- ⇒ Assessment of the case mix: type of admission, severity scores, number of organ system failures, comorbidities
- ⇒ Assessment of workload: Therapeutic Intervention Scoring System or other score
- ⇒ Nursing turnover and satisfaction
- ⇒ Cost and utilization management issues: use of blood products and expensive drugs, length of stay, cost per survivor
- ⇒ Outcomes: mortality at ICU and hospital discharge and at 6 or 12 months; quality of life and functional status at 6 or 12 months; unplanned readmissions; nosocomial events (nosocomial infections, accidental extubations, decubitus ulcers); patient and family satisfaction
- ⇒ Trainee satisfaction

Nosocomial infection rates are considered to be an accurate quality indicator [43]. Many ICUs record this type of indicator, sometimes as part of large surveillance networks (e.g., NNISS from the Center for Diseases Control [CDC], HELICS in Europe, or RESIN in France). The rates of nosocomial pneumonia, of nosocomial bacteremia, or of catheter related infections are the most widely proposed indicators in the field of ICU-acquired infections. The CDC proposes to use densities of incidence of infections, where the number of infections is the numerator, and the cumulative (for the given period) number of days for the given procedure (ventilator days, catheter days...) is the denominator. However, this is still a very crude method to adjust for risk factors for infection. The mean LOS in the given ICU, the mean length of the studied invasive procedure, the severity of illness, and the underlying diseases are determinant risk factors, which have not generally been taken into account. For these reasons, it is still difficult to use such indicators to correctly evaluate quality of care in the ICU [44].

Even using very large data bases, such as the EPIC study [45], which was a large European prevalence study involving thousands of patients in the different European countries, the significant differences in the prevalence of nosocomial infections between countries were probably not related to differences in quality of care in those countries. Again, dramatic differences in the case mix of the countries appeared. The LOS varied across countries, from 4. 5 days to 12 days, which of course modified the risk for nosocomial infections enormously. This difference in the LOS was due to the fact that what is termed an 'ICU' varies a lot between countries. For example, post-operative patients (scheduled surgery) are considered as ICU patients in some countries and not in others, where they are treated in recovery rooms, or in post-operative ICUs which were not included in the EPIC study. Sampling issues are determinant factors if we really want to understand the results with any kind of indicator of quality of care.

This is also true for other quality indicators including SMR, LOS, or cost/effectiveness ratio. It is also true for multicenter, multinational RCTs since dramatic differences in case mix, induce important center or even country effects.

Non infectious iatrogenic events occurring in the ICU (errors) could also be accurate quality indicators. Indeed, errors will probably occur far more frequently in the more severely ill patients who undergo more invasive procedures.

Assessing Risk Factors During ICU Stay to Provide Appropriate and Targeted Decisions, Including Preventive Measures

Many preventive measures should not be applied to every ICU patient, but on the contrary should be given 'à la carte' to patients who are at risk for the targeted event, in order to take the most cost beneficial decisions. Examples of such measures include stress ulcer prophylaxis, enteral and parenteral nutrition, empiric antibiotic therapies, methods to prevent nosocomial infections (selective digestive decontamination, continuous subglottic secretion suction, usage of kinetic beds), etc.

In order to select the patients who would benefit most from these techniques (which have side effects), it is necessary to use either a prospective score of the risk factors for the targeted event, or specific scores combining the risk factors in a multivariate fashion, or to use severity scoring systems which are able to predict nosocomial or iatrogenic events. However, a lot of work remains to be done in this respect, including the use of trends in severity during the first few days in the ICU [46, 47]. Obviously patients or their relatives could consider that this prospective and 'individualized' assessment of the risk for their own case, using what has been learned in groups of patients (including risk factors) is a very accurate quality indicator. The unit could use 'official guidelines' or local ones, or just decisions made for each individual using evidence and logic based algorithms. Thinking globally, but acting locally using what we know for decision making in individuals according to their particularities, specific wishes and needs are probably fundamental components of quality. The availability of local data, using an accurate clinical information system helps to improve clinical decision making, and will make patients and relatives more confident in 'their hospital'.

Using What We Know from Groups of Patients to Take Individual Decisions for Withholding and Withdrawing Care

This is a very provocative and controversial area. There are dramatic national, cultural and religious differences in withholding and withdrawing policies, which make universal guidelines useless. However, every citizen and every patient would like the 'best' decision to be made, according to his/her personal wishes, and the 'state of the art' for their particular disease. They would like the health care practitioners to take decisions based on both evidence (science), logic and ethical considerations. In these very difficult situations, it is clear that patients are at the same time individuals and members of a group (according to the disease, the culture, the religion, the country, etc). There is an extensive literature available on the concept of futility of care [48–54].

Although several authors have proposed using severity scoring systems, mainly APACHE II or III to decide when to withhold or withdraw therapy in order to avoid futility of care [48], there is a relatively strong international consensus that this is not ethical and thus not feasible [37]. In particular, the Society of Critical Care Medicine ethic's committee stated recently that "the use of scoring systems as a sole guide to make decisions about whether to initiate or continue to provide intensive care is inappropriate" [49]. Indeed it is not possible to predict death with enough accuracy with any of the available scoring systems to use it for a binary decision like whether to continue or stop supportive therapies in the ICU. No score is able to predict mortality with a more than 5 to 10 % accuracy and no score takes quality of life into account. Two studies were conducted recently in adults and children [51, 53] looking at the concept of prediction of futile therapy using severity scores; Apache II was used in the adult [53] and PRISM in the pediatric, study [51]. In the adult study, the death of no patient was so certain, based on the severity of illness score, that there was less than 1 % chance of survival. Combining the two studies, which represented 482 patients, only one patient's death was so certain that there was less than a 5 % chance of survival. In addition, a 5 % chance of survival with an excellent quality of life is more than enough to continue active care and far more reasonable than a 20 % chance of survival with a very poor quality of care. In addition, there is a very poor correlation between the different scoring systems [55]. Finally, as pointed out by Iezzoni et al. [56] predicting who dies depends on how severity is measured.

However, assessment of severity of illness, using severity scoring systems is obviously one factor which can help in decision making; in a multiparametric approach is the best one [57, 58]. The persistence of a very high level of illness severity over time during the ICU stay using daily severity scores, such as daily SOFA [11] could provide even more valuable information. We use this philosophy daily, but usually without a precise quantification of severity of illness. Daily severity scores (provided they are validated) or organ system failure scores as LOD or SOFA could easily be used to make this severity assessment ever time more evidence based.

In a group of 40 % consecutive patients, Esserman et al. [58] showed that 13 % of the patients used 32 % of the resources. A product of APACHE risk estimates on days 1 and 5 of at least 0.35, predicted 37 % of potentially ineffective care (defined as resource use in the upper 25th percentile and survival for less than 100 days) with a specificity of 98 %. In a second data set, potentially ineffective care outcome prediction had a sensitivity of 43 %, a specificity of 94 % and a positive predictive value of 80 %.

Using Severity Scores to Make Discharge Decisions More 'Evidence-Based'

Again, severity scores cannot by themselves replace a logical clinical judgement. However, they can provide interesting information which could help make discharge decisions more objective [59]. The decision between a transfer to a step down unit or the general ward could also be improved [60].

Conclusion

Most of the risk factors, prognostic factors, and quality indicators have been validated in large populations of patients and cannot be used alone for decision making in individuals. This is especially true for difficult decisions such as admission to the ICU, discharge, and, even more controversial, the withholding or withdrawing of care. Many factors have to be taken into account to in making these decisions [38, 61]. Severity scores form one of these factors. The use of the SMR to assess quality of care in the ICU must be made with extreme caution. Quality must remain a multiparametric concept, mixing many different indicators including humanity, compassion, quality of life (patients, relatives, health care professionals) and science (prognostic models). Quality of care could be summarized as the ability to use for individuals what we have learned from groups. Indeed, individuals have gained a lot from what has been learned in groups since this information, when used 'a la carte', and with logic and humanity, helps in making the best decisions for each patient during daily life.

References

1. Knaus WA, Draper EA, Wagner DP et al (1985) APACHE II: a severity of disease classification system. Crit Care Med, 13: 818–829
2. Knaus WA, Wagner DP, Draper EA, et al (1991) The APACHE III prognostic system. Risk prediction of hospital mortality for critically ill hospitalized adults. Chest 100: 1619–1636
3. Lemeshow S, Teres D, Klar J et al (1993) Mortality probability models (MPM II) based on an international cohort of intensive care unit patients. JAMA, 270: 2478–2486
4. Le Gall JR, Loirat P, Alperovitch A et al (1984) A simplified acute physiological score for ICU patients. Crit Care Med 12: 975–977
5. Le Gall JR, Lemeshow St, Saulnier F et al (1993) A new simplified acute physiology score (SAPS II) based on a European/North American multicenter study. JAMA 270: 2957–2963
6. Pollack MM, Ruttimann UE, Getson PR (1988) Pediatric risk of mortality (PRISM) score. Crit Care Med 16: 1110–1116
7. Shann F, Pearson G, Slater A, Wilkinson K (1997) Paediatric index of mortality (PIM): a mortality prediction model for children in intensive care. Intensive Care Med 23:201–207
8. Anonymous (1993) The CRIB (clinical risk index for babies) score: a tool for assessing initial neonatal risk and comparing performance of neonatal intensive care units. The International Neonatal Network. Lancet 342:193–198
9. Knaus WA, Draper EA, Wagner DP, Zimmerman JE (1985) Prognosis in acute organ-system failure. Ann Surg 202:685–693
10. Marshall JC, Cook DJ, Christou NV et al (1995) Multiple organ dysfunction score: a reliable predictor of a complex clinical outcome. Crit Care Med 23: 1638–1652

11. Vincent JL, Moreno R, Takala J et al (1996) The SOFA (Sepsis Related Organ Failure Assessment) score to describe organ dysfunction/failure. Intensive Care Med 22: 707–710
12. Le Gall JR, Klar J, Lemeshow S et al (1996) The logistic organ dysfunction system. JAMA 276: 802–810
13. Zimmerman JE, Shortell SM, Knaus WA et al (1993) Value and cost of teaching hospitals: a prospective, multicenter, inception cohort study. Crit Care Med, 21: 1432–1442
14. Knaus WA, Wagner DP, Zimmerman JE et al (1993) Variations in mortality and length of stay in intensive care units. Ann Intern Med 118: 753–761
15. Zimmerman JE, Shortell SM, Rousseau DM et al (1993) Improving intensive care: observations based on organizational case studies in nine intensive care units: a prospective, multicenter study. Crit Care Med 21: 1443–1451
16. Change RWS, Jacobs S, Lee B (1988) Predicting outcome among intensive care unit patients using computerized trend analysis of daily APACHE II scores corrected for organ system failure. Intensive Care Med 1988, 14: 558–566
17. Lemeshow S, Klar J, Teres D et al (1994) Mortality probability models for patients in the intensive care unit for 48 and 72 hours: a prospective multicenter study. Crit Care Med 22: 1351–1358
18. Ruttimann UE, Pollack MM (1991) Objective assessment of changing mortality risks in pediatric intensive care unit patients. Crit Care Med 19: 474–483
19. Wagner DP, Knaus WA, Harrell FE et al (1994) Daily prognostic estimates for critically ill adults in intensive care units: results from a prospective, multicenter, inception cohort analysis. Crit Care Med 22: 1359–1372
20. Brun-Buisson C, Doyon F, Carlet J et al (1995) Incidence, risk factors and outcome of severe sepsis and septic shock in adults: a multicenter prospective study in intensive care units. JAMA 274: 968–974
21. Cowen JS, Kelley MA (1994) Errors and bias in using predictive scoring systems. Crit Care Clin 10: 53–72
22. Kollef MH, Schuster DP (1994) Predicting intensive care unit outcome with scoring systems: underlying concepts and principles. Crit Care Med 10: 1–18
23. Le Gall JR and Loirat P (1995) Can we evaluate the performance of an intensive care unit ? Curr Opin Crit Care 1: 219–220
24. Lemeshow S, Klar J, Teres D (1995) Outcome prediction for individual care patients: useful, misused, or abused ? Intensive Care Med 21: 770–776
25. Randolph AG, Guyatt GH, Carlet J et al (1998) Understanding articles comparing outcomes among intensive care units to rate quality of care. Crit Care Med 26: 773–781
26. Naylor C, Guyatt G, for the Evidence Based Medicine Group (1996) Users' guides to the medical literature: part 10. How to use an article reporting variations in the outcomes of health services. JAMA 275: 554–557
27. Le Gall JR, Lemeshow S, Leleu G, Klar J et al (1995) Customized probability models for early severe sepsis in adult intensive care patients. JAMA 273: 644–650
28. Randolph AG, Guyatt GH, Calvin J et al (1998) Understanding articles describing clinical prediction tools. Crit Care Med 26: 1603–1612
29. Teres D, Lemeshow S (1994) Why severity models should be used with caution. Crit Care Clin 10: 93–110
30. Vassar MJ, Holcroft JW (1994) The case against using the APACHE system to predict intensive care unit outcome in trauma patients. Crit Care Clin 10: 117–126
31. Watts CM, Knaus WA (1994) Comment on "the case against using the APACHE system to predict intensive care unit outcome in trauma patients". Crit Care Clin 10: 129–134
32. Castella X, Artigas A, Bion J et al (1995) A comparison of severity of illness scoring systems for intensive care unit patients: results of a multicenter, multinational study. The European/North American Severity Study Group. Crit Care Med 23: 1327–1335
33. Gemke R, Bonsel G, Group ATP (1995) Comparative assessment of pediatric intensive care: a national multicenter study. Crit Care Med 23: 238–245
34. Rapaport J, Teres D, Barnett R et al (1995) A comparison of intensive care unit utilization in Alberta and western Massachusetts. Crit Care Med 23: 1336–1346

35. Williams J, Zimmerman J, Wagner D et al (1995) African-American and white patients admitted in the intensive care units. Crit Care Med 23: 626–636
36. Wong D, Crofts S, Gomez M et al (1995) Evaluation of predictive ability of APACHE II system and hospital outcome in Canadian intensive care unit patients. Crit Care Med 23: 1177–1183
37. Pappachan JV, Millar B, Bennett ED et al (1999) Comparison of outcome from intensive care admission after adjustment for case mix by the APACHE III prognostic system. Chest 115: 802–810
38. Randall Curtis J (1998) The "patient-centered" outcomes of critical care: what are they and how should they be used ? New Horiz 6: 26–32
39. Consensus Conference organized by the ESICM and the SRLF (1994) Predicting outcome in ICU patient. Intensive Care Med 20: 390–397
40. Sprung CL, Geber D, Eidelman LA et al (1999) Evaluation of triage decisions for intensive care admission. Crit Care Med 27: 1073–1079
41. Carlet J (1996) Quality assessment of intensive care units. Curr Opin in Crit Care 2: 319–325
42. Thijs LG and the members of the task force European Society of Intensive Care Medicine (1997) Continuous quality improvement in the ICU: general guidelines. Intensive Care Med 23: 125–127
43. The Quality Indicator Study Group (1995) An approach to the evaluation of quality indicators of the outcome of care in hospitalized patients, with a focus on nosocomial infection indicators. Infect Control Hosp Epidemiol 16: 308–316
44. National Nosocomial Infection Surveillance System Group (1991) Nosocomial infection rates for interhospital comparison: Limitations and possible solutions. Infect Control Hosp Epidemiol 12: 609–621
45. Vincent J, Bihari D, Suter P (1995) The prevalence of nosocomial infection in intensive care units in Europe: results of the European Prevalence of Infection on Intensive Care (EPIC) study. JAMA 274: 639–644
46. Girou E, Stephan F, Novara A et al (1998) Risk factors and outcome of nosocomial infections: results of a matched case-control study in ICU patients. Am J Respir Crit Care Med 157: 1151–1158
47. Soufir L, Timsit JF, Make C et al (1999) Attributable mortality and morbidity of catheter-related septicaemia in critically ill patients: a matched, risk-ajusted, cohort study. Infect Control Hosp Epid 20: 396–401
48. Atkinson S, Bihari D, Smithies M, Daly K Mason R, McColl I (1994) Identification of futility in intensive care. Lancet 344: 1203–1206
49. Ethics Committee of the Society of Critical Care Medicine (1997): Consensus statement of the Society of Critical Care Medicine's Ethics Committee regarding futile and other possibly inadvisable treatments. Crit Care Med 26: 887–891
50. Halevy A (1999) Severity of illness scales and medical futility. Curr Opin Crit Care 5: 173–175
51. Sachdeva R, Jefferson L, Coss-Bu J, brody B (1996) Resource consumption and the extent of futile care among patients in a pediatric intensive care unit setting. J Pediatr 128: 742–747
52. Schneiderman LJ, Jecker NS, Jonsen AR (1990) Medical futility. Ann Int Med 112: 949–954
53. Halevy A, Neal R, Brody B (1996) The low frequency of utility in an adult intensive care unit. Arch Intern Med 156: 100–104
54. Teres D (1997) Pushing the envelope of futility. Crit Care Med 25: 1768–1769
55. Moreno R, Miranda DR, Fidler V et al (1998) Evaluation of two outcome prediction models on an independent database. Crit Care Med 26: 50–61
56. Iezzoni LI, ASH AS, Shwartz M et al (1995) Predicting who dies depends on how severity is measured: implications for evaluating patient outcomes. Ann Intern Med 123: 763–770
57. The SUPPORT Principal Investigators (1995): a controlled trial to improve care for seriously ill hospitalized patients. JAMA 274: 1591–1598
58. Esserman L, Belkora J, Lenert L (1995) Potentially ineffective care: a new outcome to assess the limits of critical care. JAMA 274: 1544–1551

59. Zimmerman JE, Wagner DP, Draper EA et al (1994) Improving intensive care unit discharge decisions: supplementing physician judgment with predictions of next day risk for life support. Crit Care Med 22: 1373–1384
60. Auriant I, Vinatier I, Thaler F et al (1998) Simplified acute physiology score II for measuring severity of illness in intermediate care units. Crit Care Med 26: 1368–1371
61. Gemke R (1998) Clinical applications of severity scoring models. Curr Opin Crit Care 4: 133–138

Driving Improvements: Quality Management in the ICU

A. Frutiger

Learning Point

- Quality improvement is always a cyclical process involving 'closing the loop'
- The choise of methods for managing quality depends on the urgency and impact of the problem. Incident detection methods permit quick responses, while strategic health planning bodies or project groups are more appropriate for long term issues
- Quality measurement without process improvement is not worthwhile
- The Hawthorne effect must be distinguished from real improvements
- Poor process quality is expensive; well organized care processes save money

Introduction

Modern hospitals are extremely complex organizational bodies. They combine three distinct professional cultures: physicians, nurses, and administrators who all live up to different role models, and they are divided into traditionally well defended territories of specialized services having their own, sometimes insular cultures. Still, well established basic rules of quality management apply.

Quality assessment is in principle nothing more than a comparison of an observed situation with an expected or planned one. Quality improvement can be viewed as a continuous cycle called by many "quality circle":
1) a relevant problem is identified and specified
2) a standard, preferably an accurately measurable one, is set
3) quantitative data relevant to the problem are collected
4) comparisons between measurements and objectives are made
5) findings are implemented and turned into management decisions

From here on the quality circle starts anew. New, hopefully higher, standards and new objectives are set and structures and processes are refined in order to reach the goals (Fig. 1) .

Unfortunately, the attempt to improve quality quite often consists of the mere gathering of results, and is not followed by attempts to implement changes, an essential element to close the quality circle. Busy accumulation of data however,

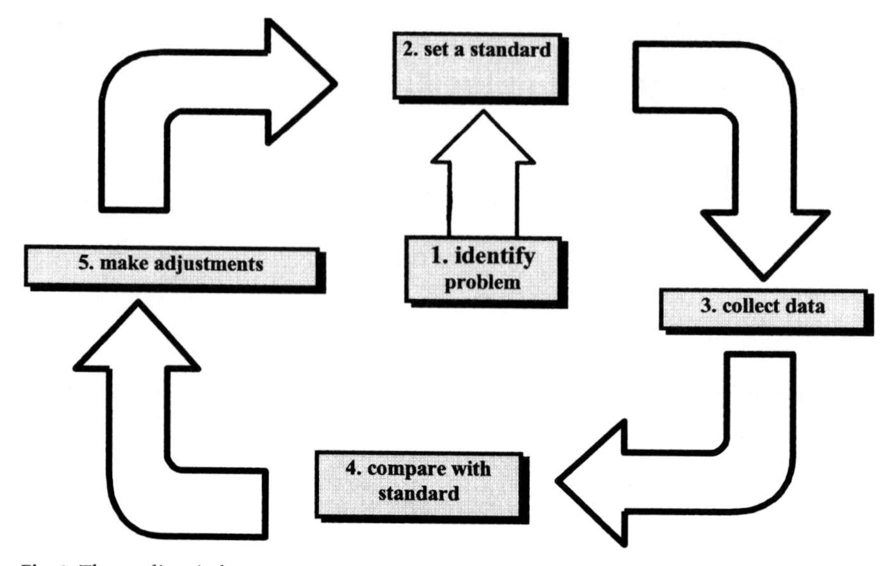

Fig. 1. The quality circle

without turning the acquired information into management decisions, does not improve quality and is not worth the effort.

One factor additionally confounding the issue is observational bias. Quite regularly, the performance of a system improves during close observation, just by looking at it (data sampling, process analysis). This beneficial observational effect is then unfortunately mistaken for a real improvement within the system. The effect is however only transitory and the system will quickly drift back to the old level of performance. This makes sense, since just looking at a process cannot permanently change it.

The preceding chapters have discussed many possible approaches to ICU observation, to the analysis of ICU use, and to the specification and quantification of the results we achieve with our patients. Additionally, evidence-based medicine (EBM) and other techniques, provide the intensivist with many good rules that should clearly be followed in running the ICU, and similarly, what would be better avoided.

The question for the ICU-practitioner is: How should all this knowledge be applied? The evidence-based gospel is clear, but what management tools are available to put the principles into action? What should be done to convert an already good ICU into an even better one? There are many ways to manage an ICU, but no matter what approach is used, it must include the basic concept of the above mentioned quality circle in order to drive improvements.

Basic Elements of Quality Control

Medical practice is undergoing major changes. Besides cost-controlling efforts and continuing advances in science and technology, the quality of care has emerged as a third important issue [1]. In fact quality improvement has the potential to bridge the gap between the ongoing progress we would like our patients to benefit from and the clearly set economic limits we are facing today.

Introduction of quality management principles into the field of medical care was advanced importantly by the work of Donabedian. His already classical definition of quality as "that kind of care which is expected to maximize an inclusive measure of patient welfare, after one has taken account of the balance of expected gains and losses that attend the process of care in all its parts." was formulated in 1980 [2]. According to his theories, overall quality comprises three areas: structures, processes and results. For each area distinct key instruments to assess and control quality are suggested [3] (Table 1).

Indicators: mainly used in the area of processes and outcomes, indicators are representative markers of performance, looking only at a segment of the processes or results, not at their totality. As surrogate markers of overall quality, indicators are used to measure outcome and to assess processes. To ensure structural quality other tools, like standards, are preferred.

In order to be useful, indicators have to:

- address a relevant issue
- evaluate a frequent situation
- ask simple questions
- give clear answers
- be easy to assess

Since outcome is dealt with in other parts of this book the present chapter will focus on those indicators reflecting process quality in the ICU. Of course some overlap is inevitable. We shall discuss mainly indicators that are suited to drive management decisions.

Process Quality and Respective Indicators

Health care is becoming so complex that the processes needed to ensure its continuity are increasingly vital [4]. This is especially true for the ICU. Process quality is the sum of all measures taken or not taken during patient care, including the timing of all activities, the total number of incidents, accidents, delays, misunderstandings, confusions and unforeseen events. The patients and their families' expectations, their satisfaction and access to intensive care are additional factors.

Table 1. Relations between quality areas and management tools

	Standards	Guidelines	Indicators
Structures	XXX	X	X
Processes	XX	XXX	XX
Results, outcomes	X	XX	XXX

At best, ICU performance can be measured indirectly [5]. When internal quality assessment is attempted, the question is asked whether the unit in question is performing better or worse than it did in the past.

Comparing the performance of one ICU with another is more difficult because of case mix and other differences. An often-cited study made comparisons between intensive care in the US and France and found some important differences [6]. American ICUs admitted older patients and resorted more frequently to invasive monitoring than their French counterparts. Severity of illness, observed mortality and therapies applied were however similar. High performance ICUs would then have lower mortalities than expected, but the assumption that severity adjusted mortality provides the basis for sound comparison does not hold true [5].

Another way to look at performance of a unit is to evaluate its management processes [6, 7] and the managerial skills of the team leader [8]. Assessment would include communications, timing of services, conflict resolution, staff satisfaction, leadership and unit culture in general. And, hopefully, organizational problems and potential means of improvement could be found.

Unit Performance

There is no formal definition of ICU performance. A high performing unit is one that admits and discharges patients rapidly and efficiently, has low severity-adjusted mortality rates, and good functional outcomes in survivors. The special care given during a hospital stay has an influence on the degree of rehabilitation after discharge. There is proof that in older patients functional outcomes in terms of activities of daily living are improved when specific care focused on a patient's independence is delivered in the hospital [9]. ICU performance seems to be linked to the degree of standardization of procedures. Results of the EURICUS-I project indicate that the higher the standardization of a unit the better its performance [10]. Whatever approach is used, there are well-established basic rules of quality management, which must be observed. If the continuous circle of identifying relevant problems, setting standards, gathering data, making comparisons, making adjustments and returning to the standards is not followed, then quality programs are not worth the effort. Meaningful activity will then turn into worthless bustle.

Guidelines

Guidelines are the main instrument to assure process quality. At best, they are evidence-based and help clinicians to directly apply the result of sound research at the bedside [11]. Guidelines will be judged by their ability to favorably affect clinical and economic outcomes. Inevitably the development, implementation and evaluation of guidelines will become an important focus of ICU research. Methods for guideline development are manifold. All will to a certain degree involve the three information sources: published scientific evidence, expert opinions, and surveys [12]. Development may occur informally or by formal methods which may involve peer groups, Delphi techniques (questionnaires circulated among experts), or formal consensus conference techniques. Since methods for guideline development are becoming increasingly sophisticated, the process itself grows more and more time consuming and expensive, as the example of a European consensus conference on selective decontamination of the digestive tract proved [13].

Until now clinical guidelines, the 'software' of medical practice, have not been subjected to the same degree of scrutiny regularly seen with health technology or 'hardware' assessment. An overview compiling published evaluations regarding the effectiveness of written clinical guidelines concluded that implementation of explicit guidelines does indeed improve clinical practice and patient outcomes [14, 15]. But, interestingly, the impact of guidelines differed in relation to the circumstances in which they were generated. Guidelines had a high probability of being effective if they were developed internally, disseminated during a specific educational intervention and when implemented in a patient-specific actual situation. A lower effectiveness was seen with guidelines developed externally at a national or international level, disseminated as state of the art publication in a journal, and implemented as a general reminder. The very process of developing and implementing guidelines within a team and close to clinical reality appears to guarantee a certain effectiveness. Busy journal authors however will be disappointed to learn how little they are listened to. ICU directors must realize that practice guidelines are crucial factors of process quality and that their development and implementation should be counted among the prominent duties.

Communication: Unit Culture

Crucial elements of process quality in a service organization are communication and timing. Shortell [16] found in a study looking at performance of 40 ICUs that units which had a team culture with supportive nursing leadership, good and timely communication, effective coordination, and collaborative problem solving approaches, were more efficient in terms of moving patients in and out of the unit, which is an indicator of process quality. These units also had a lower nurse turnover, an indicator of employee satisfaction. The authors concluded that the greater the quality of interaction among physicians and nurses in the unit, the better the unit's performance.

Physician-nurse collaboration is essential to the well functioning of a unit and continuous mutual respect and understanding are needed. The two disciplines need to define themselves in terms of their common mission [17]. Quality improvement programs have strong synergistic effects.

Computerized communication channels [18] or electronic networks are no substitute for the communication process itself, the latter being a matter of interactive human culture. A striking finding of an Israeli study investigating human errors in the ICU was the pattern of verbal communication within the ICU team [19]. Nurses were almost exclusively talking to nurses, and physicians to physicians. Only 2% of all verbal communication occurred between nurses and physicians, reflecting two parallel cultures.

Not only do health professionals continuously have to exchange information. Patients and their families also have information needs [20]. Instead of being viewed as further stressors, families should be integrated into the care process as valuable resources for patient recovery. The way an ICU takes care of the informational and emotional needs of families is an another indicator of quality.

Employee Satisfaction, ICU Burnout

Employee satisfaction is a cornerstone of the continuous quality improvement (CQI) concept. There are no ways of assessing overall staff satisfaction in ICUs, but some indirect indicators like staff sick lists or employee turnover can be used. Frequent absence is usually a clear hint of dissatisfaction. In a German ICU, sick leave rose to as high as 16% of the working time when a high rate of job dissatisfaction was present. It dropped to 6% after thorough reorganization of the unit [21].

ICU physicians are also not always satisfied with their jobs. Their tolerance to frustration may decline, causing them to think about quitting. A survey among intensivists in medical ICUs revealed a high prevalence of physician burnout, described as emotional exhaustion and depersonalization [22]. The amount of time on sick leave and nursing and physician burnout are clearly indicators of process quality.

Incident Reporting

In any quality system, routines for reporting undesirable events are key elements. Screening for adverse occurrences is a well-established method of quality control in hospitals [23]. In an epidemiological study of 51 New York hospitals there was a mean rate of adverse events caused by negligence of 3.2%, but variation among hospitals was substantial [24]. It was concluded that systematic assessment of adverse events is an important quality measure. The Harvard Medical Practice Study, looking at over 30,000 hospital records identified a 3.7% incidence of adverse events, defined as those causing disabling injuries [25]. It was concluded that systematic assessment of adverse events is an important quality measure. It appears that the careful application of available medical knowledge would bring about far more quality improvement than the continuous search for ever newer and better therapies. Nevertheless, studies dealing with adverse events, incidents or accidents in the ICU setting are not abundant. This is entirely understandable, considering that humans do not especially like to acknowledge and report their errors.

Situations, where bad rules were applied or where good rules were not used should preferably be labeled neutrally as 'incident' or 'event'. Standardized incident reporting in the ICU can become an excellent tool to monitor and improve process quality, even if such programs regularly face reluctant or hostile reactions during their introduction. Team members must agree that human errors are to be accepted as facts of life and that reporting of incidents is aimed at improvement, not at punishment. Part of the reason for the lack of spontaneous reporting may be that reporting is traditionally focused on serious or rare incidents [26]. Quite regularly the real reasons for adverse events and mistakes are 'resident pathogens' rooting deeply in the system and mostly difficult to eradicate. Incidence reporting routines combined with feedback loops to allow corrective action or adaptation of procedures should be included in every ICU quality control concept [27,28]. An Israeli study systematically investigating causes of human errors in the ICU found no less than 554 errors over a 4 month period [19]. Potentially detrimental errors occurred on average twice a day. This study clearly points out the high incidence and relative importance of human errors in the ICU.

Incident reporting at a national level has so far only been established for Australian ICUs. In a report from 1994 the authors described 390 incidents, 106 of which were actually harmful [29]. Anonymous voluntary reporting was used and reporting frequency varied considerably. Incidence monitoring as a continuous routine, and closing the loop by regularly taking corrective action, was successfully applied. The Australian Incident Monitoring Study in Intensive Care (AIMS-ICU) is a fine example of the successful introduction of a nationwide project targeted at improving processes [30, 31].

Incident reporting has also been practiced for very specific process indicators of intensive care. A large study identifying adverse drug events concluded that physicians were primarily (72%) responsible for the incidents, of which more than 50% were judged preventable [26]. Another indicator is unplanned extubation of mechanically ventilated patients. This highly undesirable incident has been reported to occur in as many as 10% of intubated patients [32]. Because of its high occurrence rate and its obvious seriousness, unplanned extubation is a worthwhile target for quality improvement [33, 34]. We submit that incident reporting should be part of any ICU quality improvement program.

Table 2 shows that, combined with a proper ICU management concept, incident reporting can become a key element in the successful management of an ICU.

The choice of indicators and how they are to be integrated into the daily practice of an ICU is very much a question of local taste. Ideally this should occur within a formal quality concept. Such programs are of much higher value if they originate and develop within the ICU team itself.

Quality Management Concepts

The recent past has seen quite a few labeled quality concepts come and go; mainly our American colleagues have been affected [35]. Peer review was favored in the 1970s, followed by 'quality assurance' and more recently by 'quality improvement'. In particular, the concept of quality assurance, a system looking for the worst performers in a group of services and taking sanctions against them (withdrawal of funding and/or recognition status), was considered as unfair and demotivating. Hospitals in the US have traditionally undertaken quality assurance activities to

Table 2. Management tools depending on the urgency of the problem

Urgency of the problem and appropriate approaches Problem	Very urgent	Relatively urgent	Mid-range	Long term
Detection	by incident reporting system	by incident reporting system assessment	by routine formal quality	by strategic health planning bodies
Response	immediate response around the clock needed	response within days to weeks	response within weeks to months needed	response within months or more
Management tools	• solution induced by current team leader (shift nurse, staff physician) • right/obligation to act is delegated to the appropriate level	• regular team meetings (unit conference) • enforcement of guidelines by sample checks • quality-conference • case-related booster teaching	• bi-annual formal quality meetings • formal process analysis by task force • audits by external peers • targeted teaching programs	• task forces • project groups • study groups
Examples	• critical equipment failure • critical incident • serious complaint (patient or relatives)	• albumin ordered despite existing prohibitve guidelines • repeat observations of inappropriate ICU admissions • serious condition undiagnosed	• ICU mortality (SMR) increasing • nosocomial infection rate above control limit • high readmission rate	• chronic bed shortage • new surgical programs planned • high refusal rate in potential organ donors

meet accreditation criteria required by the Joint Commission for the Accreditation of Health Care Organizations (JCAHO) [36].

Repeatedly, and this continues currently, quality improvement concepts have been borrowed from the industry and business world. These do not necessarily suit the needs or fit the particularities of the medical environment. If such systems are forced upon physicians and hospitals they may well sail under the flag of 'quality improvement', but are often just hidden attempts at cost containment or plain marketing.

The designation of 'centers of excellence' for instance is often a scarcely disguised attempt to negotiate low-cost packages in return for directing patients to a specific service. It is not really excellence in outcome that these negotiators are looking for. If for insurers and governments the emphasis lies on lowering costs, physicians must direct their efforts at improving quality. Physicians have to decide what role they want to play in the future of quality management [27, 28, 37, 38]. It appears far more appropriate that quality concepts for health care be developed by the health care professionals themselves and within the health system itself. This by no means excludes the wise and educated use of general principles of quality control that have already proven their value elsewhere.

Total Quality Management (TQM)

Many hospitals favor labeled concepts like TQM which is based on the three principles: continuous process improvement, employee involvement and customer (patient) satisfaction. The terms TQM and CQI are difficult to distinguish and are used alternatively in the literature. Both describe quality concepts that are mainly based on dynamic participation of all employees rather than on 'top down' management concepts. TQM is preferentially used in industrial surroundings, while CQI seems to be more appealing to service organizations and the health sector in particular. Implementing TQM in the intensive care setting involves some considerations: If the hospital has already begun TQM activities the ICU joins in by starting with a carefully chosen first project which should cover clinical and non-clinical areas [39, 40]. If the ICU is the first service to start a TQM program it may provide a starting sign for the entire hospital.

Continuous Quality Improvement (CQI)

CQI comprises a set of formal quality improvement techniques based on the collection and analysis of data generated in clinical practice in a defined setting. CQI looks for and solves problems from within the system. Fashioned after the Deming philosophy, CQI is based on the premise that employees generally have an in-depth understanding of their duties and feel valued if they are encouraged by their superiors to join in a team effort at improving quality. W. Edwards Deming was probably *THE* pioneer of the modern post war quality movement. Having served as a consultant to many Japanese industries he was disturbed to find matters not as advanced in his own home country, the United States: "We have learned to live in a world of mistakes and defective products as if it were necessary to life. It is time to adopt a new philosophy in America." [41]. The Deming philosophy comprises three key elements: customer satisfaction, employee involvement and continuous planning of action. He would condense his convictions into well-chiseled lists of phrases like 'the 14 points of management' or into easy-to-memorize action concepts, like the 'Plan-Do-Study-Act Cycle'. Deming's tireless year-long touring of the management community had its effects: a generation of managers ingested his thoughts to a considerable degree and implemented quality improvement in their daily work. His targets were factories and large business companies, not the medical world, where fabrication of products or selling of goods or services do not really apply. However, the general principle, that employees who become involved in quality improvement of their company will inevitably gain more personal satisfaction and work more productively, is certainly valid for hospitals as well. Most importantly the convincing part of the CQI-concept is its generation of a movement within a service, without dependence on outside regulatory agencies.

ISO 9000 Norms

The International Standardization Organization (ISO), mainly active in Europe, has developed quality improvement standards, first for industrial production and later for service companies [42]. ISO assists companies in the development of internal quality systems and provides a formal shell within which the rules and standards for every sector of a company's activities are defined. The formal certificate that companies are awarded after the accreditation process is generally held in high esteem and adds to the prestige of a corporation. Increasingly, there are attempts to apply the ISO 9000 concept to the hospital setting under the unproven assumption that it will work equally as well as in the industrial world. So far ISO 9000 applications in hospitals have only addressed hotel and housekeeping functions thus only scratching the surface of the problem. They have never tackled the core issues of health quality: namely cure and care. The usefulness of ISO 9000 for solving quality problems in clinical medicine must be doubted.

Other Approaches

Many ICU directors prefer to use less formal, unlabeled approaches to quality improvement. As a matter of fact to define one's institutional commitment and to design one's own quality assurance plan is a process of high quality in its own right [43]. There exist locally developed or specialty-based systems that are already considerably refined [44–46]. Their sophistication lies however more on the data acquisition side, while implementation strategies are lagging behind.

Another approach to quality of health care issues is public reporting of outcomes, already a common practice in the US. The assumption is, that public release of performance data will allow patients, purchasers and referring physicians to make educated choices [47]. The providers are then expected to become motivated to improve their performance by the known techniques of quality management. The effects of this approach are controversial. On the one hand, there is evidence that in New York public reporting of mortality after coronary-artery bypass surgery led to a 41% decline in risk-adjusted mortality [47]. On the other hand, cardiovascular surgeons in Pennsylvania are less willing to perform bypass surgery on severely ill patients since the state's reporting system began [48]. This indicates that public performance reporting can negatively affect patient's access to specific areas of care.

Common Elements in all Quality Concepts

Whatever approach is used, there are well established basic rules of quality management, which must be observed. These basic rules consist of five steps as illustrated in Fig 1. If the continuous circle of identifying relevant problems, setting standards, gathering data, making comparisons, seeking adjustments and returning to the standards is not followed, then quality programs are not worth the effort. Meaningful activity will then turn into worthless bustle.

But how these rules should be followed in daily practice is very much a question of local taste. Quality control programs are of much higher value if they originate and develop within the ICU team itself. Concepts forced on a unit by outside agencies are less well received.

Conclusions: How to set up a Quality System for an ICU?

In most ICUs, elements of a quality system have been present for a long time, if only in a more or less informal way and not labeled as such. Usually numerous rules have been written down and appear under labels like: guidelines, protocols, rules of good practice, policies, house rules, resident handbooks, etc. They are further enhanced by informal rules, the unwritten laws of the unit, which are quite often more strictly enforced than the written ones. The most natural way to start a comprehensive quality system in the ICU is to assemble all efforts and activities already in existence and to amalgamate them with the essential elements of quality management as outlined above. In order to work, the effort has to be formalized, institutionalized and forged into a quality management concept. Who belongs to the quality team, how often meetings are to be scheduled, and how audits are organized need to be defined [49].

There are some rules to be observed and a few pitfalls to be avoided:

- It would be a crucial mistake to view quality control merely as a single short interlude; it has to become a continuous and irreversible process.
- Another mistake would be to delegate quality management to external 'experts'. Health care professionals possess all the necessary knowledge to become real experts on health care quality. All they need to do is some footwork and to hang on to the rudder of the rocking boat.
- The third mistake would be to start with a system that attempts to cover everything, a goal that is too difficult and complicated to reach will end in frustration. The start should be small, simple and fast.

The aspects of structures, processes and outcomes relevant to intensive care are summarized in Table 2 of the chapter by J Carlet et al., page 314

On a more practical level, this is how we suggest that an ICU director should set up a quality system:

- As unit director you must head the quality team yourself. Attempts to delegate this task to a subordinate level or, even worse, to outsiders will cause the whole effort to fail.
- Form a quality team comprising members of all professional backgrounds and all levels of hierarchy. Inform ICU staff about the composition of this group and make it clear that quality improvement is basically the responsibility of all team members. Encourage them to take initiatives and to make suggestions for improving quality.
- Delineate the scope of care by a brief and clear summary of what your unit has to do to be a good unit or to become an even better one.
- Regularly schedule formal meetings and observe a standardized agenda by addressing the areas structures, processes and results. Have minutes carefully taken and make them available to the whole ICU staff.
- Invite peers from outside to your meetings. This will help to avoid mental inbreeding of the quality team.
- Structures: review existing standards applicable to your unit. If any kind of accreditation is available, apply for it. If there are structural aspects of your unit which are not covered by existing standards, set your own levels. Regularly compare the *de facto* state of your unit's structures with the given standards. Take corrective action if differences surface.
- Processes: regularly review the guidelines which are in effect in your unit. Have new guidelines formulated and written if an important process is poorly defined or is running with too wide a variation. Have existing guidelines removed when they become outdated or if the problem in question has become irrelevant. When introducing guidelines from outside (e.g., 'state of the art' publications), remember that the highest impact on daily practice stems from rules generated within your unit itself. Find out to what degree existing guidelines are being followed and enforced.
- Select a few processes which should stand as indicators for the overall process quality of the unit.
- Pick processes in which timing and/or communication are crucial and set the desired level of performance. The process in view must be important and frequent. The criteria as to whether the goal was attained or not must be clearly defined.
- If you find clear deviations from the set goals, take corrective action. Sometimes a formal process analysis has to be undertaken in order to find the root causes of the poor process quality in question.
- Introduce voluntary incident reporting since this tool enables you to identify trouble areas of process quality.
- Results: ICU mortality is the most important indicator of outcome quality. It is clearly defined and is the easiest to obtain. Its value is however limited if it is not combined with a diligent severity scoring. This allows calculation of severity adjusted mortality rates. Use one of the three most widely established pre-

dictive models (SAPS II, APACHE II or MPM II). Be careful to use the model only for what it is intended. If possible go beyond merely assessing mortality and get involved in morbidity or quality of life measurements in ICU survivors. Accept that the presently available tools are far from being perfect.

- Link a network with other quality groups within your hospital. The ICU is not a remote island. Most poorly running processes in a hospital have very complex interdisciplinary aspects and cannot be solved within a single unit. Make your multidisciplinary expertise as an intensivist available to the entire hospital.
- Allow a considerable amount of experimenting when you embark on a quality project, as today there is no single way towards quality control in the ICU. Avoid being constrained by too formal programs forced on your unit from outside.
- Include quality issues into your teaching activities. Make it clear to your junior staff that quality control is an integral part of patient care and not just a passing fad.
- Report your findings and approaches so that others may benefit from your experience. Be available for active participation in multicenter projects.
- Be ready to discuss quality issues openly and publicly. Accept the fact that quality control in medicine is no longer an internal affair.
- Stay ahead of government agencies, insurance companies and other regulatory bodies who might want to dictate the modalities of quality control in your unit.

References

1. Blumenthal D (1996) Quality of health care Part 1: Quality of care – What is it? N Engl J Med 335:891–895
2. Donabedian A (1980) Explorations in quality assessment and and monitoring. Vol I: The definition of quality and approaches to its assessment. Health Admin Press, Ann Arbor
3. Frutiger A, Moreno R, Thjis L, Carlet J (1998) A clinician's guide to the use of quality terminology. Intensive Care Med 24:860–863
4. Blumenthal D (1996) Quality of health care Part 4: The origins of the quality of care debate. N Engl J Med 335:1146–1149
5. Teres D, Lemeshow S (1993) Using severity measures to describe high performance intensive care units. Crit Care Clin 9: 543–554
6. Knaus WA, Le Gall JR, Wagner DP, et al (1982) A comparison of intensive care in the U.S.A. and France. Lancet I: 642–646
7. Shortell SM, Zimmerman JE, Rousseau DM, et al (1994) The performance of intensive care units: Does good management make a difference? Med Care 32: 508–525
8. Stahl LD (1985) Demystifying critical care management. Part 2. J Nurs Adm 15: 14–21
9. Landefeld CS, Palmer RM, Kresevic DM, Fortinsky RH, Kowal J (1995) A randomized trial of care in a hospital medical unit especially designed to improve the functional outcomes of acutely ill older patients. N Engl J Med 332:1338–1344
10. EURICUS-I. The effect of organization and management on the effectiveness of intensive care units in the countries of the European Community. In: Baert AE, Baig SS, Bardoux C (ed) European Union Biomedical and Health Research Vol 9. IOS Press, Amsterdam, pp 194–199
11. Cook D, Ellrodt G (1996) The potential role of clinical practice guidelines in the ICU. Curr Opin Crit Care 2:326–330

12. Roche N, Durieux P (1994) Clinical practice guidelines: from methodologic to practical issues. Intensive Care Med 20:593–601
13. Consensus Conference Report (1992) Selective digestive decontamination in intensive care unit patients. Intensive Care Med 18:182–188
14. Grimshaw JM, Russell IT (1993) Effect of clinical guidelines on medical practice:a systematic review of rigorous evaluations. Lancet 342:1317–1322
15. Grimshaw J, Freemantle N, Wallace S, et al (1995) Developing and implementing clinical practice guidelines. Qual Health Care 4:55–64
16. Shortell SM, Zimmerman JE, Gillies RR, et al (1992) Continuously improving patient care: Practical lessons and an assessment tool from the national ICU study. QRB Qual Rev Bull 18:150–155
17. Bushnell MS, Dean JM (1993) Managing the intensive care unit: physician-nurse collaboration Crit Care Med 21 (suppl 9):S389–399
18. Booth FV (1989) Effective staff communications in a large ICU. Int J Clin Monit Comput 6: 81–86
19. Donchin Y, Gopher F, Olin M, et al (1995) A look into the nature and causes of human errors in the intensive care unit. Crit Care Med 23:294–300
20. Spatt L, Ganas E, Hying S, Kirsch ER, Koch M (1986) Informational needs of families of intensive care unit patients. QRB Qual Rev Bull 12: 16–21
21. Burchardi H, Schuster HP, Zielmann S (1994) Cost containment: Europe. Germany. New Horiz 2: 364–374
22. Guntupalli KK, Fromm RE (1996) Burnout in the internist-intensivist. Intensive Care Med 22:625–630
23. Wolff AM (1995) Limited adverse occurrence screening: an effective and efficient method of medical quality control. J Qual Clin Pract 15: 221– 233
24. Brennan TA, Hebert LE, Laird NM (1991) Hospital characteristics associated with adverse events and substandard care. JAMA 265:3265–3269
25. Leape LL, Hebert LE, Laird NM, et al (1991) The nature of adverse events in hospitalized patients. Results of the Harvard Medical Practice Study II. N Engl J Med 324:377–384
26. Bates DW, Leape LL, Petrycki S (1993) Incidence and preventability of adverse drug events in hospitalized adults. J Gen Int Med 8: 289–294
27. Frutiger A (1996) Quality assessment and control in the ICU. Curr Opin Anesthesiol 9: 134–138
28. Frutiger A (1995) Le contrôle de qualité devient indispensable aux soins intensifs. Méd Hyg 53: 2041–2046
29. Hart GK, Baldwin I, Gutteridge G, Ford J (1994) Adverse incident reporting in intensive care. Anaesth Intensive Care 22:556–561
30. Beckmann U, West LF, Groombridge GJ, et al (1996) The Australian Incident Monitoring Study in Intensive Care: AIMS-ICU. The development and evaluation of an incident reporting system in intensive care. Anaesth Intensive Care 24:314–319
31. Beckmann U, Baldwin I, Hart GK, Runciman WB (1996) The Australian Incident Monitoring Study in Intensive Care: AIMS–ICU. An analysis of the first year of reporting. Anaesth Intensive Care 24:320–329
32. Maguire GP, DeLorenzo LJ, Moggio RA (1994) Unplanned extubation in the intensive care unit: a quality-of-care concern. Crit Care Nurs Q 17: 40–47
33. Sessler CN (1997) Unplanned extubations: making progress using CQI. Intensive Care Med 23:143–145
34. Chiang AA, Lee KC, Lee CC, Wie CH (1996) Effectiveness of a continuous quality improvement program aiming to reduce unplanned extubation: a prospective study. Intensive Care Med 22:1269–1271
35. Chassin MR (1996) Quality of health care Part 3: Improving the quality of care. N Engl J Med 335:1060–1063
36. Sherman JJ, Malkmus MA (1994) Integrating quality assurance and total quality management/quality improvement. J Nurs Adm 24: 37–41

37. Blumenthal D, Epstein AM (1996) Quality of health care Part 6: The role of physicians in the future of quality management. N Engl J Med 335:1328–1331
38. Linton DM, Frutiger A (1996) Intensive care standards and quality control. S Afr Med J 86:589–592
39. Buccini EP (1993) Total quality management in the critical care environment. A primer. Crit Care Clin 9:455–463
40. Lumb PD (1993) Management as the art of politics. Crit Care Clin 9:425–436
41. Deming WE (1986) Out of the crisis. Massachusetts Institute of Technology, Cambridge
42. Weaver MO (1994). ISO-9000. A building block for total quality management. Mohican Press, Loudonville
43. Booth FV (1993) ABCs of quality assurance. Crit Care Clin 9:477–489
44. Sivak ED, Perez-Trepichio A (1990) Quality assessment in the medical intensive care unit: evolution of a data model. Cleve Clin J Med 57: 273–279
45. Sivak ED, Perez-Trepichio A (1992) Quality assessment in the medical intensive care unit. Continued evolution of a data model. Qual Assur Util Rev 7: 42–49
46. Osler T, Horne L (1991) Quality assurance in the surgical intensive care unit. Where it came from and where it's going. Surg Clin North Am 71: 887–904
47. Blumenthal D, Epstein AM (1996) Quality of health care Part 6: The role of physicians in the future of quality management. N Engl J Med 335:1328–1331
48. Schneider EC, Epstein AM (1996) Influence of cardiac surgery performance reports on referral practices and access to care- a survey of cardiovascular specialists. N Engl J Med 335: 251–256
49. Macpherson D, Mann T (1992) Medical audit and quality of care – a new English initative. Qual Assur Health Care 4: 89–95

Applied Health Services Research: Translating Evidence into Practice

G. Ellrodt

Learning Points

- The 'weight' of evidence or expression of risk in abstract terms will not necessarily engage physicians. Real world expression in human terms has a greater likelihood of promoting significant evidence-based change
- The clinical improvement opportunity is easily derived from an assessment of current practice and careful review of the literature
- There are four essential steps in translating evidence into practice. These include:
  a) Prioritize opportunities
  b) Identify a multi-disciplinary team
  c) Implement the program
  d) Measure program performance and improve it
- A careful systematic assessment of barriers to implementation should be undertaken early in clinical program development
- There is a large and rigorous body of evidence to inform implementation
- Implementation programs must be custom tailored to the particular organization driven by local resources and attitudes

Scott Weingarten, MD, the director of applied health services research at a large community teaching hospital, was leading a multidisciplinary team charged with improving outcomes for patients with total hip replacement(THR). In the early 1990s there was some controversy among the practitioners about the relative effectiveness of several different approaches to deep vein thrombosis (DVT) prophylaxis in these patients.

Scott performed a comprehensive literature review and assembled a 'stack' of articles supporting the efficacy of warfarin, therapeutic heparin anticoagulation, or perhaps progressive pneumatic compression devices in these patients rather than aspirin. At the first meeting he stated that he had reviewed the literature and that there was an overwhelming amount (weight) of evidence to support warfarin or heparin and the group should therefore consistently use one of these options. The orthopedic physicians were unconvinced by Scott's presentation and stated that they had not seen the described complications in their patients.

At the next meeting Scott was more explicit and described in detail the relative risk, relative and absolute risk reductions associated with warfarin and therapeutic heparin compared to aspirin or placebo. Again the response was lukewarm at best with no consensus for change.

Undaunted, Scott returned to the literature, and reviewed current medical center practice including the number of THR performed per year and current DVT prophylaxis practice. Using the same methodology described in this chapter Scott then calculated the number of potential lives saved through a decrease in fatal pulmonary embolism if all THR patients were treated with optimal DVT prophylactic therapy. At the next meeting, which Scott feared would be his last, Scott walked the orthopedists through the calculations and demonstrated that optimal DVT prophylactic practice would save two to three lives per year at the medical center. At this point the chief of orthopedics declared that losing three lives was simply 'unacceptable' and that all patients receiving THR at the institution must from now on receive one of the literature supported (evidence-based) approaches to DVT prophylaxis. There was then unanimous agreement within the orthopedic groups. Follow-up data two months later revealed that 98% of eligible patients were receiving one of the recommended DVT prophylaxis regimens compared to 10 % prior to the intervention.

Introduction

Physicians and other healthcare practitioners face multiple challenges in caring for patients. One of the most daunting is the translation of best evidence from the medical literature into the day-to-day practice of busy clinicians. This challenge is particularly important in the complex and rapidly changing world of intensive care unit (ICU) medicine. The science of applied health services research has many definitions. For this chapter, we will define applied health services research as 'the science of translating evidence (efficacy) into practice in the real world (effectiveness)'. Applied health services research should thus be distinguished from other forms of health services research that include policy investigations and large scale studies of variation.

In this chapter, we will use a modification of existing frameworks [1, 2] to prioritize efforts, evaluate potential barriers and review applied health services approaches to overcoming challenges to evidence-based practice in the ICU. Throughout this chapter the term guideline will be used as the expression of recommendations for interventions. Readers should understand that for this chapter the terms guideline and recommendations include practice parameters, algorithms and even consensus statements. The more rigorous definition of guidelines and the operational definition for this paper is: "systematically developed statements to assist practitioner and patient decisions about appropriate health care for specific clinical circumstances" [3]. These guidelines or recommendations are but one important part of a comprehensive approach (program) to improve clinical management including dissemination, implementation, evaluation, and improvement strategies.

A Framework for Translating Evidence into Practice

Figure 1 provides an overview of the challenges and potential approaches to translating evidence into day-to-day practice in the ICU. There are four basic steps with multiple activities within each. These include:

1) Prioritize opportunities for improved performance through a systematic and quantitative approach.
2) Identify a multi-disciplinary team, that systematically assesses the potential barriers to successful implementation. It can then develop focused evidence-based recommendations, proven dissemination and implementation strategies, and the measurement system required to evaluate its impact.
3) Implement the program.
4) Measure program performance and design an improvement strategy.

In Figure 1 under the final chevron, is the probability of improved outcomes. The hypothesis is that appropriately prioritized programs, well developed and implemented, will lead to significant clinical and potentially economic improvement. Figure 3, at the end of the chapter, expresses the same framework with approaches likely to be successful according to the health services research evidence listed at the top of the columns and those less likely to be successful listed at the bottom.

Tables 1–5 and Fig. 2 are summaries that can be used by teams to assure that an appropriately rigorous approach to program development has been used. These tables can also be utilized as a diagnostic tool if an ICU program does not appear to be working as designed.

Identify and Prioritize Opportunities for Program Development

In any healthcare organization numerous opportunities for program development exist. Particularly within ICUs many competing initiatives may exist. At an institutional, departmental or unit level it is reasonable to have a group who oversee such program development and have a systematic approach to identifying and prioritizing projects. Some coordination at a level higher than the ICU is probably desirable since program impact and resource availability may be controlled at a more central level. The more centralized group setting priorities must be careful not to micro-manage. At some point priorities must be refined at the more local level (e.g., ICU). Table 1 presents some of the considerations in program selection. An advantage of an organized system is the avoidance of projects

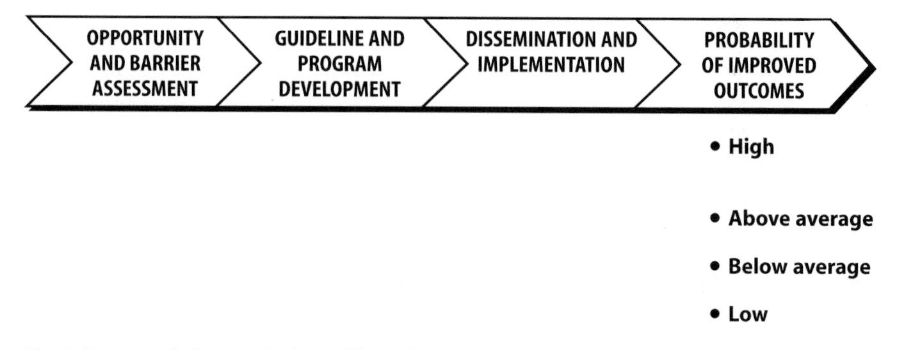

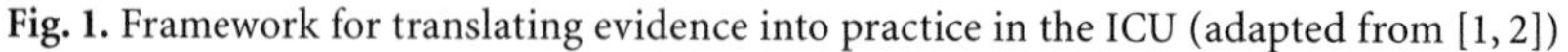
Fig. 1. Framework for translating evidence into practice in the ICU (adapted from [1, 2])

Table 1. Considerations in prioritizing ICU program development

	Considerations	Comments	Score
1.	Volume of cases	Good starting point	
2.	Burden of cases (clinical, economic)	More refined than volume alone	
3.	Assessment of current practice	May be significant challenge	
4.	Best practice from the literature or bench marking	Apply searching and critical appraisal skills	
5.	Size of gap (opportunity) between current practice and best practice explicitly expressed	Use ARR and NNT if appropriate	
6.	High level assessment of potential investment required to close gap - (human, capital)	"Back of the envelope" economic analysis	
7.	If available, use formal economic analyses to prioritize opportunities (cost effectiveness or cost benefit)	Be sure analyses use similar methodologies	
8.	External drivers of programs (e.g. regulatory or review)	Examples in US include HCFA, JCAHO, NCQA	
9.	Availability of effective leadership	Critical to success	
10.	Time frame to effect change	Immediate vs years vs decades	
11.	Community or national mandate	Important driver	

ARR: absolute risk reduction; NNT: number needed to trend; HCFA: Health Care Financing Administration; JCAHO = Joint Commission for Accreditation of Healthcare Organizations; NCAQ: National Committee for Quality Assurance.

that even when ideally executed will have minimal clinical and financial impact. A high level identification of potential barriers to success should enter into the decision making process at this time although a detailed approach to each barrier will be developed by the multidisciplinary program team. Even if a significant opportunity does exist, if the barriers to implementation are large and potentially costly to overcome, the group setting program priorities may chose another opportunity.

There are several levels of increasing sophistication in choosing a potential condition or intervention for improvement. At the most basic level the number of cases or interventions provides a reasonable starting point. If the most frequent diagnosis in an ICU is sepsis this may be a reasonable place to start but this broad and heterogeneous population may not be an optimal defined population upon which to focus. At the next level the team setting priorities may look at disease burden through a meter that includes morbidity, mortality and cost. Again sepsis may be the leading contender with this analysis but still not amenable to a focused intervention.

Further analysis might lead the prioritization team to pick a more focused topic within a condition for program development. For example, in assessing ICU utilization including septic patients the team may identify ventilator management as a significant opportunity. At this point it is reasonable to begin to assess current practice and focus on several hypotheses. For example, data from your ICU may show that your average time of mechanical ventilation is significantly above a benchmark level and that your comparatively high incidence of ventilator associated pneumonia (VAP) is contributing in part to this observation. Thus the combined input of ICU practitioners, infection control professionals, and perhaps departmental leaders may lead to the prioritization of ventilator management for a more in depth analysis. If upon preliminary review of the benchmark data, and selected articles from the literature, a significant gap exists between your current practice and 'best practice' further evaluation should be undertaken.

The size of the gap between current practice and 'best practice' may be used to drive team formation and team charge. The prioritizing team may now begin to refine its estimate of program opportunity and cost. One approach is to use well-performed clinical trials (usually randomized, controlled trials [RCTs]). If the patient population appears similar to your ICU patients and the intervention proposed is not in general use in your ICU an 'ideal' potential opportunity may be calculated based upon your number of eligible patients. For example in a RCT by E. Wesley Ely and colleagues [4], a multidisciplinary team performed daily screening of ventilated patients followed, where appropriate, by a two hour trial of spontaneous breathing. In the intervention group, physicians caring for patients who successfully completed the two-hour spontaneous breathing trial were informed of their patient's performance. For patients of physicians informed of their weaning trial success a statistically significant reduction of time on mechanical ventilation from a mean of 6 to 4.5 days was seen. In addition complications including patient removal of tube, reintubation, tracheostomy, and prolonged mechanical ventilation were reduced from 41% to 20% of patients. Total ICU costs were $5,150 lower for protocol patients.

Using a simple approach based upon the principle of absolute risk reduction (ARR) and number needed to treat (NNT) [5] the team can assess the opportunity in a more quantitative manner. Using the information from Ely's article [4] and current practice the team could calculate the potential benefits of such a program. For example:

If 200 mechanically ventilated patients per year are cared for in your ICU the team might anticipate:

200 patients x 1.5 fewer days per patient = 300 fewer ventilator days.

And: 200 patients x (ARR of complications with intervention) =
200 x (41% risk without intervention – 20% risk with intervention)
= 200 x 0.21 = 42 fewer complications per year

And: 200 patients x $5,150 lower Total ICU costs per patient =
$1,030,000 lower total ICU costs.

A number of caveats must be considered in using this approach:

1) The article upon which the estimates are based must be strong methodologically and applicable to your patients and environment.
2) The opportunity is an ideal estimate based upon compliance observed in the original article.
3) The cost estimates are for total costs not direct variables. In other words it is unlikely that your ICU and institution will actually recover all these dollars.

4) There is no estimate of the cost of setting up and operating the program. High level estimates, however, would suggest that the costs are not prohibitive since the personnel are already employed and a re-design of work flow might be all that is required to operationalize the program.

In the Ely article [4] no mention is made of the VAP rate. One might predict, however, that since the duration of ventilation is reduced with the intervention the risk might decrease. The team prioritizing issues or the actual multidisciplinary team developing the program might perform an additional analysis to assess the potential impact of an intervention aimed directly at decreasing the risk of VAP. The number of patients might be different for this evaluation since the entry criteria for the relevant study may be different. In addition some patients may already be managed in the semi-recumbent position based upon physician preference or incomplete adherence with an ICU policy or guideline. For example: In an article by Drakulovic and colleagues [6] the use of a semi-recumbent position for patients undergoing mechanical ventilation reduced the rate of clinically suspected VAP from 34% to 8% and for microbiologically confirmed pnemonia from 23% to 5%. This represents an ARR of 26% for clinically suspected VAP and 18% for microbiologically confirmed pneumonia. For this example one can calculate the potential opportunity using a modification of the ARR approach.

If we assume that 200 patients might be eligible for this intervention we can calculate the potential impact by:

200 eligible patients x (100-percentage of patients already managed in semi-recumbent position – number of patients with contraindications to position)/100) x ARR = predicted number of patients not developing VAP.

In this calculation several of the realities of improved management are incorporated. This includes the fact that often some, but not all, patients are already managed according to best practice recommendations and some patients (in this example those with C-spine injuries and hypotension) have contraindications to the proposed intervention.

If 200 patients are mechanically ventilated

And: 25% of patients are already managed in the semirecumbent position

And: 5% of patients have a contraindication to this position (e.g. due to hypotension)

Then: 200 eligible patients x (100% - 25% already managed in position – 5% of patients with contraindications/100) x .26 ARR for clinically suspected VAP = number of episodes of VAP prevented.

And: 200 x (.70) x .26 = 36 fewer episodes of clinically suspected VAP per year.

(For further in-depth discussion of interventions to reduce the risk of VAP please see the chapter by Deborah J. Cook, page 185).

Identify the Multidisciplinary Team to Address Potential Barriers and Develop Program

Assemble Multidisciplinary Team

Once a condition or intervention has been identified and prioritized a multidisciplinary team should be assembled. The composition of such a team will vary. The following principles may be useful:
1) Keep the numbers small and manageable
2) Assure representation from disciplines that will be central to implementation
3) Chose opinion leaders to chair and participate
4) In recruiting potential members make clear why the program has been selected, expressed in real world clinical terms. For example the potential to save 10 lives per year will be more compelling than the possibility of saving dollars.

It is important that the team understands that their responsibility is not just to develop guidelines or other forms of clinical recommendations but also to design a comprehensive program that will address barriers to success, dissemination and implementation strategies, and an evaluation system. The steps the team should undertake are summarized in Table 2.

Assess Potential Barriers to Successful Implementation

As the multidisciplinary team begins design of the ICU program it should perform an inventory of potential barriers to implementation. Many, but not all of these will center upon physicians. A recent systematic review by Cabana and colleagues may be helpful as a checklist to assess potential barriers and as a guide to program design. The chapter focuses on physician adherence to 'guidelines'. How-

Table 2. Developing programs in the ICU

Step	Steps in Development	Comments
1.	Develop multidisciplinary team	Include opinion leaders
2.	Assess potential barriers to success	See Figure 2
3.	Determine the key areas upon which to focus and perform/updated literature review	Seek evidence-based guidelines, consensus statement, and systematic reviews where available
4.	Grade recommendations	Consider ACCP approach (see text & Table 3)
5.	Use rigorous process to develop recommendations and express in clear, concise actionable terms	If vague terms used and weak recommendations made, impact may be minimal
6.	Develop dissemination and implementation strategies	Choose from strategies that 'work'
7.	Develop measurement strategy	Few key measurements. Consider intermediate outcomes

ever, the term guideline is broadly defined in this article and may include guidelines, practice parameters, clinical policies, or national consensus statements [7]. The ICU team must remember that the framework for barrier assessment was developed around outpatient and non-acute care interventions. In addition, its applicability to the ICU and utility in improving performance have not been tested. A summary of the Cabana framework is presented in Figure 2. The framework is based upon a sequence of behavior change from knowledge, through attitudes to behavior. Although there are several such approaches this seems logical and potentially useful. Further validation of the framework and real world utility will be required. As the team develops recommendations and designs dissemination and implementation strategies, referral back to the checklist may be helpful to assure that the development team has addressed most or all issues.

Identify those Few Key Interventions that will Lead to Improved Outcomes

A significant challenge for any team is to remain focused on those critical interventions for which a clear relationship exists between an improved process and a better outcome. Some of the current criticism of clinical pathways may arise from the inclusion of multiple interventions some of which are of significant importance in changing outcomes, but many of which are not. Physicians seem overwhelmed by the shear mass of information. Thus the multidisciplinary development team needs to focus its efforts on several key interventions ('key aspects of care'). To choose these the team can:

1) Utilize existing systems that have reviewed the clinical literature and identified 'key aspects of care'. One such system, oriented to the inpatient and ICU environment, is the 'Evidence-based Forecaster' from Zynx Health of Cedars-Sinai Health System [8].

Table 3. ACCP evidence grading system (from [11] with permission)

A: Methods strong, results consistent – RCTs, no heterogeneity*
1: Effect clear – Clear that benefits do (or do not) outweigh risks

A: Methods strong, results consistent – RCTs, no heterogeneity
2: Effect equivocal – Uncertainty whether benefits outweigh risks

B: Methods strong, results inconsistent – RCTs, heterogeneity present
1: Effect clear – Clear that benefits do (or do not) outweigh risks

B: Methods strong, results inconsistent – RCTs, heterogeneity present
2: Effect equivocal – Uncertainty whether benefits outweigh risks

C: Methods weak – Observational studies
1: Effect clear – Clear that benefits do (or do not) outweigh risks

C: Methods weak – Observational studies
2: Effect equivocal – Uncertainty whether benefits outweigh risks

*Heterogeneity describes the situation when several RCTs yield widely differing estimates of treatment effect for which there is no explanation.

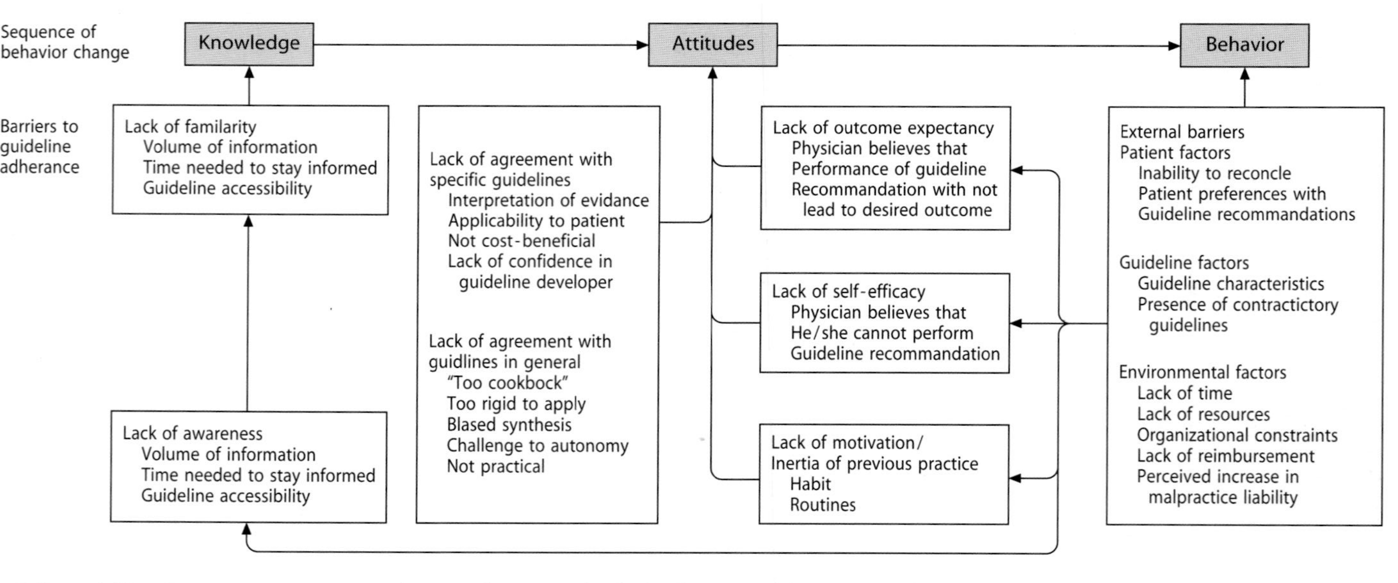

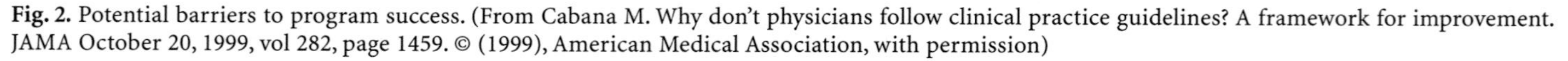
Fig. 2. Potential barriers to program success. (From Cabana M. Why don't physicians follow clinical practice guidelines? A framework for improvement. JAMA October 20, 1999, vol 282, page 1459. © (1999), American Medical Association, with permission)

2) Identify, by consensus, the potential key interventions. Using a systematic search strategy and critical appraisal of identified articles the team can use evidence-based medicine (EBM) principles to estimate potential impact. The team should search for economic analyses of interventions thought to be potentially advantageous. These more formal analyses including cost-benefit and cost effectiveness studies may be helpful in further refining selection of 'key aspects of care'.

These few critical interventions now form the clinical basis for your program. For example, the team developing recommendations for ventilator management may choose three key interventions based upon the literature identified during the program prioritization process and program development process. These might include:

1) Daily review of mechanically ventilated patients by a multidisciplinary team to determine eligibility for extubation/weaning [4].
2) Placing all patients without contraindications in the 45-degree semi-recumbent position to decrease the incidence of VAP [6].
3) Weaning by a single protocol. For example T-piece/flow-by or pressure support ventilation (PSV) rather than synchronized intermittent mandatory ventilation (SIMV) [9].

The third recommendation above raises an interesting question for guideline program development. A recent systematic review of the literature suggests that few trials exist to determine the superiority of one weaning approach over another. The best evidence suggests that either T-piece or PSV is superior to SIMV. Which of these two suggested approaches is superior is unknown at this time. What may be more important to the success of weaning is the system by which weaning is applied rather than the mode itself. [9, 10] In other words, the systematic approach to weaning using a protocol and team approach rather than multiple individuals using multiple different modes in different manners. This re-emphasizes that guidelines (even when based upon best evidence) are but a part of a complex program for management.

Grade the Recommendations

When the team has selected the few key interventions it may wish to express the strength of recommendations in some manner. Multiple systems have been proposed for grading the strength of evidence and recommendations for treatment or prevention. Many of these systems are cumbersome and may not fulfill the goal of informing practitioners of the rigor of evidence, the degree of disagreement, and the trade-offs of benefits and risks.

The grading system used by the American College of Chest Physicians (ACCP) [11] integrates strength of evidence, heterogeneity in study results and trade-offs between benefit and harm. As such it is a major step forward in clarifying the potential impact of guideline recommendations on patients. The letter grade refers to the strength of study design (methodological rigor) and consistency of results (heterogeneity). The numeric grade refers to the certainty regarding the trade-off between benefits and risks associated with a given recommendation (Table 3).

Table 4. Summary of effectiveness of dissemination strategies: results of systematic reviews (from [14] with permission)

Intervention	Comments	Effectiveness	References
Interactive educational meeting	Includes active discussions and role playing	+	[2,13,15-17]
Case based CME	Use clinical scenarios	+	[18,19]
Academic detailing	'Outreach visits'	+	[13,15,20,21]
Opinion leaders	Variable impact Positive in AMI care	+/–	[13,15,20,22,23]
Printed educational material	Not useful unless coupled with other interventions	+/–	[2,15,20,24]
Traditional CME	Consistently ineffective	–	[2,13,15,20,25-28]

+: all or at least 75% of systematic reviews demonstrate effectiveness; +/–: most (>50%, <75%) of systematic reviews demonstrate effectiveness; –: some (<50 %) systemic reviews demonstrate effectiveness. CME: continuing medical education; AMI: acute myocardial infarction.

Using the ACCP grading system the team might conclude the following. For the recommendation to have a team systematically review each mechanically ventilated patient each day and feedback to the clinician or team the results of their evaluation [4] the grade would be A1. The methods are strong (RCT) and since only one study has been performed there is no heterogeneity. Therefore, A is appropriate. In addition since the benefits, including shorter duration of mechanical ventilation, are coupled with a reduction in risks the recommendation is clearly A1.

For the recommendation to have a protocol for weaning using T-piece rather than PSV or SIMV the recommendation could be graded B1. Here the methods are strong including RCTs and a high quality systematic review [9], but there is significant heterogeneity (T-piece versus PSV). In addition, there appears to be a clear benefit without additional risks of using T-piece or PSV weaning versus SIMV.

For the final recommendation, positioning patients in the 45° semi-prone position the recommendation should be A1. The methods are strong (RCT), there are no conflicting results between trials regarding the benefit of this intervention, and the benefits for properly selected patients clearly outweigh the risks.

Use a Rigorous, Locally Driven Process to Develop Clear Actionable Recommendations

The process by which the team determines which recommendations it will make, the rigor of the development process, and strength of evidence may well determine acceptability by clinicians. Several studies have addressed the issue of guideline content and development process. Although these did not specifically address ICU guideline programs the observations may be transferable. Studies have concluded that:

1) Guidelines are more likely to be followed if they are evidence-based [12]
2) Guidelines are less likely to be followed if they are controversial, incompatible with current values, and vague and non-specific [12]

3) Guidelines are less likely to be followed if they demand extra resources and require new knowledge and skills, or provoke negative patient reactions [12]
4) Guidelines developed internally have a higher probability of being effective than external local or national guidelines [2, 13].

Thus there is support from both observational studies [12] and systematic reviews [2, 13] that the process of guideline development is important. The development team should keep in mind that local development does not mean ignoring national recommendations from credible organizations that are evidence-based. It does imply, however, that these national recommendations require local review and endorsement before they will be broadly accepted. A summary of these observations is shown in Figure 3 under the development chevron. We have attempted to show the impact of evidence and local influence by the hierarchy of listing. More rigorous approaches are listed at the top and align with a higher probability of improved outcomes under the final chevron. Following development of focused and prioritized recommendations and before design of the dissemination and implementation programs the team may wish to assess its current recommendations. For the three interventions recommended thus far, and assuming specific and explicit expressions of these recommendations have been written, the team may review the barrier list of Figure 2 and determine how many, if any, of the barriers have been addressed and which barriers remain.

Develop Dissemination and Implementation Strategies

The development team has multiple options for disseminating and implementing their recommendations (guidelines). The simple reminder that "guidelines do not implement themselves" [3] should serve as a warning that the hard work of making guidelines work has now begun. Several different approaches to categorizing

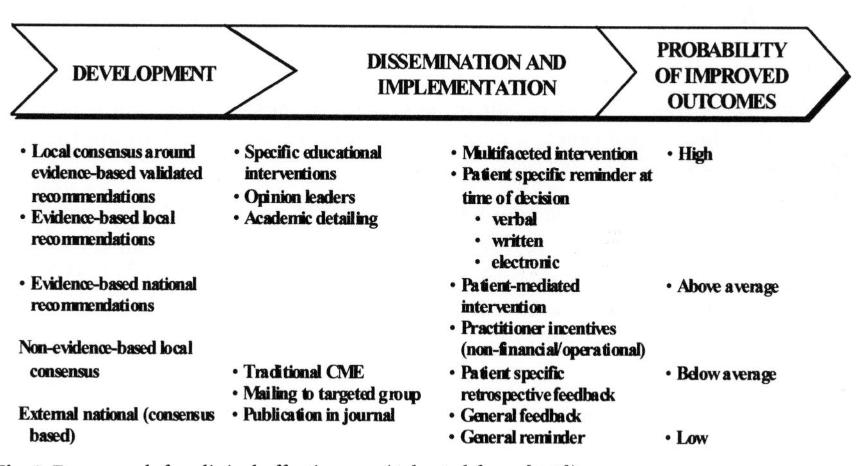

Fig. 3. Framework for clinical effectiveness (Adapted from [1, 2])

interventions have been developed. Grimshaw and Russell [2] have separated dissemination and implementation strategies. In this approach, dissemination includes getting the word out to the front line practitioners in a manner that is likely to actually change behavior. Implementation can be considered more reinforcing and active. In reality potential interventions are probably along a spectrum and are often used in combination. There is an extensive literature around dissemination and implementation. The focus has been on changing practitioner behavior (not just physicians), and includes many well-designed trials. Tables 4 and 5 summarize the findings of systematic reviews of studies evaluating the impact of various approaches to improving practitioner performance [14].

There are several caveats in applying the results of these systematic reviews to the ICU setting:

1) Most interventions to improve performance have not been performed in the ICU setting
2) The ICU presents certain unique challenges including the amount of information to be integrated and the time in which decisions must be made
3) ICUs have different organizational structures and therefore what may be applicable to one ICU may not be useful in another
4) ICUs may have only several practitioners (e.g., a closed unit) or multiple practitioners
5) ICUs are often part of a teaching program and therefore issues of housestaff training including autonomy, frequent turnover and varying levels of skill and sophistication must be addressed.

At this time, as the multidisciplinary team designs strategies to improve practitioner performance, it may be useful to return to the list of barriers. Since the team knows which critical interventions will be implemented it can custom tailor its dissemination and implementation strategies for the practitioners and systems predicted to be essential to success. The team can choose from the following interventions for dissemination:

Interactive educational meetings: These sessions include active discussion, role-playing and training exercises in a conference setting. Such sessions have consistently demonstrated effectiveness in promoting behavior change [2, 13, 15–17].

Case-based continuing medical education (CME): In these sessions information is provided to healthcare practitioners as clinical case scenarios. This approach is consistently effective [18, 19].

Academic detailing: In this adaptation of pharmaceutical industry detailing, trained persons meet with providers in their own practice environment to provide information and promote discussion. This approach has proved consistently effective in North America in changing prescribing habits. The identification and targeting of barriers to change may be useful [13, 15, 20, 21].

Local opinion leaders: These individuals are influential, and well respected providers who support the program. They encourage their colleagues to participate. Although their impact has not been consistent in the literature they may improve adherence to process of care measures. Their impact on outcomes is less

Table 5. Summary of effectiveness of implementation strategies: results of RCTs and systematic review (from [14] with permission)

Intervention	Comments	Effectiveness	References
Multifaceted	Multiple dissemination and implementation strategies	+	[13, 15, 20, 25, 29]
Concurrent reminders	Written or computerized	+	[2, 15, 20, 21, 30–32]
Computerized tools	Significant investment may be required	+	[30, 33–37]
Patient targeted	Patients stimulate provider change	+	[13, 15, 20]
Operational incentives	System changes including standing orders	+	[38–41]
Complementary practitioner	Non-physicians such as nurses and respiratory therapists	+	[4, 10, 42]
Case management	Coordinate, facilitate nd manage care	+/–	[43, 44]
Audit and feedback	Retrospective feedback about performance	+/–	[2, 13, 15, 20, 21, 32, 45]

+: all or at least 75% of systematic reviews demonstrate effectiveness; +/–: most (>50%, <75%) of systematic reviews demonstrate effectiveness; –: some (<50 %) systemic reviews demonstrate effectiveness.

clear [13, 15, 20, 22]. In one study of particular interest to intensivists a RCT of opinion leaders was conducted in 37 Minnesota hospitals. These individuals were selected using a validated tool. They focused on barriers to change, and comparative performance for aspirin, beta-blockers, lidocaine and thrombolytic use in acute myocardial infarction. In the opinion leader group their was a statistically significant improvement in appropriate use of beta-blockers and aspirin but no change in the use of thrombolytics or lidocaine [23].

Printed educational materials: These include recommendations or guidelines that are mailed, hand-delivered, electronically or audio-visually presented to providers. Alone these materials have not been shown to change practice. When used as one component of a multifaceted intervention, however, they have been successful [2, 15, 20, 24].

Traditional CME: Traditional CME which uses didactic lectures to convey information to health care providers has not been shown to improve clinical outcomes. This does not mean that a team should not consider this approach as part of a more comprehensive strategy, but traditional CME alone will not result in improved performance [2, 13, 15, 20, 25–28].

In addition the multidisciplinary team should chose from the following implementation strategies. If the team foresees multiple significant barriers to successful implementation a multifaceted approach should be considered. If the team diagnoses a few focused barriers, a more 'surgical' approach using a single implementation strategy may be appropriate. Table 5 summarizes the effectiveness of these potential implementation strategies as assessed by systematic reviews.

Again the caveat that many of these strategies have not been tested in the ICU setting must be kept in mind. Possible implementation strategies include:

Multifaceted approach: This strategy employs a combination of approaches to influence provider behavior. These may include dissemination strategies linked to implementation strategies. An example might be an opinion leader using concurrent feedback during rounds. A multifaceted approach has consistently demonstrated effectiveness. It is unclear, however which combination of strategies is most effective [13, 15, 20, 25, 29].

Concurrent reminders: Reminders are messages to providers to perform a given task. They may be delivered manually (in writing or verbally), or in a computerized format. Guidelines using patient specific reminders at the time of consultation are likely to be effective. Written and electronic reminders appear to be equally effective. Verbal reminders have not been as well studied [2, 15, 20, 21, 30–32].

Computerized tools: Computerized tools involve feedback, provision of guidelines or algorithms, computer assisted diagnosis and medical record keeping. Computerized reminders have been most completely studied in the outpatient setting and have been shown to be effective. Computerized drug algorithms are effective in improving physician prescribing. Computer based clinical decision support systems for diagnosis have not been effective [30, 33–36]. A computer assisted management program for antimicrobials has been studied in the ICU [37]. This computerized decision support system integrated hospital epidemiological information with patient specific data and presented the physician real time antimicrobial prescribing advice. Use of the program resulted in clinically and statistically significant reductions in: 1) the prescription of drugs to which the patient was allergic; 2) excess drug dosages; 3) antibiotic susceptibility mismatches; and 4) adverse drug events. In addition adherence to the recommendations of the computerized antimicrobial support system resulted in significantly lower: 1) antimicrobial drug costs; 2) hospital length of stay; and 3) total hospital costs [38]. Despite the great promise of this program it is unclear whether it can be exported to other institutions and have similar impact.

Patient targeted interventions: This approach has also been referred to as patient mediated interventions. Specific information is sought from or given to patients who then stimulate change in their provider. This approach has been used by the pharmaceutical industry in their direct to consumer marketing. Although some variability in effectiveness has been seen in trials and systematic reviews this is in general an effective approach [13, 15, 20]. This approach is not appropriate for the ICU patient but might be considered in improving follow-up care in areas such as adherence to medication regimens at home.

Non-financial operational incentives: These include changes in the patient care system that enable the provider to improve patient care. Such approaches may include total quality management/continuous quality improvement (TQM/CQI) programs involving a multidisciplinary team using a systematic approach. They may implement system, policy or procedure changes in care. Changes that include standing orders have been effective, but other interventions surrounding the standing orders were included in the trials. In general these studies have focused on improved provision of preventive services rather than ICU interventions

[38–41]. The potential use of nursing policy modification for the management of mechanically ventilated patients in the semirecumbent position is promising (see the chapter by D.J. Cook, page 185).

Complementary practitioners: These are non-physicians who take a major role in patient management. A limited number of studies support the expanded role of pharmacists in patient counseling and physician education [42]. In the randomized trial of protocol-directed weaning versus physician directed weaning from mechanical ventilation by Kollef et al. [10], nurses and respiratory therapists initiated and managed the weaning process with improved results. In the study by Ely and colleagues [4] a multidisciplinary team including physicians, nurses, and respiratory therapists screened potentially eligible patients for weaning suitability. It is unclear exactly what role the respiratory therapists and nurses played in this intervention.

Case management: This is the coordination, facilitation, and management of care delivery across the healthcare continuum. Since case management is almost always performed by non-physicians, there is overlap between this literature and that on effectiveness of complementary providers. Studies of case management have demonstrated variable effectiveness in improving patient outcomes and decreasing costs. A positive effect may be related to disease condition and specialty training of case managers [43, 44].

Audit and feedback: This implementation strategy involves the provision of retrospective feedback of clinical performance to providers. It may include comparisons with other providers and/or specific recommendations for improvement. Studies have demonstrated variable effectiveness. Audit and feedback alone modestly improves provider prescribing and test ordering behavior [2, 13, 15, 20, 21, 32, 45].

The multidisciplinary team can select from the above dissemination and implementation options to custom tailor a strategy based upon effectiveness of interventions, barriers within their organization and resources available to the team. If the organization has not engaged in these types of activities in the past, or if no such efforts have been made in the ICU a multifaceted approach should be considered. Since the three potential interventions proposed for illustrative purposes in this chapter are tightly linked, the following strategy might be considered. Obviously many approaches are possible.

1) Review barriers: If they include several of the typical challenges including:
   a) Lack of awareness and familiarity with screening and protocol directed weaning evidence on the part of ICU attendees and perhaps housestaff
   b) Self efficacy and motivation issues centered around habit.
   c) Behavior barriers including the potential complexity of the recommendations (e.g., the exact criteria for weaning eligibility) and environmental factors including organizational constraints and lack of time

2) Then:
   a) Identify an opinion leader in the ICU (may or may not be the director) who agrees with the recommendations. This person has presumably been on the development team and actively supported the recommendations.

b) Have opinion leader provide academic detailing to other attendings
c) Hold small group interactive educational sessions with respiratory therapy, nurses and physicians. This session might include critical appraisal of the supporting articles
d) Gain support for a multidisciplinary team approach to weaning eligibility as was done by Ely and colleagues [4] coupled with a weaning team similar to that described by Koleff et al. [10]
e) Gain nursing support for a policy to place all patients on mechanical ventilation (who do not have a contraindication) in the semirecumbent position.

Develop Measurement Strategy

The multidisciplinary team may be tempted to measure multiple process and outcome variables. It must, in some way avoid this temptation to make accurate and useful measurement possible. The team should at least ask the following questions in selecting variables, and determining how data will drive evaluation and determination of success.

- Is this variable of absolute importance in determining the success or failure of the program?
- Are there reasonable intermediate outcomes that are easier to measure? For example in the prevention of VAP using the semirecumbent position does the team need to measure hospital mortality or just the frequency of clinical suspected pneumonia using explicit criteria?
- Is the information needed to evaluate the program already available somewhere in the system? For example, can it be found in some administrative or financial database?
- Have we adequately defined the variable to encourage reliable recording?
- Who is going to measure the selected variable?
- In what database is the variable to be entered?
- Who will enter the data?
- Who will be responsible for data integrity?
- Who will be responsible for data evaluation?
- At what interval will we evaluate the program?
- To whom will interim results be reported and by whom?
- Who will act upon the results?
- What are the criteria for success?

Disseminate and Implement Program

The multidisciplinary team is now ready to begin implementation. It is reasonable to assume that all will not go smoothly at the beginning of the program. Therefore the team must be vigilant and sensitive to barriers that were either not recognized or not adequately addressed. The team should not assume all is going well without hands on experience patient by patient. The strategies selected for dissemination and implementation may require modification. A summary of dissemination and implementation strategies is expressed in Figure 3. This integrates Tables 4 and 5 with recommendation development and probability of improved outcomes. It thus represents the right side of Figure 1 with focus on dissemination and implementation.

Evaluate Program and Improve Performance

If the team has selected an appropriate condition or intervention for improvement, has focused its efforts on a few key interventions and utilized effective dissemination and implementation strategies, it is likely that the program will be successful. However, ongoing evaluation and improvement will be required. As outlined above in the measurement and implementation sections, the team must be vigilant. In evaluating the program and improving it the team should consider the following:

1) How well have we implemented our new processes of care? For example, are we screening all eligible patients for extubation or weaning.
2) Do our outcomes, compared to baseline, appear to be improving? For example, is average time on the ventilator decreasing? Is our VAP rate falling? What is our new cost per case or ICU length of stay? Have we had an unexpected downstream impact on care? For example, has our ICU length of stay fallen but our total hospital length of stay increased? Why did this occur?
3) Is there new information from the literature that needs to be incorporated into our recommendations? For example, is it now clear from a new RCT that pressure support weaning is better than T-piece?

The multidisciplinary team should evaluate this information on a regular basis and be ready to improve the program as required.

Conclusion

We have presented an approach to improving clinical and financial outcomes in the ICU that integrates clinical trial information with applied health services literature to effectively translate best practice into day-to- day care in the ICU. This approach is based upon current evidence and can be used at any healthcare organization, even with limited resources.

We have emphasized the importance of the following:

- Prioritize programs based upon opportunity, leadership, and external factors
- Use a multidisciplinary team and the literature to determine the few key areas upon which to focus within a program
- Select from dissemination and implementation strategies that have been proven effective. Remember that many of these strategies are less rigorously studied in the ICU literature and therefore extrapolation to the critical care setting must be undertaken with caution
- Measure a few key process and outcome measures
- Evaluate the program frequently and be ready to intervene to improve performance.

Using this approach an organization should be able to effectively translate efficacy information from the literature into clinically effective practice for the ICU and institution.

References

1. Ellrodt G, Cook DJ, Lee J, Cho M, Hunt D, Weingarten S (1997) Evidence-based disease management. JAMA 278:1687–1692
2. Grimshaw JM, Russell IT (1993) Effect of clinical guidelines of medical practice: a systematic review of rigorous evaluations. Lancet 342:1317–1322
3. Field MJ, Lohr MJ (1990) Clinical practice guidelines: directions for a new program. National Academy Press, Washington DC
4. Ely EW, Baker AM, Dunagan DP, et al (1996) Effect on the duration of mechanical ventilation of identifying patients capable of breathing spontaneously. N Engl J Med 335:1864–1869
5. Guyatt GH, Sackett DL, Cook DJ for the Evidence-Based Medicine Working Group (1994) Users' Guides to the medical literature. II. How to use an article about therapy or prevention. B. What were the results and will they help me in caring for my patients? JAMA 2741:59–63
6. Drakulovic MB, Torres A, Bauer TT, Nicolas JM, Nogué S, Ferrer M (1999) Supine body position as a risk factor for nosocomial pneumonia in mechanically ventilated patients: a randomised trial. Lancet 354:1851–1858
7. Cabana MD, Rand CS, Powe NR, et al (1999) Why don't physicians follow clinical practice guidelines? JAMA 282:1458–1465
8. Zynx Evidence-Based Forecaster. Zynx Health Incorporated Web site. Available at: http://www.zynx.com/ebf
9. Butler R, Keenan SP, Inman KJ, Sibbald WJ, Block G (1999) Is there a preferred technique for weaning the dfficult-to-wean patient? A systematic review of the literature. Crit care Med 27:2331–2236
10. Kollef MH, Shapiro SD, Silver P, et al (1997) A randomized, controlled trial of protocol-directed versus physician-directed weaning from mechanical ventilation. Crit Care Med 25:567–574
11. Guyatt GH, Cook DJ, Sackett DL, Eckmann M, Pauker S (1998) Grades of recommendations for antithrombotic agents. Chest 114:441S–444S
12 Grol R, Dalhuisen J, Thomas S, Veld C, Rutten G, Mokkink H (1998) Attributes of clinical guidelines that influence use of guidelines in general practice: observational study. Br Med J 317:858–861
13. Oxman AD, Thomas MA, Davis DA, Haynes RB (1995) No magic bullets: a systematic review of 102 trials of interventions to improve professional practice. Can Med Assoc J 153:1423–1431
14. Ellrodt G, Rhew D, Stone E (1999) Improving Practitioner Performance: What Works. VHA, Clinical Advantage Program, VHA Inc Irving
15. Bero LA, Grilli R, Grimshaw JM, Harvey E, Oxman AD, Thomson MA (1998) Closing the gap between research and practice: an overview of system reviews of interventions to promote the implementation of research findings. The Cochrane Effective Practice and Organization of Care Review Group. Br Med J 317:465–468
16. Silagy C, Lancaster T, Gray S, Fowler G (1994) Effectiveness of training health professionals to provide smoking cessation interventions: systematic review of randomized controlled trials. Qual Health Care 3:193–198
17. Smith RC, Marshall AA, Cohen-Cole SA (1994) The efficacy of intensive biopsychosocial teaching programs for residents: a review of the literature and guidelines for teaching. J Gen Intern Med 9:390–396
18. Gifford DR, Mittman BS, Fink A, Lanti AB, Lee ML, Vickrey BG (1996) Can a specialty society educate its members to think differently about clinical decisions? Results of a randomized trial. J Gen Intern Med 11:664–672

19. Wilkes MS, Usatine R, Slavin S, Hoffman JR (1998) Doctoring: University of California, Los Angeles. Acad Med 73:32–40
20. Davis DA, TAylor-Vaisey A (1997) Translating guidelines into practice. A systematic review of theoretic concepts, practical experience and research evidence in the adoption of clinical practice guidelines. Can Med Assoc J 157:408–416
21. Yano EM, Fink A, Hirsch SH, Robbins AS, Rubenstein LV (1995) Helping practices reach primary care goals. Lessons from the literature. Arch Intern Med 155:1146–1156
22. Thomson O'Brien MA, Oxman AD, Haynes RB, Davis DA, Freemantle N, Harvey EL (1998) Local opinion leaders: effects on professional practice and health care outcomes. The Cochrane Library, Issue 2, 2000. Update Software, Oxford
23. Soumerai SB, McLaughlin TJ, Gurwitz JH, et al. (1998) Effect of local medical opinion leaders on quality of care for actue myocardial infarction: a randomized controlled trial. JAMA 279:1358–1363
24. Freemantle N, Harvey EL, Wolf F, Grimshaw JM, Grilli R, Bero LA (1998) Printed educational materials: effects on professional practice and health care outcomes (Cochrane Review). The Cochrane Library, Issue 2, 2000. Update Software, Oxford
25. Davis DA, Thomson MA, Oxman AD, Haynes RB (1995) Changing physician performance. A systematic review of the effect of continuing medical education strategies. JAMA 274:700–705
26. Davis DA, Thomson MA, Oxman AD, Haynes RB (1992) Evidence for the effectiveness of CME. A review of 50 randomized controlled trials. JAMA 268:1111-1117
27. Haynes RB, Davis DA, McKibbon A, Tugwell P (1984) A critical appraisal of the efficacy of continuing medical education. JAMA 251:61–64
28. Bertram DA, Brooks-Bertram PA (1977) The evaluation of continuing medical education: a literature review. Health Educ Monog 5:330–362
29. Wensing M, Grol R (1994) SIngle and combined strategies for implementing changes in primary care: a literature review. Int J Qual Health Care 6:115–132
30. Balas EA, Austin SM, Mitchell JA, Ewigman BG, Bopp KD, Brown GD (1996) The clinical value of computerized information services. A review of 98 randomized clinical trials. Arch Fam Med 5:271–278
31. Austin SM, Balas EA, Mitchell JA, Ewigman BG (1994) Effect of physician reminders on preventive care: meta-analysis of randomized clinical trials. Proc Annu Symp Comput Appl Med Care 121–124
32. Buntinx F, Winkens R, Grol R, Knottnerus JA (1993) Influencing diagnosis and preventive performance in ambulatory care by feedback and reminders. A review. Fam Prac 10:219–228
33. Hunt DL, Haynes RB, Hanna SE, Smith K (1998) Effects of computer-based clinical decision support systems on physician performance and patient outcomes: a systematic review. JAMA 280:1339–1346
34. Johnston ME, Langton KB, Haynes RB, Mathieu A (1994) Effects of computer-based clinical decision support systems on clinician performance and patient outcome. A critical appraisal of research. Ann Intern Med 120:135–142
35. Langton KB, Johnston ME, Haynes RB, Mathieu A (1992) A critical appraisal of the literature on the effects of computer-based clinical decision support systems on clinician performance and patient outcomes. Proc Annu Symp Comput Appl Med Care 626–630
36. Shiffman RN, Liaw Y, Brandt CA, Corb GJ (1999) Computer-based guideline implementation systems: a systematic review of functionality and effectiveness. J Am Med Inform Assoc 6:104–114
37. Evans RS, Pestotnik SL, Classen DC et al. (1998) A computer-assisted management program for antibiotic and other antiinfective agents. N Engl J Med 338:232–238
38. Herman CJ, Speroff T, Cebul RD (1995) Improving compliance with breast cancer screening in older women. Results of a randomized controlled trial. Arch Intern Med 155:717–722
39. Herman CJ, Speroff T, Cebul RD (1994) Improving compliance with immunization in the older adult: results of a randomized cohort study. J Am Geriatr Soc 42:1154–1159

40. Margolis KL, Nichol KL, Wuorenman J, Von Sternberg TL (1992) Exporting a successful influenza vaccination program from a teaching hospital to a community outpatient setting. J Am Geriatr Soc 40:1021–1023
41. Margolis KL, Lofgren RP, Korn JE (1988) Organizational strategies to improve influenza vaccine delivery. A standing order in a general medicine clinic. Arch Intern Med 148:2205–2207
42. Bero LA, Mays NB, Barjesteh K, Bond C (1997) Expanding the roles of outpatients pharmacists. Effects on health services utilisation, costs, and patient outcomes. (Cochrane Review) The Cochrane Library, Issue 2, 2000. Update Software, Oxford
43. Fergusjon J, Weinberger M (1998) Case management programs in primary care. J Gen Intern Med 13:123–126
44. Marshall M, Gray A, Lockwood A, Green R (1997) Case management for people with severe mental disorders (Cochrane Review). The Cochrane Library, Issue 2, 2000. Update Software, Oxford
45. Thomson O'B, Oxman AD, Davis DA, Haynes RB, Freemantle N, Harvey EL (1997) Audit and feedback versus alternative strategies: effects on professional practice and health care outcomes (Cochrane Review). The Cochrane Library, Issue 2, 2000. Update Software, Oxford

Translating the Evidence: Creating and Sustaining Change

W. J. Sibbald and G. K. Webster

Learning Points

- The ability to change clinical practice patterns to reflect new evidence is essential to the provision of high quality critical care
- The development of change strategies should be informed by a relevant theoretical framework
- There are many examples of change strategies in both the health and business sectors
- When selecting a priority area requiring change in healthcare, data-based benchmarking can be used in the absence of high level research evidence
- Change strategies should be locally relevant to maximize the likelihood of success
- Inadequate attention to inter-personal issues is a frequent barrier to the success of change strategies
- It is imperative to evaluate the impact of change initiatives and report results to participants

Before summarizing the models and tools used to drive changes in clinical practice patterns, we offer the following account of one of our own successful change initiatives:

Intensive care patients are at increased risk for the development of pressure ulcers which are both clinically significant and costly to treat [1]. Awareness of this fact, combined with the availability of new types of surfaces for preventing pressure ulcers, led us to carry out a baseline prevalence study of pressure ulcers in the intensive care units (ICUs) of our hospital to determine the magnitude of the pressure ulcer problem. This initial survey showed that the prevalence in our ICU population was higher than the national average for acute care settings. Using the national acute care average as our 'change target' (i.e., a benchmark), we set out to reduce the prevalence and severity of pressure ulcers.

To achieve this goal we carried out a randomized controlled trial (RCT) to determine if assigning at risk patients to receive air suspension surfaces (intervention) resulted in fewer and less severe pressure ulcers than among the control patients who received standard care [1]. Based on this RCT, it was determined that assignment to the more expensive air suspension surfaces reduced the prevalence and severity of pressure ulcers (i.e., increased outputs), and was more cost-effective (i.e., reduced inputs) than standard care. The assignment of patients at risk to these more appropriate surfaces was then introduced as a standard of care in our ICU.

Since it is known that most health care environments do not provide optimal care to all patients, we then set out to determine if there was a need for improvement in the management of pressure ulcers in all of the acute care wards of the hospital. We elected to carry out the prevalence and risk assessment using hand-held computer devices and noted the prevalence in our acute care wards was also above the national average. Our original intervention was then expanded to include a broader range of surfaces outside the ICU. A change strategy was designed, implemented and evaluated as a before/after study. Our change goal was achieved and a long term follow up survey found that the changes had been sustained even after the intervention was over.

The next steps in this continuous change cycle will be to introduce an evidence-based algorithm for the prevention and treatment of pressure ulcers across the continuum of care (i.e., in acute care, long-term care and home care), to close the gap between the current practice patterns and what is supported by the evidence. A final phase will include improving the coordination of care between the different sectors.

After presenting the models and tools for driving change in this chapter, our pressure ulcer change strategy will be re-examined to highlight the components that led to its success.

Introduction

The ability to change clinical practice patterns is a major determinant of clinical effectiveness in intensive care medicine, a discipline with a rapidly evolving knowledge base. A broad range of strategies can be used to translate evidence into practice, many of which have been evaluated using rigorous study designs. Before discussing how to change practice patterns, it is important to understand why changes in practices are needed and the pressures that make change a priority for critical care managers. It is also useful to identify those change strategies described in the business literature that may be useful to consider for improving clinical practice patterns.

The need for change in any clinical environment usually has one of two objectives: 1) to increase outputs (i.e., proportion of high quality outcomes) with the minimum required inputs (i.e., level of intervention or cost to system); or 2) to decrease inputs (e.g., drug costs) without compromising outputs (e.g., ICU length of stay or mortality). Figure 1 is a schematic of the relationship between inputs and outputs, and highlights that changing the processes of care (e.g., drugs recommended for sedation) can critically alter outputs.

Pressures that require change management originate from internal and external sources [2]. Examples of external forces include changes in the age and clinical characteristics of the population, advances in technology, the publication of new research evidence, utilization or performance reports, media attention, and

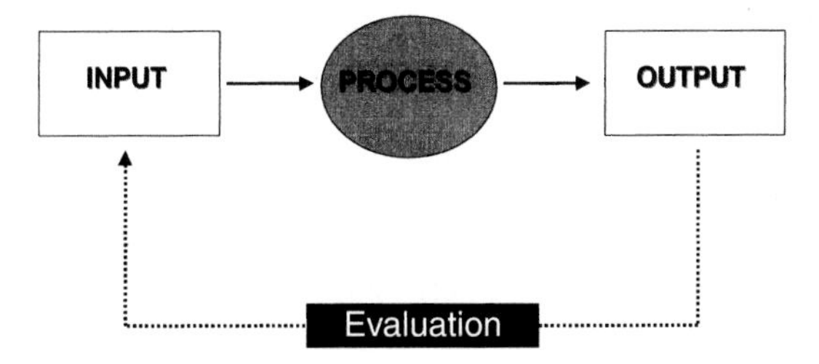

Fig. 1. Schematic of the relationship between inputs and outputs

Table 1. Change pressures currently present in the ICU environment

External pressures for change	Internal pressures for change
Increased pressure to contain costs	Expanding and changing roles of providers working in ICUs
Increasing and aging population leading to increased volumes	Introduction of new staff (e.g., physicians with an evidence-based emphasis)
Longer life expectancy means seeing an older patient population	Quality and/or cost conscious managers or new operational strategies
Innovations which require the use of new techniques and/or increase the probability and length of survival	Reliance on multi-disciplinary teams maintains the momentum of an evolving knowledge base in the ICU
Increased access to systematic summaries of the research evidence	Increased availability of clinicians trained in intensive care
Increasing demands of patient/families resulting from their increased access to medical information through the Internet	Increased concern over multi-resistant bacteria

changes in government policies. Managers are typically responsible for scanning the environment for these external forces, and their interpretation of the external environment has a large impact on whether or not they believe change is a priority. Internal forces of change refers to those factors which are occurring within an organization, and include such issues as a new strategic plan for a department or hospital, increased or decreased availability of human and structural resources, new or existing staff committed to implementing change within the organization on a large or small scale. Table 1 lists some of the pressures currently present in the ICU environment.

When assessing whether or not there is a need to improve the processes of care, it is important to evaluate the presence of gaps between current practices and what is determined to be a best practice, for example, by identifying relevant evidence-based recommendations or data-based benchmarks [3]. The process of identifying and grading research-based evidence is described in an earlier chapter by Cook and Giacomini. If there is an absence of strong research-based evidence on what should be done, it is then necessary to identify a benchmark or indicator of the best available outcomes that can be achieved. The identification of benchmarks or indicators requires data, usually from more than one provider and preferably from several institutions [3]. Once the best achievable outcome is determined (i.e., the benchmark), internal processes of care can be evaluated by comparing their outcomes against the benchmark. Knowledge and technology in critical care are so dynamic that there is continuous pressure for changing practices to provide the best possible care based on the available evidence (i.e., from data and published research).

Efforts to improve the quality and effectiveness of health care require the translation of evidence into practice, otherwise changes in practice patterns will not keep pace with changes in research findings, even when the research findings are convincing and the information is widely distributed. For example, despite strong evidence from several RCTs that the early provision of beta-blockers for acute myocardial infarction reduced mortality, only 53% of eligible patients receive beta-blockers [4]. One review of the quality of care received by Americans estimates that only 60% of patients with chronic conditions receive the recommended care [5]. As outlined later, even with concerted and well-planned efforts, the translation of evidence into better practice patterns is challenging and does not always achieve optimal results. For example, we know that there is underutilization of many ICU practices that have been shown to be effective (e.g., DVT prophylaxis, selective digestive decontamination [SDD], and early enteral nutritional support).

The chapter begins with a description of several models which offer different pathways to changing behavior. This section is followed by an overview of change strategies used in the healthcare and business sectors, barriers to change and how to evaluate change initiatives. The chapter is intended to provide the reader with an insight into practical issues surrounding the implementation of changes in practice patterns in the ICU environment.

Models for Changing Practice Behavior

We recommend that at least one of the models for changing behavior described below be used to guide the development of implementation strategies to translate evidence into practice. To start with, however, it is apparent that most published works on translating research into practice do not describe the change strategy and its impacts within the context of a model for explaining change. For example, a random sample of 54 research studies on changing health professionals' behavior found that only two of these studies indicated that the choice of change strategy was informed by theory or a formal body of knowledge [6]. By identifying specific challenges associated with a change initiative, developers can use change models to determine the rationale they should apply when selecting individual change tools, and when assembling a multi-faceted implementation strategy. Using theory to inform the development of implementation strategies should improve the effectiveness and efficiency of these strategies, by ensuring all necessary barriers are targeted and minimizing the use of ineffective strategies.

Several individual-based and organizational-based models of change are described below. This is followed by an introduction to the 'Social Marketing' [7] and the 'Precede-Proceed' [8] planning frameworks, both of which provide systematic approaches to using theory to guide the development of implementation strategies.

One of the most widely applied individual-based models is the information deficit model. This model proposes that simply providing the proper information to the provider is sufficient to bring about a desired change in behavior. However, this model is now viewed as an inadequate explanation of the factors that change behavior. Many researchers concerned with translating research into practice claim that while getting the right information to practitioners is an important component of producing change, it is rarely sufficient to change behavior when used in isolation [6]. This claim is supported by several rigorous studies, all of which concluded that passive learning, such as lectures and mailings of educational material, have limited impact on practitioner behavior [9,10].

The psychology literature provides several examples of how to influence the behavior of individuals, and models therein include: learning theory, social cognition, stages of change, and receptivity to change.

Learning theory emphasizes the use of positive and negative consequences to change behavior [11]. According to this model, behaviors that are accompanied by positive consequences (i.e., reinforcers) are more likely to be repeated, and those accompanied by negative consequences are less likely to be repeated. When applying learning theory to change practice patterns it is, therefore, important to ensure that the desired practices are reinforced with the most positive consequences and that any negative consequences associated with the desired practices are mitigated. In these cases, a qualitative investigation, such as a focus group with ICU physicians on fluid management practices, may provide the necessary insight into the incentives and disincentives that are driving the current practice patterns.

For example, the multi-disciplinary team approach found in many ICUs can be a negative reinforcer of poor performance if superiors criticize staff who point out potential problem areas. If, however, the environment is supportive of staff identifying the need for improvements, then the team culture becomes a positive reinforcer of improving the quality of care. Another example of a positive reinforcer is when staff are rewarded for upgrading their skills through the pursuit of additional training.

Social cognition models promote the perspective that how a person thinks about a situation has an important influence on how they will behave [6]. These models emphasize three types of beliefs that influence how people behave, including:

1) perceived benefits weighed against perceived barriers to the action
2) perceptions of the attitudes of others towards the behavior
3) sense of self-efficacy, or belief in one's ability to perform a behavior

An example of this model in the ICU comes from the pressure ulcer project, described previously. By benchmarking against the national average, we demonstrated that patients could benefit from improvements in the processes of care. The RCT we carried out established the clinical and resource benefits associated with assigning at risk patients to air suspension surfaces, therefore, providing the clinicians with the confidence that their change in practices would be deemed justified by peers and also that they had the self-efficacy required to assign patients to appropriate surfaces.

Stage models of change are adaptations of the social cognition models described, above. One of these models includes the following stages: precontemplation; contemplation; preparation; action; and maintenance [12]. According to proponents of these models, individuals pass through several stages before changing, and the interventions must address the stage-specific needs and barriers at each stage. However, evidence supporting the assumption that people must progress through each stage in a linear manner is lacking [6].

A receptivity to change model classifies individuals as innovators, early-adopters, early-majority, late majority and laggards, depending on how quickly they change their behavior [13]. Each of these sub-groups may require different levels of intervention to change behavior and change at different rates. Implementation strategies can be designed to take advantage of variances in receptivity to change, for example, by recruiting early adopters to train and motivate members of the early and late majority groups.

Organizational change is also thought to progress through a series of stages. One model describes the processes of unfreezing existing patterns, changing to a new pattern, and refreezing of new attitudes and practices, through reinforcement and support [12]. Other issues considered important in organizational change include:
1) Context: why and when change should occur
2) Process: how the changes should occur
3) Content: what changes should occur

Applying Change Models within a Planning Framework

Models of change may be most useful when used within a planning framework [12]. Using a planning framework helps ensure all the necessary steps are followed. The social marketing and the precede-proceed frameworks have been used for the development, implementation and evaluation of interventions to change health behaviors [12].

Social marketing provides a framework for identifying factors that drive change [7] and it includes the following steps:
1) Planning and strategy
2) Specification of program structure and outcomes; and define sub-groups
3) Develop and pilot test materials with target audience
4) Implementation
5) Evaluation
6) Feedback

The precede-proceed model outlines the steps which should precede the intervention and how to proceed with the implementation of the strategy and its evaluation

[8]. The precede stage focuses on problem specification and contributing factors. Priorities for the intervention are determined by a process that ranks the importance and amenability to change of predisposing, enabling and reinforcing factors:
1) Predisposing factors include attitudes, beliefs and perceptions
2) Enabling factors include resources, skills and facilities
3) Reinforcing factors include rewards and incentives such as positive feedback

Strategies to Change Practice Behavior

Change Strategies Identified in the Medical Literature

A review of the literature on changing the practices of health care providers produced a large number of RCTs and systematic reviews. Given the limited number of ICU-specific studies, the search was expanded to include all areas of medicine. The literature search was limited to RCTs and systematic reviews as this approach allowed us to focus on the studies with the highest levels of evidence. The search employed the terms similar to those used by the Cochrane Review Group on Effective Practice and Organization of Care (EPOC) to identify studies for a recent publication on translating research into practice [12]. Our search terms included: Physician's practice patterns/standards[mesh]; professional practice/standards[mesh]; intensive care units/standards[mesh]; critical care[mesh]; randomized controlled trial[mesh]; medical audit[mesh]; practice[all fields]; outreach[tw]; academic detailing[all fields]; feedback[all fields]; written material[tw]; reminder-systems[all fields]; continuing medical education[mesh]; comparative study[all fields]; intervention[all fields]; practice guideline[tw]; impact[tw]; quality of health care[all fields]; quality assurance[tw]. These terms were used in several different combinations. We also searched the references from the Cochrane Collaboration EPOC group's systematic reviews of interventions to change professional practice and our personal holdings.
The articles identified describe a broad range of tools that have been evaluated for their ability to change practice patterns. Although few of these were specific to changing practices in the critical care setting, many of the tools evaluated in other settings should be transferable to the critical setting. Table 2 provides a list of selected articles describing research transfer efforts in the critical care setting. As a result of the limited number of critical care studies, change strategies evaluated in all health care setting are described along with reports of their effectiveness.

Formal Continuing Medical Education (CME) has been described as "highly variable, ranging from passive, didactic, large-group presentations to highly interactive learning methods, such as workshops, small groups, and individualized training sessions" [10]. The objective of formal CME is to improve and maintain the performance of health care providers, most often physicians [14]. Reviews of these highly variable activities consistently report that it has little impact on changing physician behavior.

In a recent review of 14 RCTs examining the impact of formal CME activities, Davis et al. [10] classified the delivery format into one of the following cate-

Table 2. Selected articles describing research transfer efforts in the critical care setting

Brook AD, Ahrens TS, Schaiff R, et al (1999) Effect of a nursing-implemented sedation protocol on the duration of mechanical ventilation. Crit Care Med 27:2609-2615
Kern H, Kox WJ (1999) Impact of standard procedures and clinical standards on cost-effectiveness and intensive care unit performance in adult patients after cardiac surgery. Intensive Care Med 25:1367-1373
Price J, Eckleberry A, Grover A, et al (1999) Evaluation of clinical practice guidelines on outcome of infection in patients in the surgical intensive care unit. Crit Care Med 27:2118-2124
Clemmer TP, Spuhler VJ, Oniki TA, Horn SD (1999) Results of a collaborative quality improvement program on outcomes and costs in a tertiary critical care unit. Crit Care Med 27:1768-1774
Sinuff T, Cook DJ, Peterson JC, Fuller HD (1999) Development, implementation, and evaluation of a ketoconazole practice guideline for ARDS prophylaxis. J Crit Care 14:1-6
Vukic M, Negovetic L, Kovac D, Ghajar J, Glavic Z, Gopcevic A (1999) The effect of implementation of guidelines for the management of severe head injury on patient treatment and outcome. Acta Neurochir (Wien) 141:1203-1208
Sandison AJ, Wyncoll DL, Edmondson RC, Van Heerden N, Beale RJ, Taylor PR (1998) ICU protocol may affect the outcome of non-elective abdominal aortic aneurysm repair. Eur J Vasc Endovasc Surg 1998 Oct;16(4):356-61.
Hendryx MS, Fieselmann JF, Bock MJ, Wakefield DS, Helms CM, Bentler SE (1998) Outreach education to improve quality of rural ICU care. Results of a randomized trial. Am J Respir Crit Care Med 158:418-423
Pitimana-aree S, Forrest D, Brown G, Anis A, Wang XH, Dodek P (1998) Implementation of a clinical practice guideline for stress ulcer prophylaxis increases appropriateness and decreases cost of care. Intensive Care Med 24:217-223
Devlin JW, Holbrook AM, Fuller HD (1997) The effect of ICU sedation guidelines and pharmacist interventions on clinical outcomes and drug cost. Ann Pharmacother 31:689-695
Keenan SP, Doig GS, Martin CM, Inman KJ, Sibbald WJ (1997) Assessing the efficiency of the admission process to a critical care unit: does the literature allow the use of benchmarking? Intensive Care Med 23:574-580
Chiang AA, Lee KC, Lee JC, Wei CH (1996) Effectiveness of a continuous quality improvement program aiming to reduce unplanned extubation: a prospective study. Intensive Care Med 22:1269-1271
Hoey LL, Nahum A, Vance-Bryan K (1994) A prospective evaluation of benzodiazepine guidelines in the management of patients hospitalized for alcohol withdrawal. Pharmacotherapy 14:579-585

gories: didactic, interactive, or mixed. Didactic sessions included lectures or presentations with minimal audience involvement. Interactive formats included role-play, discussion groups, hands-on training, problem solving, or case solving. Mixed formats included both passive and interactive elements. In order to isolate the impact of these three approaches to CME, the review was limited to RCTs of CME activities that were intended to be persuasive rather than coercive or incentive-based and were not delivered as part of a multi-faceted strategy. None of the four didactic interventions altered physician performance. Four of the six interactive interventions were successful. Five of the seven mixed interventions were successful. The authors also compared single session interventions to those offered as a series and found that two of the seven single sessions were successful compared to seven of the ten interventions offered as a series. Group size was not found to be a predictor of success, but customization efforts did appear to increase the likelihood of positive results. Therefore, when this type of strategy is used, preferably in conjunction with other strategies, it is important to ensure that the content is relevant for the participants. This can be done by determining the learning needs before developing the actual learning material.

Audit and feedback is defined "as any summary of clinical performance of health care over a specified period of time" [15]. The summary may also include recommendations for clinical action. The information may be given in a written, electronic or verbal format. The feedback will be either group or individual-based feedback and be either passive (unsolicited) or actively involve clinicians. It may also include blinded or non-blinded peer-based comparisons.

A systematic review of audit and feedback RCTs reported that it is sometimes effective, but the effects are typically small to moderate when it does work [15]. Audit and feedback was most effective for changing prescribing and diagnostic test ordering practices. The authors emphasize that the approaches to audit and feedback were not uniform and that this may explain the inconsistent findings. Other things which may influence the impact of audit and feedback include the content of the message, mode of delivery, and target audience. Based on a review of 36 published studies, Mugford et al. [16] claimed that feedback is likely to be most effective when it is presented in a timely manner and when clinicians have agreed to a review of their practices. Thomson et al. [17] emphasize that feedback must be delivered in a way that extends beyond the simple diffusion of information, since it has been shown that diffusion alone is insufficient to change practices. However, definitive trials which demonstrate the importance of timely data are lacking. There is also insufficient evidence on which to make recommendations regarding the content, format, mode, source and frequency of feedback. Theoretically, feedback that is personalized, peer-based, timely, frequent and delivered in a one-to-one format should be more effective. Feedback is also likely to be more effective if it is bundled with complementary strategies.

Local opinion leaders are educationally influential providers who are identified by their colleagues as being effective communicators and clinical experts [18]. Local opinion leaders are positioned to influence the attitudes and perceptions of colleagues through effective communication and leading by example. Local opinion leaders may also increase perceived self-efficacy by providing options for care, particularly where there is uncertainty [19]. Evaluations of the influence of local opinion leaders has produced mixed results [19] with just 2/13 trials [20, 21] providing strong evidence of a clinically meaningful effect. Soumerai [21] reported that combining local opinion leaders with audit and feedback was more effective than providing audit and feedback alone. The large variance between individual local opinion leaders combined with the absence of any standardized approaches for acting as a local opinion leader likely contributes to the mixed effects of this strategy for influencing practice behavior.

Reminders are any intervention, manual or computerized, that prompt the health care provider to perform a clinical action [19]. Reminders can help care providers change old habits and sustain new ones, especially if they are provided at the time of decision-making. Systematic reviews support the use of reminders as an effective practice change strategy in a broad range of clinical circumstances and environments [22]. Reminders can have implicit or explicit suggestions, be generic or patient-specific, and may require response from the provider. Other variations include the targeted behavior, the source of the reminder, if it was locally developed and whether or not it is computer-based. A review of 68 studies found that the use of computerized reminders can lead to improvements in decisions on drug dosage, the provision of preventive care and the general clinical management of patients, but not diagnosis [12]. Using a one-month alternating time series design, reminders significantly increased adherence to an evidence-based guideline for early (two day) discharge of low-risk chest pain patients [23]. Structured written reminders were placed on the patient charts on day one and were followed up with a structured phone message if a low risk patient was in hospital for more than 24 hours, to remind the physician they could be discharged before day three.

Academic detailing/educational outreach visits involve a trained person who meets face-to-face with a provider in their practice settings to provide information with the intent of changing the provider's performance [24]. The information given may include feedback on the provider's performance. Educational outreach visits have been evaluated primarily for their impact on prescribing practices. This strategy does have an impact on prescribing practices, especially when combined with social marketing strategies (e.g., local promotional activities) [24]. It has also increased the provision of a range of preventive practices. It is unclear how educational outreach compares to other strategies and it may be most effective when used in conjunction with other strategies. The importance of repeat visits also requires further investigation. Although there are no cost effectiveness studies on using educational outreach visits to change practices, the people developing the implementation strategies need to be aware that it can require a significant time investment on the part of the detailer if they are making multiple visits to several practitioners.

Educational outreach has improved the quality of care in a group of rural ICUs in the mid-west US [25]. A university-based multi-disciplinary team provided face-to-face personalized feedback on-site to their rural peers. Control hospitals did not receive an intervention. The objective of the detailing session was to improve the processes of care for patients receiving mechanical ventilation. Compliance with most of the recommended processes of care increased significantly for the intervention hospitals compared to the control hospitals. Most outcomes and resource measures had non-significant improvements in the intervention group compared to the control group. One exception was for mortality, which improved non-significantly in the control group and deteriorated slightly in the intervention group. This study [25] suggests that a multi-disciplinary educational outreach approach that includes personalized feedback may be a useful approach to improving the processes of care in rural ICUs. It also highlights the need to use an adequate sample size and to monitor the impact of the intervention on relevant outcomes.

Local consensus processes: Inclusion of participating providers in a discussion to ensure that they agreed that the chosen clinical problem was important and the approach to managing the problem was adequate [19]. This consultative approach at the pre-implementation stage increases the likelihood that the recommendations will be compatible with the providers and the health care setting. According to Davis et al. [26] these are both noneducational variables affecting the adoption of clinical practice guidelines. Local consensus processes also fit with the social cognition model, by providing an opportunity for providers to change their perceptions of what treatments are most effective and to observe peer acceptance of the final recommendations.

Distribution of printed educational materials including clinical practice guidelines has limited impact when used alone. Freemantle et al. [27] found this approach to have very little effect on practice behavior. Grilli and Lomas [28] reviewed 23 studies and found that less complicated guidelines were more effectively adopted. Davis et al. [26] have identified several noneducational variables affecting adoption of guidelines (quality, the provider, the practice setting, incentives, regulations and patient factors). These same authors [26] also identified attributes that affect adoption of guidelines (relative advantage, compatibility, complexity, trialability, and observability). Typically, the distribution of guidelines and recommendations is insufficient to change practice behavior, unless it is accompanied by another change strategy; even with active dissemination, guideline adherence is less than optimal [29].

The terms Quality Improvement (QI) and Continuous Quality Improvement (CQI) refer to a broad range of approaches to changing practice behavior. Typically, a CQI intervention will include problem specification, solution identification and pilot testing followed by widespread implementation. Based on a review of 54 studies of CQI by Shortell et al. [30], it is still not known whether or not CQI is effective. Several non-randomized studies reported positive results, but the three randomized studies found no positive effect from CQI interventions.

The results of a before-after quasi-experimentally designed trial using historical controls indicate that a collaborative quality improvement program that emphasized team culture and skills development had positive effects [31]. Significant improvements were reported for a several practices (e.g., use of enteral feeding, antibiotic use and appropriate use of sedation) and overall hospital costs. Of particular interest is that the severity of patients increased during the five year study period, but hospital costs declined. It was not possible to determine if these changes were a result of the QI project.

Another popular approach is a model for improvement developed by Langley, Nolan and Nolan [32]. This model asks the following three questions:
1) What are we trying to accomplish?
2) How will we know that a change is an improvement?
3) What change can we make that will result in an improvement ?

The model recommends applying the Plan-Do-Study-Act (PDSA) Cycle to promote rapid cycle inductive learning as a daily activity for all health professionals. The PDSA approach also emphasizes the importance of changing systems, as well as individual behavior. Both CQI and PDSA are associated with variations in the way change is implemented and may benefit from developing theory-informed evidence-based change strategies.

Change Strategies Identified in the Business Literature

The current emphasis on quality improvement in health care has its roots in American industry which in turn adopted its emphasis from W. Edwards Deming's influence on Japanese manufacturing practices [33]. The healthcare sector tends to focus on just two of Deming's fourteen principles of quality improvement, statistical measurement and standardization [31]. The remaining twelve principles emphasize the importance of building safe, collaborative environments and leveraging the knowledge and skills of workers, empowering them to be the foundation for improvement. [34].

In a review of change initiatives carried out in several different sectors, Kotter and Schlesinger [35] also identified several environment factors that influence whether or not change strategies will be successful. They recommend choosing change strategies based on the following three criteria:
1) the length of time before the change must be achieved;
2) clarity of the plan of action; and
3) the amount of involvement required from employees.

In addition, four situational factors to consider are:
1) The amount and kind of resistance that is anticipated;
2) The position of the initiator relative to the resistors with regard to power;
3) Who has access to the data for designing the change and the energy for implementing it; and
4) The urgency and risks involved.

Kotter and Schlesinger [35] recommend choosing one or more of the following change strategies when attempting to implement change:
1) Education and communication
2) Participation and involvement
3) Facilitation and support
4) Negotiation and agreement
5) Manipulation and co-optation
6) Explicit and implicit coercion

Once again, the strategies selected and how they are designed should be informed by the criteria and situational factors described above.

Identifying and Overcoming Local Barriers to Change

Before developing and implementing a change strategy, it is wise to identify potential barriers to success. One approach to identifying barriers, identified in the health literature, is to undertake a 'diagnostic analysis' [12]. This involves identifying the groups affected by and influencing the changes, assessment of the change in practice, assessment of the preparedness of the team (e.g., do the providers have the motivation and training required to change their practices?), identify structural and systemic barriers, and identify enabling resources (e.g., local opinion leader and early adopters).

A similar approach, called 'diagnosing resistance', was identified in the business literature [35]. This process helps managers predict what types of resistance they might encounter. Four common reasons for resistance are listed:

1) self-interest or fear of losing something of value;
2) misunderstanding of the implications of the change and lack of trust;
3) different assessment of the need for change and/or the value of the change strategy; and
4) a low tolerance for change.

Regardless of the approach to identifying barriers, it is critical that the implementation strategy be customized to increase the chance of success and effective use of resources.

Boyle and Callahan [36] used a structured interview format to learn why physicians often resist applying new clinical practice guidelines based on outcomes data. They discovered that some of this resistance could be explained by moral and quasi-moral concerns experienced by the physicians. They grouped these concerns into the following three categories:

1) Skepticism about the source, reliability and objectivity of outcomes data, including the validity of inferences drawn from the data used to construct practice guidelines.
2) Objections or hesitations based not on the reliability of the data or guidelines but on contrary patient preferences, clinical experience, and legal worries.
3) Tacit motivation, rarely apparent in the sociological literature and/or admitted hesitatingly by physicians. These motives included ego, economics and convenience. The authors noted that these factors are endemic to most professions and are hard to completely overcome.

Bolye and Callahan [36] emphasize that the successful adoption of practice guidelines is highly dependent on whether or not physicians can change their practice patterns and still believe they are acting in a morally justifiable way.

Barriers can be classified as being individual, team, hospital, or research and development factors [37]. Theory can inform which strategy is most likely to be useful in overcoming the barrier (e.g., if information overload is an issue, computer-assisted reminders can reduce the likelihood of forgetting to use the new practice). Many barriers are best addressed by non-physicians which is a good reason to involve multi-disciplinary teams. Competing priorities can also impede the translation of research into practice [38]. Improvements in computer technology make it possible for physicians to have access to electronic databases that can be searched for high-quality evidence-based recommendations at the bedside [39]. Physicians with access to these resources are better equipped to apply research findings in the clinical setting.

Once the local barriers have been identified, the team can begin to plan how to overcome these barriers. The most effective way to overcome the barriers to changing practice behavior is to develop a multi-faceted, evidence-based implementation strategy. The inclusion of individual change strategies in a multi-faceted strategy should be justified by at least one of the theoretical models of change, described above. Table 3 links these individual-based theoretical models for changing behavior with the change strategies described above. This table is a guide for selecting a change strategy that addresses the nature of barriers identified. For example, improving an inappropriately low rate of prescribing of beta-blockers at discharge for patients hospitalized following an acute myocardial infarction is likely the result of physicians not appreciating the benefits of this practice to the patients. In this case, the information deficit can be addressed through dissemination of guidelines and followed up with the more effective face-to-face educational outreach/academic detailing and reinforced using reminders. In another situation, you might be challenged with increasing the use of a superior but complex surgical technique. In this situation your multi-faceted intervention should also include a training component to improve self-efficacy among the surgeons who will be changing their techniques. Models of organizational change are described in an earlier chapter.

In the business literature, Kotter [40] recommends eight steps that will increase the probability of overcoming resistance to a change initiative. These steps are:

1) Establish a sense of urgency
2) Form a powerful guiding coalition
3) Create a vision
4) Communicate the vision
5) Empower others to act on the vision

Table 3. Linking Learning Theory and Social Cognition Theory with strategies for changing practice behavior

Model	Emphasis based on theory	Change strategy
Learning Theory	positive and negative consequences	– reward/supports for desirable practices – remove rewards/supports for undesirable practices – include disincentives for undesirable practices (e.g., require justification)
Social Cognition Model	perceived benefits over risks	– information dissemination – educational outreach
	how perceived by others	– local opinion leaders – local consensus process – audit and feedback
	self-efficacy	– educational outreach – training (e.g., new surgical technique) – provide reminders – educational meeting with opportunities for role practicing

6) Plan for and create short-term wins
7) Consolidate improvements and produce still more change
8) Institutionalize new approaches

Sustaining Change

The ability to sustain change is important in terms of promoting long term clinical effectiveness. It is also important to know what resources must by provided to sustain change in an efficient manner. Unfortunately, there is an absence of high level evidence to determine how to sustain changes once they are achieved. The early discharge protocol for low-risk chest pain patients, described above, used reminders in an alternating time series design and found that within a month of stopping the reminders, their impact had diminished [23]. This is another reason to look for low cost change strategies that can be maintained if necessary.

Evaluating Change Strategies

It is important to plan the evaluation before implementation begins, to ensure proper baseline information is collected for the intervention and control groups. There may be limited resources shared between the intervention and evaluation in which case the implementation resources or design should not be eroded to benefit the evaluation process. It makes no sense to carry out a rigorous evaluation of an under-resourced implementation strategy. The evaluation can be organized according to Kirkpatrick's four-level evaluation hierarchy of: participant satisfaction; participant learning; change in practices; and change in outcomes [41]. As a minimum, change in processes of care and outcomes should be measured when evaluating a change strategy.

Translating research into practice programs are often delivered to groups of providers at the same institution, so the normal RCT design is not applicable. In these settings it is appropriate to undertake a cluster randomization design when allocating units to intervention and control groups for the evaluation. This approach requires a sample size inflation factor to compensate for the intra-class correlations within each cluster. Rigorous evaluations are only required when new approaches are being implemented for the first time.

Conclusion: Re-Examining our Pressure Ulcer Change Initiative

We can now review the pressure ulcer success story from the perspective of the change models and tools described above. The most applicable model in this situation is the social cognition model which focuses on individual perceptions of benefits versus harms, perceptions of peers, and sense of self-efficacy. The change tools used were audit and feedback (prevalence surveys) and academic detailing (one-to-one training). Initially, a senior clinician and a health services researcher introduced the need for a baseline study to determine if improvements were necessary and the need for an RCT to determine whether or not improving surfaces could solve the problem in a cost effective manner. The baseline study convinced staff that there really was a need for improvement (i.e., potential for benefits). Using an RCT to demonstrate that assigning at-risk patients to air suspension surfaces reduced the prevalence and severity of pressure ulcers provided the credibility needed to support a change in standard practice (i.e., peers will look favorably upon decisions based on an RCT), and demonstrated that the practice was doing more good than harm. Academic detailing was used to train staff in risk assessment and surface assignment and use (i.e., self-efficacy was increased). Feedback from the initial follow-up prevalence survey reinforced to staff that their efforts resulted in clinical improvements and this reinforcement likely contributed to the sustained change that was observed in the long term follow up prevalence survey. By creating a safe, collaborative environment, clinical teams will be more receptive to change and welcome improving processes of care as a rewarding aspect of their clinical work.

References

1. Inman K, Sibbald WJ, Rutledge FS, Clark BJ (1993). Clinical utility and cost-effectiveness of an air suspension bed in the prevention of pressure ulcers. JAMA 269:1139–1143
2. Rakich JS, Longest BB Jr, Darr K (1992) Managing Health Services Organizations, Third Edition. Health Professions Press, Toronto
3. Keenan SP, Martin CM, Kossuth JD, Eberhard J, Sibbald WJ (1999) The Critical Care Research Network: A partnership in community-based research and research transfer. J Eval Clin Pract 5:1–8
4. McLaughlin TJ, Soumerai SB, Willison DJ, et al (1996) Adherence to national guideline for drug treatment of suspected acute myocardial infarction: Evidence for under treatment in women and the elderly. Arch Intern Med 156:799–805
5. Schuster MA, McGlynn E, Brook RH. (1998) How good is the quality of health care in the United States ? Milbank Q 76:517–563
6. Marteau, T, Sowden A, Armstrong D (1998) Implementing research findings into practice: beyond the information deficit model. In: Haines A, Donald A (eds) Getting research into practice. BMJ Books, London, pp 36–42
7. Kotler P (1984) Social marketing of health behavior. In: Frederiksen LW, Solomon LJ, Brehony KA (eds) Marketing health behavior: principles, techniques and applications. Plenum Press, New York, pp 23–39
8. Green LW, Kreuter MW, Deeds SG, et al. (1980) Health education Planning: a diagnostic approach. Mayfield Publishing Company, California.
9. Bero LA, Grilli R, Grimshaw JM, Harvey E, Oxman A, Thomson MA (1998) Closing the gap between research and practice: an overview of systematic reviews of interventions to promote the implementation of research findings. The Cochrane Effective Practice and Organization of Care Review Group. Br Med J 317:465–468
10. Davis D, Thomson O'Brien MA, Freemantle N, Wolf FM, Mazmanian P, Taylor–Vaisey A (1999) Impact of formal continuing medical education – Do conferences, workshops, rounds and other traditional continuing education activities change physician behavior or health care outcomes? JAMA 282:867–874
11. Skinner BF (1953) Science and human behavior. Macmillan, New York.
12. The Cochrane Review Group on Effective Practice and Organisation of Care (EPOC) (1999) Getting evidence into practice. Effective Health Care Bulletin 5:1–16

13. Rogers E (1983) Diffusion of Innovations. Free Press, New York
14. Davis DA, Thomson MA, Oxman AD, Haynes RB (1995) Changing physician performance. A systematic review of the effect of continuing medical education strategies. JAMA 274:700–705
15. Thomson MA, Oxman AD, Davis DA, Haynes RB, Freemantle N, Harvey EL (1997) Audit and feedback: effects on professional practice and health care outcomes (Part I). The Cochrane Library, Issue 1, 1999. Update Software, Oxford
16. Mugford M, Banfield P, O'Hanlon M (1991) Effects of feedback of information on clinical practice: a review. Br Med J 303:398–402
17. Thomson MA, Oxman AD, Davis DA, Haynes RB, Freemantle N, Harvey EL (1997) Audit and feedback versus alternative strategies: effects on professional practice and health care outcomes (Part II). The Cochrane Library, Issue 1, 1999. Update Software, Oxford
18. Flottorp S, Oxman A, Bjornal A (1998) The limits of leadership: opinion leaders in general practice. J Health Serv Res Policy 3:197–202
19. Thomson O'Brien MA, Oxman AD, Haynes RB, Davis DA, Freemantle N, Harvey EL (1998) Local opinion leaders: effects on professional practice and health care outcomes. The Cochrane Library, Issue 3, 1999. Update Software, Oxford
20. Lomas J, Enkin M, Anderson GM, Hannah WJ, Vayda E, Singer J (1991) Opinion leaders vs audit and feedback to implement practice guidelines. Delivery after previous cesarean section. JAMA 265:2202–2207
21. Soumerai SB, McLaughlin TJ, Gurwitz JH, et al (1998) Effect of local medical opinion leaders on quality of care for acute myocardial infarction: a randomized controlled trial. JAMA 279:1358–1363
22. Oxman AD, Thomson MA, Davis DA, Haynes RB (1995) No magic bullets: a systematic review of 102 trials of interventions to improve professional practice. Can Med Assoc J 153:1423–1431
23. Weingarten SR, Riedinger MS, Conner L, et al (1994) Practice guidelines and reminders to reduce duration of hospital stay for patients with chest pain. An intervention trial. Ann Intern Med 120:257–263
24. Thomson O'Brien MA, Oxman AD, Davis DA, Haynes RB, Freemantle N, Harvey EL (1997) Educational outreach visits: effects on professional practice and health care outcomes. The Cochrane Library, Issue 4, 1999. Update Software, Oxford
25. Hendryx MS, Fieselmann JF, Bock MJ, Wakefield DS, Helms CM, Bentler SE (1998) Outreach education to improve quality of rural ICU care. Results of a randomized trial. Am J Respir Crit Care Med 158:418–423
26. Davis DA and Taylor–Vaisey A (1997) Translating guidelines into practice: a systematic review of theoretical concepts, practical experience and research evidence in the adoption of clinical practice guidelines. Can Med Assoc J 157:408–416
27. Freemantle N, Harvey EL, Wolf F, Grimshaw JM, Grilli R, Bero LA (1997) Printed educational materials: effects on professional practice and health care outcomes. The Cochrane Library, Issue 3, 1999. Update Software, Oxford
28. Grilli R, Lomas J (1994) Evaluating the message: the relationship between compliance rate and the subject of practice guidelines. Med Care 32:202–2.13
29. Cameron C, Naylor D (1999) No impact from active dissemination of the Ottawa Ankle Rules: further evidence of the need for local implementation of practice guidelines. Can Med Assoc J 160:1165–1168
30. Shortell SM, Bennett CL, Byck GR (1998) Assessing the impact of continuous quality improvement on clinical practice: what will it take to accelerate progress. MilBank Q 76:593–624
31. Clemmer TP, Spuhler VJ, Oniki TA, Horn SD (1999) Results of a collaborative quality improvement program on outcomes and costs in a tertiary critical care unit. Crit Care Med 27:1768–1774
32. Berwick DM (1996) A primer on leading the improvement of systems. Br Med J 312:619–622
33. Gabor A (1990) The man who discovered quality: How W. Edwards Deming brought the quality revolution to America. Penguin Books, New York.

34. Walton M (1990) Deming management at work. Perigree Books, New York.
35. Kotter JP, Schlesinger LA (1979) Choosing strategies for change. Harvard Business Review March–April:4–11
36. Boyle PJ, Callahan D (1998) Physicians' use of outcomes data: Moral conflicts and potential resolutions. In: Boyle PJ (eds) Getting doctors to listen: Ethics and outcomes data in context. Georgetown University Press, Washington
37. Donald A, Milne R (1998) Implementing research findings in clinical practice. In: Haines A, Donald A (eds) Getting research into practice. BMJ Med J Books, London, pp 52–62
38. Marshall MN (1999) Improving quality in general practice: qualitative case study of barriers faced by health authorities. Br Med J 319:164–167
39. Haynes RB, Sackett DL, Guyatt GH, Cook DJ, Gray JA (1997) Transferring evidence from research into practice: 4. Overcoming barriers to application [editorial]. ACP J Club 126:A14–A15
40. Kotter JP (1995) Leading change: Why transformation efforts fail. Harvard Business Review March–April:59–67
41. Hutchinson L (1999) Evaluating and researching the effectiveness of educational interventions. Br Med J 318:1267–1269

Subject Index